Medical education and training
From theory to delivery

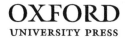

2L7 CAR (B)

Professor of General Practice and Primary Care,
Dean of Warwick Medical School and
Pro-Vice-Chancellor (Regional Engagement),
The University of Warwick, UK

Neil Jackson

Dean of Postgraduate General Practice,
The London Deanery, University of London,
and Honorary Professor of Medical Education,
Queen Mary School of Medicine and Dentistry,
University of London, UK

OXFORD
UNIVERSITY PRESS

OXFORD

UNIVERSITY PRESS

Great Clarendon Street, Oxford OX2 6DP

Oxford University Press is a department of the University of Oxford.
It furthers the University's objective of excellence in research, scholarship,
and education by publishing worldwide in

Oxford New York

Auckland Cape Town Dar es Salaam Hong Kong Karachi
Kuala Lumpur Madrid Melbourne Mexico City Nairobi
New Delhi Shanghai Taipei Toronto

With offices in

Argentina Austria Brazil Chile Czech Republic France Greece
Guatemala Hungary Italy Japan Poland Portugal Singapore
South Korea Switzerland Thailand Turkey Ukraine Vietnam

Oxford is a registered trade mark of Oxford University Press
in the UK and in certain other countries

Published in the United States
by Oxford University Press Inc., New York

British Library Cataloguing in Publication Data

Data available

Library of Congress Cataloging-in-Publication-Data

Data available

Typeset by Cepha Imaging Private Ltd., Bangalore, India
Printed in Great Britain
on acid-free paper by
Biddles Ltd., King's Lynn, Norfolk
ISBN 978–0–19–923421–9

1 3 5 7 9 10 8 6 4 2

Whilst every effort has been made to ensure that the contents of this book are as complete,
accurate and up-to-date as possible at the date of writing, Oxford University Press is not
able to give any guarantee or assurance that such is the case. Readers are urged to take
appropriately qualified medical advice in all cases. The information in this book is
intended to be useful to the general reader, but should not be used as a means of
self-diagnosis or for the prescription of medication.

Foreword

Sir Liam Donaldson

The challenges facing young doctors seem to increase exponentially. Not only does the body of knowledge grow but also the skill set expected of the clinicians is constantly expanding. Patients rightly want their doctor to have breadth of knowledge, depth of compassion, supreme communication skills, and, perhaps above all, plentiful empathy.

How we create individuals who meet these requirements, how we take young men and women and guide them to strive to achieve these aims, and to be able to cope with new challenges is what medical education is ultimately about. This book is a wonderful guide to how to accomplish this. By encompassing not just the classical aspects of medical education, but going far beyond this to explore topics such as learning in the community, medical leadership, and maturing learners, I believe that this book will provide important insight for many into this critical phase of medical development.

At the heart of this book is the definition of what it means to be a medical professional in the twenty-first century. It is fundamental that as this understanding evolves we ensure that this is adequately communicated to future doctors. Time spent at medical school is crammed with learning, and perhaps most importantly self-development. However, it is here that the opportunity lies to set future clinicians on to a clear, defined pathway where their vision is always to ensure the best possible care for their patients. But to do so while understanding that modern times demand that this excellence is not only routinely demonstrated on a day-to-day basis but can be proven and certified to maintain public acceptance.

We have much to learn still. Methods to assess medical knowledge and skills are changing rapidly, for example improved information technology has permitted the creation of modalities such as computer simulation, and how this is utilized is not clear in all specialities yet. Equally, we may have not, to date, found the perfect mechanisms to select potential clinicians; while striving to move away from old systems we must ensure that new ones are rigorous and evidence based.

Ultimately this book will, I am sure, become a guide for many in medical education. It will help to ensure that future generations of doctors are trained to meet the changing needs of our population. As the book so clearly identifies, medical education is a lifelong process. Looking back over my career in medicine, it is clear to me that while my time at medical school laid the foundations for my future, so much of my training and development occurred after medical school, and through the generosity of clinicians with their expertise, knowledge, and time. This book is an extension of this attribute of clinicians – the desire to always learn and perhaps even more so to constantly teach.

Preface

We are both experienced medical educators of both undergraduates and post-graduates and have demonstrated a long-standing commitment to multiprofessional education and training. After collaborating closely in London for 6 years, we edited our first book together entitled *Guide to Education and Training in Primary Care* in 2002. Oxford University Press approached us at the end of 2006 and asked if we had considered compiling a second edition. Predictably this initial conversation provoked an enthusiastic discussion about the overarching theme for a new book and we actively debated whether to again selectively focus on primary care or to be more generic in our approach. For this new venture, we have gathered together over the last year what we consider to be an impressive array of contributors with a wide variety of experience across diverse academic, service and lay backgrounds. We hope that this book conveys the excitement and enthusiasm we both feel for our subject. We set out to provide both theoretical and practical guidance for those planning, delivering, and receiving education and training in ever changing healthcare environments. Our aim is also to provide a useful resource to countries outside the UK, with a range of higher education and healthcare models.

The book aims to provide a comprehensive, up-to-date review of medical education and training with a seamless approach across the undergraduate/postgraduate years. Recent changes in medical education and training have been highlighted. It is anticipated that the readership of this book will extend to healthcare professionals in primary, community, and secondary care settings and organizations, including NHS trusts, Strategic Health Authorities, Postgraduate Deaneries, and University Departments of Medical/Clinical Education. We hope that teachers, students, and clinicians will all find it useful. We also seek through the process of medical education and training to promote professionalism, leadership, and a culture of lifelong learning and reflective practice for all doctors and healthcare professionals working in our NHS. This will in turn enable them to meet the challenge of a fast-changing world, medical advances, new technologies, and new approaches to patient care.

Stay ahead with online updates!

Make sure you have the latest information on medical education and training to hand – visit our dedicated website at www.oup.com/uk/gmet to download online updates from our author team.

Contents

Contributors

Michael J Bannon
Postgraduate Dean,
Oxford Postgraduate Medical and
Dental Education,
University of Oxford, UK

Rex Bird
PMETB Lay Visitor,
Birmingham, UK

Isobel Bowler
Independent Research Consultant,
London Deanery, UK

Jonathan Burton
Retired GP and former
Associate Director,
Department of Postgraduate
GP Education,
London Deanery, UK

Peter Cantillon
Senior Lecturer,
Department of General Practice,
Clinical Science Institute,
National University of Ireland,
Ireland

Victoria Carr
Consultant Psychologist,
Work Psychology Group,
Nottingham, UK

Yvonne Carter
Professor of General Practice and
Primary Care, Dean of Warwick
Medical School, Pro-Vice-Chancellor
(Regional Engagement),
The University of Warwick, UK

John Clark
Director of Medical Leadership and
International Relations,
NHS Institute for Innovation and
Improvement, UK

Angela Coulter
Chief Executive, Picker Institute
Europe, UK

David Davies
Associate Professor (Reader),
Institute of Clinical Education,
University of Warwick, UK

Helena Davies
Sheffield Children's Trust, UK

Isobel Down
Independent Consultant,
NHS Institute for Innovation and
Improvement, UK

Liam Glynn
Lecturer, Department of General
Practice, Clinical Science Institute,
National University of Ireland,
Ireland

Michael J Goldacre
Professor of Public Health,
Unit of Health-Care Epidemiology,
Department of Public Health,
University of Oxford, UK

Anne Hastie
Director of Postgraduate General
Practice Education,
London Deanery, UK

Richard Hays
Professor of Medical Education and
Head of School of Medicine,
Keele University Medical School,
UK

Gareth Holsgrove
Gareth Holgrove Ltd.,
Cambridgeshire, UK

Sir Donald Irvine
Chairman of Picker Institute Europe,
UK

Neil Jackson
Postgraduate Dean, Department of
Postgraduate GP Education,
London Deanery, UK

Neil Johnson
Associate Dean for Teaching,
Institute of Clinical Education,
Warwick Medical School,
University of Warwick,
UK

Pat Lane
Director of Postgraduate
General Practice Education,
South Yorkshire and South Humber
GP Deanery, UK

Chris McManus
Professor of Psychology and
Medical Education,
University College London, UK

Geoff Meads
Past Chair of UK Centre for
Advancement of Interprofessional
Learning (CAIPE), Warwick Medical
School, UK

Sue Morrison
Associate Director of Postgraduate
General Practice Education,
London Deanery, UK

Fiona Patterson
Professor of Organisational
Psychology, City University
London, UK

Ed Peile
Professor Emeritus of Medical
Education, Institute of Clinical
Education, Warwick Medical School,
University of Warwick, UK

Anne Slowther
Associate Professor Clinical Ethics,
Institute of Clinical Education,
Warwick Medical School, UK

John Spencer
Professor, School of Medical
Education Development, Newcastle
University upon Tyne Medical
School, UK

John Spicer
Associate Director in Postgraduate
GP Education, London Deanery, UK
and Senior Lecturer in Clinical
Ethics and Law, St George's
University of London, UK

Cees van der Vleuten
Professor of Education,
Department of Educational
Development and Research,
University of Maastricht,
The Netherlands

David Wall
Deputy Regional Postgraduate Dean,
West Midlands Deanery,
Birmingham, UK

Val Wass
Professor of Community Based
Medical Education,
Manchester Medical School,
University of Manchester, UK

Chapter 1

Professionalism and professional regulation

Sir Donald Irvine

Over a hundred years ago Sir William Osler, writing about being a doctor, said, 'The physician needs a clear head and a kind heart. His work is arduous and complex requiring the exercise of the very highest faculties of the mind, whilst constantly appealing to the emotions and finer feelings'.[1] Today Osler would see that the science and practice of medicine and the society within which doctors work have changed out of all recognition. Yet, for all that, some things do not change. When illness strikes, we the public still want doctors who are technically excellent and who at the same time are able and willing to relate to us and care for us, to help us through our trouble.

This book is about medical education. My introductory chapter is about providing context by relating the opportunities for medical education to the professionalism that lies at the heart of doctoring, and to the associated regulatory framework within which doctors must practise.

Medical professionalism

When people think they are ill they go to a doctor to find out what is wrong with them and what can be done to make them better. They expect to see a 'good' doctor,[2] someone they can trust without even having to think about it.

Recent studies[3–7] have shown what 'goodness' in a doctor means from the public's point of view. Patients and their relatives think of it in terms of up to date medical knowledge and clinical skill, clinical experience, sound judgement, wisdom, reliability, thoroughness, honesty, and general integrity. Good doctors respect their patients' autonomy, are able and willing to form a satisfactory relationship with them, and will always put their patients' interests first. They are interested in their patients, listen to them, and know how to communicate with them effectively. They are kind, courteous, considerate, empathetic, and caring. They go out of their way to find out what makes their patients tick, what their feelings, fears, and preferences are. They will always try to protect their patients from harm. When clinical teamwork is appropriate for the patient they become effective team players.

All these attributes matter to patients because they know perfectly well that what their doctor does can make the difference between life and death, or between enjoying a full recovery and suffering serious disability. Together they epitomize the patients' views of what doctors' professionalism means to them.

This understanding was captured recently by the Royal College of Physicians of London, which summarized medical professionalism as 'a set of values, behaviours and relationships that underpins the trust the public has in doctors'.[8] It is reflected in more detail in the latest edition of the UK General Medical Council's (GMC) *Good Medical Practice*[9] and the North American sister document, *Good Medical Practice – USA*.[10] These two statements are the most authoritative and comprehensive descriptions of the modern doctor's duties and responsibilities in use today.

It is doctors' extensive training and experience in diagnosis that distinguishes them from other healthcare professionals. Patients know this, which is why they see doctors as ultimately responsible for their care. Diagnosis, and much of modern medical treatment, are founded on scientific and technical knowledge, which change and expand with terrifying speed. They often involve complex clinical problem solving and decision-making, which in turn depend on powers of observation, analytical, technical and interpersonal skills, experience, critical judgement, and honesty. This is the reason why the medical profession insists on recruiting high achievers, why they are given a rigorous and lengthy training in the science, practice, and ethics of medicine, and why in future the established doctor's continuing professional development will have to be equally systematic and rigorous.[2]

By its very nature much of medical practice is unsupervised. Sustaining day-to-day optimum performance is therefore still very much a matter of individual conscience and self-discipline – literally self-regulation.[11] This is true even though the scope for discretion by individual practitioners has become more circumscribed recently by evidence-based medicine, practice guidelines, and the much greater scrutiny of clinical results by peer review, informally and through regulation. Conscientiously maintaining and improving practising performance, and indeed striving constantly for excellence, are hallmarks of true professionalism.

For most of the twentieth century notions of medical professionalism were the product of the thinking of doctors themselves.[12] Doctors alone controlled access to the knowledge base of medicine and much about the clinical process was enveloped in mystery and shielded from public view. Doctors had huge autonomy and patients little.

However, in the last decade this situation has been changing dramatically. For the first time information technology and the Internet have given members of the public direct access to the database of medicine. These facilities, in the hands of a much more educated population living in the consumer world, are altering the power dynamics of the doctor–patient relationship towards the patient. For example, more people now want more say in clinical decisions that are going to affect their lives; and they are more likely to want to know that their own doctors (and nurses) are up to the mark, and that they can be sure of the quality and safety of their healthcare at the time they are using the service.[13,14]

In response a new, more patient-centred form of professionalism has been evolving that recognizes that patient autonomy is pre-eminent – it is the patient who has the illness and who has to manage and live with the consequences.[8,11,15–17] This fundamental change is proving to be quite a challenge to many doctors and professional institutions still used to thinking and acting along traditional doctor-centred lines.[12]

The professionalism of doctors cannot be seen in isolation from their workplace. Most doctors today work in organizations such as the UK National Health Service (NHS) or managed care systems in the USA, where they are either employed by, or in contract with, an institutional provider. Institutions can enhance doctors' professionalism by, for example, ensuring that doctors have adequate time for their patients and that they are practising in an institutional culture that understands and nurtures the relationship between professionalism and high performance. They can support doctors' professional development by providing the sophisticated clinical data systems essential for giving optimal comparative feedback on personal and team performance.

However, institutions can also undermine professionalism. For example, they may have workplace practices – such as institutionalized clinical micromanagement – that diminish doctors' sense of responsibility, and therefore demotivate and demoralize them. Similarly, an institution may organize its patient services in ways that make it difficult for doctors to maintain the degree of continuity of patient care needed to establish a relationship of trust. Or there may be institutional policies, as on the availability and choice of drugs, that may conflict with doctors' judgements of what is best for their individual patients.

We are used to thinking about medical professionalism in relation to individual doctors and their personal performance in the consulting room and within the clinical team. Certainly, doctors themselves are primarily responsible for the quality of their own performance and ethical conduct. However, the medical profession has hitherto assumed collective responsible for making sure that all patients are served by good doctors, and that the population is therefore protected from doctors who are incompetent or just not good enough. So, professionalism has both personal and group dimensions.

In the British Commonwealth and the USA in particular it is this collective responsibility that has been the basis of self-regulation. It has not been as effective as it could and should be, which is why change is in the air.

Professional regulation

Professional regulation should be founded on values and standards of practice shared by doctors and the public. It is the basis for the profession's contract with the public.[18,19] Medical education is the principal (but not the only) means whereby such values and standards are taught, learnt, digested, internalized, and continually refreshed at all stages in a doctor's career. That is why from the earliest days of the modern medical profession, the relationship between medical education and medical professionalism and regulation has been so fundamental.

Klein[20] put his finger on the nub of the relationship between public policy and professional regulation when he said 'the aim of public policy is to make the medical profession collectively more accountable for its performance. The aim of professional self-regulation is to make individual practitioners more accountable to their peers. Control over the medical profession collectively is a complement to – not a substitute for – control by the medical profession of its members. The precise balance between the two will depend on the extent to which the medical profession can be trusted to deliver its part of the bargain'.

The basic instrument of professional regulation is licensure. Licensing authorities are statutory bodies to which legislatures have delegated the responsibility of ensuring that only people they consider to be properly qualified are allowed to practise medicine. Thus the GMC is the national licensing authority in the UK. It discharges its basic statutory functions by maintaining registers of practitioners whom it has authorised to practise. In Canada, Australia, and the USA licensure is the responsibility of states or provinces, but the function is the same.

Specialist certification may or may not be statutory. In the USA, for example, the specialty boards are private professional certificating organizations whose members are appointed for their knowledge and experience of education and assessment in their field. In the UK the Royal medical colleges are charitable membership organizations responsible for the content and standards of education and training needed for entry to their respective specialties. However, it is the government-appointed Postgraduate Medical Education and Training

Board (PMETB), shortly to be absorbed into the GMC, which at the moment certificates doctors who have completed training satisfactorily. These doctors' names are then placed on the specialist or general practice registers held by the GMC.

Accreditation is the process through which designated authorities approve the educational experience and standards of training offered by post-graduate organizations. In the UK the GMC accredits basic medical education in UK medical schools, and is likely to do this for postgraduate training in future.

These, then, are the basic principles and mechanisms that inform the governance of the medical profession. Every doctor and medical student has a duty to understand them and to uphold the standards expected of them personally and in cooperation with colleagues. Any action that damages a doctor's personal integrity damages the integrity of the whole profession.[21]

Evolving professional regulation

Historically, professional regulation has tended to follow changes in practice and medical education. Thus the licensing of doctors began in the nineteenth century with state recognition of the emerging modern medical profession. The early focus was on medical education,[16] partly to distinguish those who were deemed by doctors' organizations of the day to have been properly trained from those who had not, and partly to close down or overhaul educational institutions whose training of medical students was simply inadequate. Accelerating specialization in the mid-twentieth century spawned programmes of graduate training, which in turn led to the introduction of specialist certification.

Throughout this long period of time international medical regulation was passive and reactive. It was mainly concerned with making students into doctors, and generic doctors into specialists and family practitioners. Doctors, once trained, were assumed to be practising well and keeping themselves up to date according to standards they themselves determined. Action by regulators on a doctor's registration could only be triggered by a complaint, usually about some form of gross misconduct, not about poor clinical practice. Whistleblowing by doctors about colleagues' poor practice was virtually taboo.

In the last 20 years or so medical regulation has come under increasing public scrutiny for three main reasons.[12,16] First and most important, consumer interests and the media began to criticize doctors' regulators for being overly complacent about the profession's habit of turning a blind eye to poor clinical practice, at the expense of patient safety. Secondly, the public sensed that, in the energetic pursuit of scientific medicine and research, the medical profession was losing sight of the human dimensions of medical practice, especially the need for doctors to be able to communicate properly with their patients and form meaningful relationships with them. And third, some policy makers and doctors' leaders could see that medical regulation was in a backwater, inward looking, isolated from the real world, and largely unaware of the significance for it of the quality movement gathering pace across healthcare. All in all, professional self-regulation as practised was not making the contribution it should to patient safety and the quality of care, and was therefore undermining the very professionalism it was supposed to foster and protect.

In this climate of growing public unease, more recent embarrassing, well-publicized medical disasters in the USA, Canada, New Zealand, and the UK compelled action. For the public the question now was whether the profession and its regulators had the stomach to deal effectively with poorly performing doctors. While patients' trust in individual doctors remained high where their personal experience was good, the hitherto unquestioning confidence in the medical regulators was replaced by a demand for more rigorous protection from poorly performing doctors, concrete evidence of all doctors' ongoing fitness to practise, more public involvement in regulation, more explicit and transparent accountability, and less self-interested protectiveness. It became clear that in future, trust in the collective profession must be founded on a truly patient-centred culture of medical practice, and a system of professional regulation and medical education that put the interests of patients unequivocally first.[12,16]

Doctors thus found themselves with two basic options.[12] They could accept the public's criticisms of their stewardship of self-regulation with good grace, wholeheartedly adapt their ideas of professionalism and professional responsibility to meet society's new expectations, and so re-build and strengthen the relationship of trust both parties want. That option has the potential for giving the best results for everyone because of the level of commitment it implies. Or they could do little, forcing the state (usually reluctantly) to take more direct managerial control itself. In the event the jury is still out. The profession has inclined to the first option, although progress has varied according to the degree of internal resistance.[22] There have been three main strands – the introduction of explicit professional standards, new arrangements for dealing with poorly performing doctors, and revalidation using measures that should ensure the ongoing competence of established doctors.

The key thing today is to recognize that modern healthcare is a complex system in which the behaviour of doctors is critical to the safety, effectiveness, and acceptability of medical care. So, the public has every reason to expect consistently good performance and zero tolerance of poor performance, as it does with aircrew in the civil aviation industry. Hence the object of modern professional regulation – to make sure that every patient has a good doctor.[2]

The new UK model of professional regulation

The UK is an instructive case study because, there, public loss of confidence, precipitated by the failure of paediatric cardiac surgery at the Bristol Royal Infirmary in the early 1990s, galvanized both the government and the profession to think radically.[12,23,24] They decided to abandon reactive regulation in favour of a proactive model aligning professional regulation more closely with clinical governance at the workplace and wider systems of quality improvement and quality assurance. The changes have been led by informal alliances between reforming doctors – many of them leading teachers – and progressive patient organizations, managers, policy makers, and politicians. The transition phase has been slow because of some continuing professional resistance to meaningful change.

The new UK approach starts with patient autonomy, sees patients and the public as partners with the medical profession, and is based on values and standards agreed by the public and the profession together. Doctors are expected to internalize these standards mainly through medical education. The standards are to be underwritten by licensure, certification, and contracts of employment. All doctors become personally responsible for demonstrating that they remain fully fit to practise throughout their active professional lives, through revalidation. Doctors who fall below the required standards will have the opportunity to remediate under supervision, but if they cannot, they will have to stop practising.

There is to be more lay involvement in the governance of the profession and the replacement of doctors elected by the profession with doctors appointed by an independent commission. The full dimensions of the changes are set out in the report *Good doctors, safer patients* published by Sir Liam Donaldson, the Chief Medical Officer for England,[25] and more recently in a Bill now before Parliament.

The standards

The values and standards expected of every doctor on the medical register are described in the GMC's *Good Medical Practice*. Some 60 generic standards capture the essence of what the public and doctors together think makes a good doctor. They are to be complemented by specialty-specific standards now being developed by the Royal colleges. Persistent failure to practise in accordance with the standards will put a doctor's licence to practise at risk. Work is therefore underway to define the criteria, thresholds, competencies, and sources of evidence needed to make Good Medical Practice ready for full operational use in licensure, certification, revalidation, and fitness to practise arrangements.

However, there is a serious and highly sensitive unresolved question.[2,24] There are still many doctors who see such standards as aspirational. The public, on the other hand, while remarkably tolerant of minor lapses,[3] nevertheless expect broad compliance with standards of conduct and competence on which they can rely. In the UK today there is still a very wide gap between good and not good enough to remain on the register, despite full exposure of the problem at the Shipman Inquiry.[26]

How has this come about? Historically the profession has rightly insisted on high standards for initial licensure and subsequent admission to the specialist register, but has tolerated much lower standards from some established doctors before concerns about their practice trigger regulatory action. The Bell Curve has a long downside.[2,27] One result is that there are still doctors practising today whom colleagues would not accept as good enough to treat their own families. This is not a tenable ethical position.

It may be that at the end of the day it will be outside pressure, caused by the regular publication and public scrutiny of the results of revalidation, that forces closure of the gap.

Revalidation

Revalidation is the process whereby doctors demonstrate regularly that they are fit to practise in their chosen field.[28] There is to be a two-strand model embracing re-licensure by the GMC and re-certification by the Royal colleges. Ideally, the two processes will be complementary.[25]

Assessment will be against the standards set by the GMC and the Royal colleges through *Good Medical Practice*[13] Revalidation is to be underpinned by the GMC's fitness to practise procedures that will be used to decide what to do about doctors whose performance is not up to scratch. Arrangements for retraining such doctors where necessary are already in place.

The public has strong views about revalidation. In Britain, a 2005 Mori Social Research Institute survey[13] showed that nine out of 10 members of the public thought it important that doctors' competence should be checked every few years. Nearly half the sample thought that these assessments happen already, and that they should be every year. The public is most concerned about the doctor being up-to-date, having a high success rate with treatments, getting high satisfaction ratings from patients, and having good communication skills.

Re-licensure will be every 5 years and will usually involve satisfactory participation in annual appraisal at the workplace, informed by standardized multi-source feedback, and the satisfactory resolution of any issues affecting a doctor's conduct or competence known to a GMC affiliate (agent) in the local area.

Re-certification, also normally 5-yearly, will involve everyone on the specialist or general practitioner registers held by the GMC. Each specialty is to design methods for assessing performance against the specialty-specific standards.

It remains to be seen whether the UK medical profession has the will to make sure that revalidation achieves its purpose.[24,26,29]

The new challenge for medical education

This brings me to education, the subject of the book. From this chapter it must be obvious to readers that attention in future will focus much more on established doctors and how they can sustain optimal performance throughout their professional lives. That is what the public will be watching for. Their expectation brings new challenges and opportunities for medical educators. The big issue is with institutional cultures and hidden curricula in our educational establishments. These can have a huge impact on doctors' attitudes, which are crucial to good practice. I make three points here.

The first is about professional values and standards. It will fall primarily to the educational system to help all students and doctors to internalize the profession's standards, and to aspire to excellence.[2,30] All doctors, whether trained in the UK or elsewhere, need to take full ownership of the standards, to understand the obligations and responsibilities they carry, to equate them with their professional identity, and to be committed, in conscience, to practising in accordance with them. They ought to know why they should feel proud to be members of a highly respected profession, and understand their role in maintaining that respect. This is the essence of personal self-regulation. Seen in this light, regulation may be seen as supportive rather than oppressive, with revalidation a welcome recognition of excellence sustained rather than the marker of a minimum standard attained with as little effort as possible.

Done well, there are big gains in this for doctors as well as patients. For example, doctors should have greater peace of mind and the self-confidence that comes from knowing, and being able to show others, that they are on top of the job, absolutely reliable and trustworthy. Doctors who are self-confident and self-aware are more able to take control of their own professional lives, and not to feel that they are being driven by the system as so many do today. Self-confidence, self-respect, and self-control beget high morale.[2]

The second point is about teachers. The educational system cannot respond adequately to the new task until it gives far more attention to sustaining the highest quality clinical teachers in the future. Medical education is heavily dependent, rightly, on experiential learning. Everyone knows that teachers' influence, by deed as much as word, is critical. They lead through the example of their own practice, and have a responsibility to show what excellence in practice, and in their approach to their own learning, means in everyday life. Indeed their collective example is the nub of the hidden curriculum, the living embodiment of what an educational institution stands for. So medical teachers are an institution's most precious asset, the gold in the bank. Thus their importance must be recognized accordingly and their practice, professional development, and the accompanying support networks, move centre stage.

Thirdly, it is interesting that while the public eye is fixed firmly on the established doctor, the whole edifice of medical education has been built around preparing doctors for independent practice. By and large basic and specialist training have been innovative and professionally done in the UK. The same cannot be said of continuing professional development, for reasons explained earlier. That is the historic legacy, from which we must now move away. As structured, medical education will find it difficult to achieve the enhancement and professionalization of continuing professional development now necessary. A mindset change, which translates into significant system redesign, is needed urgently.

And finally

At the end of the day it all comes down to leadership. Perhaps the greatest challenge for the institutions of the medical profession is whether they have the imagination and courage to overcome the tribalism and professional self-interest that so often bedevils innovation, progress, and proper protection of the public.[12] On this, the leadership given by medical educators will be critical. They are the front line. They have the opportunity of a lifetime.

References

1. Osler W. Teaching and thinking. In: *Aequanimitas*. Philadelphia, PA: P Blakiston's Son and Co., 1904, pp. 132–3.
2. Irvine DH. Everyone is entitled to a good doctor. Abridged version of the 30thWilliam Osler Lecture delivered at McGill University November 2006. *Med J Aust* 2007; **186**: 256–61.
3. Chisholm A, Cairncross L, Askham J. *Setting standards: the views of members of the public and doctors on the standards of care they expect from doctors.* Oxford: Picker Institute Europe, 2006. http://www.pickereurope.org/Filestore/Publications/Setting_Standards_Final.pdf Accessed October 2007.

4. Hasman A, Graham C, Reeves R, Askham J. *What do patients and relatives see as key competencies for intensive care doctors?* Oxford: Picker Institute Europe, 2006. http://www.pickereurope.org/Filestore/Publications/CobatriceFull_report_with_isbn_web_(2).pdf Accessed October2007.

5. Coulter A. What do patients want from primary care? *BMJ* 2005; **331**: 1199–2001.

6. Wensing M, Jung HP, Mainz J, Olesen F, Grol R.A systematic review of the literature on patient priorities for general practice care. 1. Description of the research domain. *Soc Sci Med* 1998; **47**: 1573–88.

7. Bendapudi NM, Berry LL, Frey KA, Parish JT, Rayburn WL. Patient perspectives on ideal physician behaviours. *Mayo Clinic Proc* 2006; **81**: 338–44.

8. Royal College of Physicians of London. *Doctors in society: medical professionalism in a changing world*. Report of College Working Party on Medical Professionalism. London: RCP, 2005.

9. General Medical Council. *Good medical practice*, 4th edn. London: GMC, 2006. http://www.gmc-uk.org/guidance/good_medical_practice Accessed October 2007.

10. Alliance for Physician Competence. *Good medical practice-USA*, 2007. https://gmpusa.org/Docs/Good%20Medical%20Practice%20-%20USA %20version%200.1%20final.pdf Accessed October 2007.

11. Cruess R, Cruess SR, Johnston SE. Professionalism: an ideal to be sustained. *Lancet* 2000; **356**: 156–9.

12. Irvine DH. *The doctors' tale: professionalism and public trust*. Oxford: Radcliffe Medical Press, 2003.

13. MORI. *Attitudes to revalidation and regulation of doctors*. London: Department of Health, 2005.

14. College of Physicians of Ontario. Revalidation consultation summary. April 7 2006. The Gallup Organisation for the American Board of Internal Medicine. *Awareness of and attitudes towards board certification of physicians*. Princeton NJ: The Gallup Organisation, 2003.

15. Freidson E. *Professionalism reborn: theory, prophecy, policy*. Cambridge: Polity Press, 1994.

16. Stacey M. *Regulating British medicine: the General Medical Council*. Chichester, UK: Wiley, 1992.

17. Rosen R, Dewar S. *On being a doctor: refining medical professionalism for better patient care*. London: King's Fund, 2004.

18. Cruess SR. Professionalism and medicine's social contract with society. 2006; **449**: 170–6.

19. Irvine DH. The performance of doctors.1. Professionalism and self-regulation in a changing world. *BMJ* 1997; **314**: 1540–2.

20. Kline R. *Regulating the medical profession: doctors and the public interest. Healthcare 1997/1998*. London: King's Fund, 1998, p. 163.

21. Horton R, Gilmore I. *Lancet* 2006; **368**: 1750–1.

22. Allsop J, Jones K. Protecting patients: international trends in professional governance. In *Rethinking governance, remaking the professions: international trends in healthcare* (Eds Kuhlmann E, Saks M). Bristol: Policy Press, 2007.

23. Bristol Royal Infirmary Inquiry. *Learning from Bristol: the report of the public inquiry into childrens' heart surgery at the Bristol Royal Infirmary 1994–1995*. London: Stationary Office, 2001.

24. Irvine DH. A short history of the General Medical Council. *Med Educ* 2006; **40**: 202–11.

25. Donaldson L, Chief Medical Officer. *Good doctors, safer patients*. London: Department of Health, 2006.

26. The Shipman Inquiry. *Safeguarding patients: lessons from the past, proposals for the future*. London: Stationary Office, 2004.

27. Gawande A. The Bell Curve. In *Better: surgeon's notes on performance*. London: Profile Books, 2007.

28. General Medical Council. *Revalidating doctors: ensuring standards, securing the future*. London: GMC, 2000.

29. Pringle M. *Revalidation of doctors: the credibility challenge*. London: The Nuffield Trust, 2005.

30. Cruess R. Teaching professionalism. *Clin Orthop* 2006; **449**: 177–85.

Chapter 2

Measuring professionalism

Richard Hays

Introduction

Not so long ago, the focus of medical education was on the immense breadth
(and at times considerable depth) of the knowledge required for individuals to
develop into sound medical practitioners. This is no easy task, as medical
practice is underpinned by a wide range of biomedical, behavioural, and social
sciences, and research makes almost daily additions to the understanding
of human structure and function, mechanisms of disease and potentially
effective interventions that can improve quantity and quality of life. The pace
of development is fast, and the challenge for medical education is to produce
graduates who not only have a current knowledge and skills base, but can
adapt to change and maintain their currency of practice, translating new
knowledge and skills into effective clinical practice over a potentially long
career.

However, there are other challenges for medical education that reflect
changes in the way society functions. It is also not so long since doctors were
regarded as *the* experts in healthcare. They were recognized as academically
strong, highly trained, hard working people who did the best that was possible
in the circumstances. Honesty and reliability were taken for granted. Mistakes
were regarded as sad but inevitable events and poor outcomes were rarely
challenged. Where a doctor made an error, it was often understood to be due
to overwork or within an 'acceptable' range, as doctors are human and
inevitably make mistakes. Community trust in doctors was high. This land-
scape has also changed, perhaps dramatically, as doctors have been shown
to be fallible and analyses of critical errors shows that quality improvement
methods are relevant and effective in medical practice.[1] All patients want
and expect competent medical care,[2] and reactions to poor outcomes
are now more likely to include anger and probing questions, sometimes with
a high media profile, and careers of doctors involved in errors can be in
jeopardy.

A final challenge is to ensure that doctors always act in the best interests of patients, not themselves. Even if we assume that correct clinical decisions are made most of the time, the care of individual patients has to be within the capacity of individual doctors; this requires a degree of continuing self-awareness, or insight.[3] The provision of care must also fall within a legal framework that is designed to safeguard those who are vulnerable through illness. There have been only a few instances of deceitful and criminal behaviour by doctors,[4,5] but these instances have had a profound effect on the practice of medicine and the way that society regards doctors. A strong patient safety and quality of care agenda has emerged. In response, doctors must now regularly demonstrate that they are meeting professional behaviour requirements. In the UK this is managed through annual performance appraisal that looks much more broadly than clinical outcomes.

Most of the public concern about professionalism of doctors involves experienced doctors, most whom would not have been taught or assessed on professionalism during their undergraduate or postgraduate training. Yet there is evidence that poor behaviour as a student may predict later professional behaviour problems,[6] a finding that may have most influenced medical education by confirming the need to formally consider professionalism as a core curriculum issue at all levels of medical education.

During the 1990s, a majority of medical schools began to include in their curricula some information about humanistic values, ethics and responding to societal needs, but these topics were infrequently assessed.[7] As community expectations grew, so too has the response by medical educators, who now devote considerable resources to the development of doctors as professional people who not only have the requisite knowledge and skills to provide clinical care, but the capacity to provide high-quality care in a professional manner throughout their careers.[8] Professionalism is now regarded as something requiring life-long development, maintenance, and monitoring. All medical curricula, both undergraduate and postgraduate, now include substantial components that aim to produce the rounded professional, and these are reviewed by medical school and postgraduate course accreditation organizations.

Because this rapid development has occurred at a time of continuing change in community expectations and legal frameworks, it is probable that it has happened in advance of our ability to fully understand how to develop professionalism and demonstrate that doctors have achieved the desired level.[9] This chapter explores the development of professionalism through medical education, and does this from the perspective of how professionalism can be measured.

Defining professionalism

The idea of professionalism is not new. The best recorded early expression of the role of doctors as professionals is in the Hippocratic Oath, which originated in the fourth century BC; although professionalism almost certainly evolved over time. Hilton and Southgate provide an excellent summary of this evolution and the current understanding of underpinning values of professionalism and concepts such as 'phronesis', 'mindful practice', and reflective practice', describing a learner's progress through 'proto-professionalism' to mature professionalism.[10] Building on this improved understanding of professionalism, several nations have recently developed and adopted rather similar codes of practice for doctors, from medical students to experienced clinicians, that are broader than the traditional clinical focus of the past; examples include Canada, the USA, the UK, and Australia.[11-14] The most explicit is arguably Good Medical Practice,[13] originally developed in the UK but now adopted more widely, in which three of the seven themes are 'Working with colleagues', 'Probity', and 'Health'. Table 2.1 summarizes the principles associated with these three themes, taken from the General Medical Council (GMC) website. Note the words 'you must' precede most statements, allowing little room for debate. The result is that providers of medical education now have much more guidance on what to include in medical curricula to assist graduates achieve learning objectives based on these formerly un-taught and un-assessed attributes of medial practice.

These themes are equally relevant at postgraduate level, where changing work practices make working with colleagues even more important.

The teaching and learning of professionalism

Translating even the more recent and more explicit understanding of medical professionalism into a curriculum is a significant challenge. Curricula at all levels are already overcrowded, as they attempt to cope with the ever-expanding body of knowledge and the increasing range of technical skills that are required for medical practice. Freeing up time to devote to professionalism generally makes for interesting curriculum planning meetings! However, a feature of the elements of professionalism is that they are by nature less suitable for didactic teaching and learning, and more suitable for 'learning by seeing and doing'. The essential outcome is that learners not only know about the appropriate professional values, attitudes, and behaviours, but that they become aware of their own values, attitudes, and behaviours, observe these in the doctors they are exposed to, and can make judgements about what is right. There are stages of development of proto-professionalism, from novice

Table 2.1 A summary of 'probity' and 'health' within *Good Medical Practice*.[13]

Working with colleagues	*Working with teams:* respect, ensure communication, regularly review practice and support colleagues
	Conduct and performance of colleagues: protect patients, inform relevant authorities about concerns, have systems to manage colleagues with poor performance
	Respect for colleagues: treat with respect, not bully or make unfounded criticisms
	Arranging cover: ensure patients medical care is provided during absences
	Taking up and ending appointments: complete contractual notice periods in changing employment
	Delegation and referral: be satisfied that delegations and referrals are to appropriately qualified doctors
	Sharing information with colleagues*: share all relevant information for safe healthcare (if necessary obtain formal consent)
Probity	*Being honest and trustworthy:* inform the GMC without delay about charges for criminal offences, professional registration problems or suspension from work anywhere in the world
	Providing and publishing information about yourself: publish accurate information; not make unjustifiable claims about quality and outcomes
	Writing reports and curriculum vitaes: be honest and trustworthy when writing documents; always be honest about your experience, qualifications and positions
	Research: act with honesty and integrity, protect patient's interests and follow national governance guidelines
	Financial and commercial dealings: be open and honest in any financial arrangements with patients
	Conflict of interest: act in the patients' best interests when making referrals or providing care; neither seek nor accept gifts that may be seen to affect the way you manage patients; not allow any financial interest in a healthcare provider influence clinical decisions and you must tell the patient about any such interests.
Health	*Personal health and risk to others:* consult a suitably qualified colleague if ill and a risk to yourself or patients and follow their advice; be registered with a GP outside of your family to ensure access to independent and objective healthcare and not treat yourself*; be immunized against common serious communicable diseases where vaccines are available*

Those marked with an * are a should rather than a must.

medical student to mature professional, and all undergraduate and postgraduate medical curricula should contribute to this developmental pathway.[10] In the UK the GMC has recently published guidance on professionalism and fitness to practise for medical students, indicating the differences in standards expected of medical compared with other university students.[15] There is also an interesting debate about how developing as a professional might lead to a degree of callousness or hardening in order to cope with the role,[16] as there is some evidence that empathy (as measured) falls during medical education.[17]

The traditional way that medical students and recent graduates have learned professional values, attitudes, and behaviours has been based largely on role modelling. This is a powerful method, but inappropriate role modelling is as powerful as appropriate role modelling. Hence the most important influences on the learning of appropriate medical professionalism are for all clinical teaching staff to: *understand* and *agree* with the curriculum content listed under professionalism; *demonstrate* appropriate medical professional behaviour to students in their clinical work; *highlight* and *discuss* any issues related to professionalism as they arise in clinical cases; and *provide feedback* to students on how they think and behave with respect to professional issues.

Two recent research papers highlight the importance of teacher behaviour in teaching health professional students. The first is the finding that the professional 'lapses' of medical students are similar to those of their teachers,[18] and the second is that students (in nursing) regard the professional misbehaviour of their teachers (e.g. failing to show for a scheduled lecture) as being just as serious as any they might exhibit.[19] Just as students are expected to conform to raising standards of professionalism, so too are their teachers. Professional 'lapses' are likely to occur in both student and teacher groups, and the key issue may be that this is acknowledged and discussed openly, rather than teachers being allowed to escape scrutiny. Any sign of respected teachers and clinicians demonstrating poor values, attitudes, and behaviours is a powerful 'hidden curriculum' that leads some learners to believe that the professionalism in the curriculum is 'false' or not to be taken seriously.

Hence the real challenge for medical educators is the selection of appropriate role models as clinical teachers. This is partly addressed by teacher training, using tools such as standardized videos of problem student behaviour to improve agreement on and detection of problem behaviours in students.[20] Ideally, only those clinicians who demonstrate appropriate professional behaviour should be recruited as teachers. However, as medical education expands and needs to utilize almost all clinical resources, this is becoming both more difficult and more important.

Assessment of professionalism

The assessment of professionalism falls into the 'hard to measure' category, for several reasons. The first is that there is still not widespread agreement on exactly what is professionalism, despite the more explicit definitions described above. Medical practice has evolved over the last two decades from a position where the doctor often worked alone, was always the leader of any group, and was generally forgiven any 'mistakes', to one where doctors are part of multi-professional teams, do not necessarily lead teams, and are under close scrutiny about their performance. Patients want to be, and often are, much better informed about their options and many expect to have some choice about what is best for them. Failure to provide high-quality care – a judgement that is evolving towards higher standards – can be a criminal offence. Depending on one's viewpoint, these are either major or somewhat subtle changes in the way doctors work, away from individual and towards group and systems functions. Included in this change are interprofessional communication, ethical frameworks, and legal issues, all topics that were not included in the basic medical curricula of most current clinical teachers. As with most topics in medical education, there is a set of knowledge, skills, and attitudes that make up the notion of professionalism.

The second reason is that it is difficult to be precise about precisely what can be expected of students and registrars as they progress through 'proto-professionalism'.[10] Many medical students are young, and poor behaviour can be blamed on 'high spirits' or immaturity. Many experienced clinical teachers would question the fairness of making negative comments about some behaviours in student files, perhaps because they either observed similar behaviours in peers who have developed into very good doctors, or they did similar things themselves. Should maturity be considered in making a judgement? If so, how is maturity defined and measured? The evidence about predictive validity of poor behaviour in medical students is still not strong. While doctors presenting to a Medical Board with professional problems were found more likely to have records of poor behaviours in student files, not all students with such records demonstrated professional problems.[6] There is even less in the literature about postgraduate trainees, perhaps because professional concerns about registered medical practitioners have to be managed within the constraints of potentially adversarial legal frameworks. Further research is needed to determine which behaviours in both medical students and postgraduate trainees better predict subsequent problems. This is a key issue in standard setting.

The third reason is the unwillingness of clinical teachers to make what could be regarded as 'harsh' judgements about learners who transgress professional boundaries. There is generally a wide area of 'grey' between the clearly poor and the clearly acceptable students. Many clinical teachers wonder if it is not just a personality clash, and are reluctant to make adverse comments as 'I might be the only person who thinks this of this student'. It is also common for clinical teachers to see less of learners, particularly undergraduate students, than they would like and therefore to not feel uncomfortable about making a judgement based on only brief 'snapshots'.

The fourth reason is that students and recent graduates may be reluctant to inform teachers about peers whose behaviour causes them concern. Here lies a combination of loyalty to friends and a tacit agreement that friends do not tell tales about each other. Further, while peer assessment can have a positive influence on learner behaviour, this requires a combination of experience and training.[21] Hence peer assessment has to be used with caution, particularly in summative assessment.

Assessment of professional behaviours should therefore be designed as a predominantly positive, empowering process that models and rewards appropriate professional behaviour in students, following an evidence-based approach that considers validity, reliability, practicality, efficiency, acceptability, and educational impact.[22] If personal qualities are considered in student selection, it is likely that the great majority of entering medical students will be highly motivated to do well and to aspire to be exemplary doctors. Hence they should have the attitudinal foundation necessary to be sound professionals. Basic medical education should then focus on providing them with the necessary knowledge and skills to be sound professionals, through a combination of knowledge provision, skills training, and role modelling. The majority of the assessment should be formative, so that medical students learn to reflect on their own professional behaviour, as well as those of their peers and teachers, in a way that improves self- and mutual awareness and guides progression through proto-professionalism to mature professionalism. Within this formative assessment, a small proportion of individuals will be identified raising concerns. The bar should arguably be set low for this, to increase the *sensitivity* of the assessment, as this allows for wide discussion about behaviours and 'where the line should be drawn'. Such discussions should be useful for all students and staff as they may narrow the 'grey' area of judgement, guide future personal development for all, and trigger early interventions for a minority.

The most important indicator of a potential 'problem' student, postgraduate trainee, or experienced clinician may be repetition of poor behaviours, with several different observers, in different situations, and over a period of time. An even stronger indicator may be that the individual does not learn from discussion about the poor behaviours, and stronger still, one that cannot accept that there is a problem despite mounting evidence from several different observers and situations; these may indicate poor insight and limited chance of improvement.[3] While the latter are a small minority, it is only by collecting judgments from several sources that any pattern of problem behaviour will become apparent. There may be debate about how many incidents of which kind constitutes a pattern, and this is usually a judgement call by experienced education managers. When a serious problem arises with a 'problem' senior student, it is not unusual for other students and staff to quietly say 'I am not surprised that student is in trouble, as this has been happening for a while'. This represents a failure of the system, as it is likely that early intervention could have either corrected the behaviour or resulted in earlier disciplinary action. One strategy is to implement a 'yellow card/red card' or 'three strikes and you are out' system, as these provide warning to transgressors that behaviour change is necessary to avoid serious consequences, and allows for earlier formal intervention.

Assuming the above system works well, then postgraduate medical learners should all have the necessary knowledge and skills to be competent professionals, and the focus of professional development should be on gaining experience, reflecting on the meaning of those experiences, and developing a set of 'mature' professional behaviours that can be role modelled to more junior colleagues.

Assessment tools

Many of the traditional assessment tools have not proven to be useful in assessing professionalism,[23,24] and many focus on only certain components of the more recently broadened definitions. Knowledge about professional behaviours can be assessed in written tests involving simulated cases, and professional skills and behaviours can be assessed in OSCE stations as part of integrated clinical assessment.[20] However, these assessments may miss 'problem' students as it s possible to know enough about and be able to perform well enough under observation, but then behave poorly when not observed. The contribution of Miller's pyramid (adapted in Figure 2.1) is the concept that it is what doctors *do*, not what they *can do*, that matters.[25] While all clinical assessment should include true performance assessment (what doctors *do*), the case for assessing professional behaviours in the workplace is particularly strong at both undergraduate and postgraduate levels.

Hence the most appropriate assessment tools for professional behaviours are those that provide judgements about student behaviour in clinical contexts, ideally from several different perspectives, in several different situations and on several different occasions.[26] This means assessments by peers, tutors, patients, and other members of the healthcare team. Students may prefer to provide the information anonymously.[26] Such assessment can be made individually, relating to specific placements or group activities, or can be made together as a 360 degree or multi-source feedback (MSF) assessment.[27]

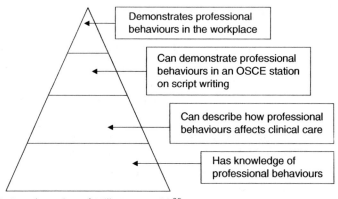

Fig. 2.1 An adaptation of Miller's pyramid.[25]

The latter offer the advantage that the simultaneous views of the different groups can be compared, leading to useful discussions about how professional behaviours are viewed by different stakeholders. MSF is gaining acceptance as a standard inclusion in regular performance appraisals that are now common in the health professions and university management and so it may be wise to introduce medical students to this process early. There is evidence that students prefer immediate feedback,[26] and the feedback also makes an ideal contribution to Learning Portfolios, as a trigger for reflection and personal growth.

There are problems using observational ratings such as those in MSF. As stated above, individuals filling them in may be unwilling to express concerns in a formal assessment process, particularly about behaviours. There are three ways of addressing this. The first is to use rating forms that seek information on learners' performances in a range of components of competence, including clinical knowledge and clinical skills.[26] Indeed it makes sense to assess professional behaviours only in the context of an integrated clinical assessment. The second is to provide space for observers to describe any behaviour that caused concern. It may be easier to describe behaviours rather than make a judgement about it, leaving the medical education office to make the judgement, particularly if there is more than one described concerning behaviour and a pattern is evident. For example, writing 'on some occasions failed to introduce himself to patients and on one occasion (an 84-year-old man with lung cancer) volunteered that treatment would not be worthwhile at his age' may be easier for an observer than to provide a score out of 10 for 'communication with patients'. Hence observer rating forms should include space for comments that should be monitored and, where necessary, compiled as a 'track record' in case a formal response is required. Appendix 1 provides an illustrative example of a rating form for medical students and early postgraduates that addresses the recent GMC initiative.[15] The addition of non-professional assessment to this form may strengthen its value in assessment by closely aligning professionalism and clinical performance.[26]

The third way if improving compliance is to make the collection of observer ratings a frequent event, such that staff and students become accustomed to their use. It is possible to require observer ratings, from at least the tutor perspective, at the completion of every clinical placement. Patient assessments are less valuable in contributing to a score, as most are glowing, but are useful because they send the message to staff and students that the views of patients are important. Self-assessments can also be useful, as they provoke discussion with learners about the concordance of their and others' views,[28] but can also be done less frequently.

In addition to the routine collection of mostly positive judgements about learner performance, it is worth considering instituting a form of incident reporting to notify programme managers of examples of both exemplary and poor professional behaviour exhibited by learners. This to some extent assures clinical teachers who feel that they have too little time with individual students to form a judgement over time, as they are free to submit at any stage a report that becomes part of the longitudinal record of the learner, and hence help programme managers recognize any patterns that may emerge.[29] Note the inclusion again of the positive reporting – a system that is seen to report only faults may be used less willingly. As an example, a student who goes to the trouble of personally escorting an anxious patient through some investigations might merit a mention by either the patient or the tutor, and this should be fed back formally and recorded in the student's record or portfolio as an example of exemplary professional behaviour. Care must be taken not to simply reward students who cynically pursue such opportunities knowing that a letter of commendation would follow. At the other end of the scale, a student who is observed to do something reprehensible, even on one occasion, such as arriving at a ward round smelling of alcohol, might merit (as well as being sent away) an incident report that triggers a letter of warning and referral for a health assessment.

Scoring and reporting issues

One of the objectives of assessment tools is to produce a score that can be interpreted as 'safe to proceed' (pass) or 'not safe to proceed without further learning and assessment' (fail). In almost all assessments the major uncertainty is the margin for error at the borderline of these two categories. As stated above, this grey zone may be larger when assessing professional behaviours.

Standard setting processes are the best way of narrowing this grey zone,[30] but may be more difficult with professionalism until there is stronger agreement on what is acceptable. The rating form in Appendix 1 demonstrates two other ways in which this is attempted. The first is that there is an 11-point scale (0–10) for each statement, and these can be added together to produce an overall score. This is a method for deriving a numerical score from ratings that fits measurement theory, but suffers from all the problems of any rating scale. The assessors may not use the scales appropriately (e.g. scoring everyone in the middle), although this can be addressed through assessor training. The second is that the last statement is an overall or *global* rating of the student's performance. Global ratings by experienced assessors are often more accurate than component scores.[31] It is possible that poor scores against one or two of the statements can be 'masked' by good scores against other statements, and global ratings are a useful check to ensure that serious but isolated problems are not easily overlooked.

It is also worth considering the relative merits of graded and non-graded reporting systems for scores for professionalism. Given the greater uncertainty about what professionalism includes, the notion that staff and students both have 'lapses' and that this is a set of attributes that evolves and requires effort to maintain over a long career, it may be better to adopt an non-graded satis-factory/unsatisfactory model. The key issue is that appropriate professional behaviours are recognized and the rest referred for closer analysis.

Conclusions

The modelling and measurement of professionalism in medical students, trainees, and experienced clinicians remain significant challenges to both educators and employers. The definition of professionalism is less clear than is necessary, and continues to develop amidst pressures from changing work-force models, changing community expectations and increasing interest in the safety and quality of healthcare. For example, it is not clear what the impact on safety will be from the more fluid and diverse team membership models that are likely to be providing more of the healthcare. Further, how normal professionalism develops in learners is uncertain. Professionalism may not be 'teachable', although still 'learnable', and learners are subject to many influences external to formal learning. Still further, the measurement of professionalism is less precise than necessary, and risks focusing on more easily identified, but perhaps less serious concerns. The stakes may be high, as poor professionalism is now part of the regular assessment and perform-ance review of all medical practitioners, from students to leaders of the profession, whether engaged in clinical, teaching, research, or management roles.

Despite workforce shortages, serious or persistent minor professional lapses are likely to become serious barriers to career progress, regardless of knowledge and technical expertise. However, medical educators cannot wait for the still substantial research agenda on professionalism to be realized and must proceed with the task of fostering appropriate professional behaviour, based on the best available evidence.

Further reading

Stern DTE (Ed.). *Measuring professionalism*. Oxford: Oxford University Press, 2006.

References

1. Katz JN, Kessler CL, O'Connell A, Levine SA. Professionalism and evolving concepts of quality. *J Gen Intern Med* 2007; **22**: 137–9.
2. Irvine DH. Everyone is entitled to a good doctor. *Med J Aust* 2007 **186**: 256–61.
3. Hays RB, Jolly BJ, Caldon LJM *et al.* (2002). Is insight important? Measuring the capacity to change. *Med Educ* 2002; **3**: 965–71.
4. The Shipman Inquiry. http://www.the-shipman-inquiry.org.uk (accessed December 2006)
5. Bundaberg Hospital Commission of Enquiry. http://www.bhci.qld.gov.au (accessed December 2006)
6. Papadakis MA, Hodgson CS, Tehrani A, Kohatsu ND. Unprofessional behaviour in medical schools associated with subsequent disciplinary action by a State Medical Board. *Acad Med* 2004; **74**: 980–99.
7. Swick HM, Szenas P, Danoff D, Whitcomb M. Teaching professionalism in undergraduate medical education. *JAMA* 1999; **282**: 830–2.
8. Cohen JJ. Professionalism in medical education, an American perspective: from evidence to accountability. *Med Educ* 2006; **40**: 607–17.
9. Saultz JW. Are we serious about teaching professionalism in medicine? *Acad Med* 2007; **82**: 574–86.
10. Hilton S, Southgate L. Professionalism in medical education. *Teach Teach Educ* 2007; **23**: 265–79.
11. Frank JR, Jabbour M, Tugwell P, *et al.* Skills for the new millenium: report of the societal needs working group, CanMEDS 2000 Project. *Ann R Coll Physicians Surg Can* 1996; **29**: 206–16.
12. Medical Board of Queensland. *Good medical practice, 2006*. Online at: http://www.medicalboard.qld.gov.au/Publications/Publications_files/Good%20Medical%20Practice.pdf (accessed September 2007)
13. General Medical Council. *Good Medical Practice, 2006 Edition*. Online at http://www.gmc-uk.org/guidance/good_medical_practice/index.asp (accessed September 2007).
14. Accreditation Committee on Graduate Medical Education. *Educational outcomes for medical practice*. At http://www.acgme.org/outcome/comp/compFull.asp (accessed September 2007)

15. General Medical Council *Medical students: professional behaviour and fitness to practise.* http://www.gmc-uk.org/education/undergraduate/undergraduate_policy/professional_behaviour.asp (accessed September 2007)

16. Rentmeester CA. Should a good healthcare professional be (at least a little) callous? *J Med Philos* 2007; **32**: 43–64.

17. West CP, Huntington JL, Huschka MM *et al.* A prospective study of the relationship between medical knowledge and professionalism among internal medicine residents. *Acad Med* 2007; **82**: 587–91.

18. Ainsworth MA, Szauter KM. Medical student professionalism: are we developing the right behaviours? A comparison of professional lapses by students and physicians. *Acad Med* 2006; **81**: S83–6.

19. Clark CM, Springer PJ. Incivility in nursing education: a descriptive study of definitions and prevalence. *J Nurs Educ* 2007; **46**: 7–14.

20. Srinivasan M, Litzelman D, Seshadri R *et al.* Developing an OSTE to address lapses in learners' professional behaviour and an instrument to code educators' responses. *Acad Med* 2004; **79**: 888–96.

21. Schonrock-Adema J, Heijne-Pwnninga M, Van Duijn MA, Geertsma J, Cohen-Schotanus J. Assessment of professional behaviour in undergraduate medical education: peer assessment enhances performance. *Med Educ* 2007; **41**: 836–42.

22. Van der Vleuten CPM. The assessment of professional competence: developments, research and practical implications. *Adv Health Sci Educ* 1996; **1**: 41–67.

23. Veloski JJ, Fields SK, Boex JR, Blank LL. Measuring professionalism: a review of studies with instruments reported in the literature between 1982 and 2002. *Acad Med* 2005; **80**: 366–70.

24. Jha V, Bekker HL, Duffy SRG, Roberts TE. A systematic review of studies assessing and facilitating attitudes towards professionalism in medicine. *Med Educ* 2007; **41**: 822–9.

25. Miller G. The assessment of clinical skills/competence/performance. *Acad Med* 1990; **65**: S63–7.

26. Arnold L. Shue CK, Kalishman S *et al.* Can there be a single system for peer assessment of professionalism among medical students? A multi-institutional study. *Acad Med* 2007; **82**: 578–86.

27. Wood L, Hassell A, Whitehouse A, Bullock A, Wall D. A literature review of multi-course feedback systems within and without healthcare services, leading to 10 tips for their successful design. *Med Teach* 2006; **28**: 185–91.

28. Hays RB. Self-evaluation of videotaped consultations. *Teach Learn Med* 1990; **2**: 232–6.

29. Papadakis M, Loeser H. Using clinical incident reports and longitudinal observations to assess professionalism. In *Measuring Medical professionalism* (Ed. Stern D). Oxford: Oxford University Press, 2006; 159–173.

30. Norcini JJ. Setting standards on educational tests. *Med Educ* 2003; **37**: 464–9.

31. Cohen R, Rothman AI, Poldre P, Ross J. Validity and generalisability of global ratings in an objective structured clinical examination. *Acad Med* 1991; **66**: 545–8.

Appendix 1: **Example student professionalism rating form**

Student name:	**Number:**

For each of the following desirable attributes of (appropriate level of learners in medicine), please circle the number from 0 to 10 that best matches your judgement of how this student has performed during this academic year.

1. Maintaining good medical practice

Attendance at learning sessions, submission on time of coursework, awareness of curriculum requirement, respect for teachers.

0	1	2	3	4	5	6	7	8	9	10
Nil	Very poor		Poor		Just enough		Sufficient	Sound		Excellent

Comments:

Responsibility for own learning, reflection on feedback, constructive response.

0	1	2	3	4	5	6	7	8	9	10
Nil	Very poor		Poor		Just enough		Sufficient	Sound		Excellent

Comments:

2. Teaching, appraising, and assessing

Basic teaching skills, awareness of principles of medical education, contribution to learning of others.

0	1	2	3	4	5	6	7	8	9	10
Nil	Very poor		Poor		Just enough		Sufficient	Sound		Excellent

Comments:

3. Relationships with patients

Awareness of limitations, honesty about position and abilities, appropriate clinical supervision.

0	1	2	3	4	5	6	7	8	9	10
Nil	Very poor		Poor		Just enough		Sufficient	Sound		Excellent

Comments:

Respect for patients' right and decisions, focus on patient priorities, absence of discrimination.

0	1	2	3	4	5	6	7	8	9	10
Nil	Very poor		Poor		Just enough		Sufficient	Sound		Excellent

Comments:

4. Working with colleagues

Teamwork with others in medicine, nurses, allied health professionals, etc., leadership.

0	1	2	3	4	5	6	7	8	9	10
Nil	Very poor		Poor		Just enough		Sufficient	Sound		Excellent

Comments:

Management of uncertainty readiness to raise concerns over work of colleagues if patients are at risk.

0	1	2	3	4	5	6	7	8	9	10
Nil	Very poor		Poor		Just enough		Sufficient	Sound		Excellent

Comments:

5. Probity

Honesty about problems in clinical work, research, writing reports and CVs, financial dealing.

0	1	2	3	4	5	6	7	8	9	10
Nil	Very poor		Poor		Just enough		Sufficient	Sound		Excellent

Comments:

6. Health

Awareness of personal health problems and risks for patients, seeking of appropriate medical advice, awareness of Ethics, Personal, and Professional (EPP) issues

0	1	2	3	4	5	6	7	8	9	10
Nil	Very poor		Poor		Just enough		Sufficient	Sound		Excellent

Comments:

7. Overall judgement about the professionalism demonstrated by this developing medical practitioner.

0	1	2	3	4	5	6	7	8	9	10
Nil	Very poor		Poor		Just enough		Sufficient	Sound		Excellent

Comments:

I am a Tutor/Peer (please circle one) _____ TOTAL SCORE: _____

Chapter 3

Educational standards

Yvonne Carter and Neil Jackson

Undergraduate medical education

The first section of this chapter on educational standards focuses on how the General Medical Council (GMC) sets and monitors standards in undergraduate medical education in the UK. This covers undergraduate education and the first year of training after graduation. A medical degree from one of the UK medical schools, is recognized for the purposes of registration with the GMC. In order to ensure that medical schools maintain these standards the GMC runs a quality assurance programme that involves regular monitoring and visits to schools and their partner institutions. A valuable part in the process of developing and delivering undergraduate curricula has been the ongoing and developing partnerships between medical schools and the NHS. This programme is called Quality Assurance of Basic Medical Education (QABME).

The undergraduate curriculum is recognized as the first stage of medical education. It provides an underpinning for future learning and practice as a first year foundation year doctor (FY1) and beyond. Graduates who have gone through this process must be aware of, and meet, the principles of professional practice set out in the GMC's publication *Good Medical Practice*.[1] These principles make clear to the public the standards of practice and care they should expect (see Box 3.1).

The GMC also produces joint guidance with Medical Schools Council on professional behaviour and fitness to practise (see Chapter 18). The Education Committee established a joint working group with the Medical Schools Council in 2005. The aim of the working group was to consider constructive ways of improving student fitness to practise in the UK. The working group have consulted widely and the result is new joint guidance, *Medical Students: Professional Behavior and Fitness to Practise*.[2] The guidance is aimed at medical students and all those involved in medical education. It covers:

- professional behaviour expected of medical students
- areas of misconduct and the sanctions available
- the key elements in student fitness to practise arrangements

Box 3.1 The duties of a doctor registered with the General Medical Council

Patients must be able to trust doctors with their lives and well-being. To justify that trust, we as a profession have a duty to maintain a good standard of practice and care and to show respect for human life. In particular as a doctor you must:

- make the care of your patient your first concern
- treat every patient politely and considerately
- respect patients' dignity and privacy
- listen to patients and respect their views
- give patients information in a way they can understand
- respect the rights of patients to be fully involved in decisions about their care
- keep your professional knowledge and skills up to date
- recognize the limits of your professional competence
- be honest and trustworthy
- respect and protect confidential information
- make sure that your personal beliefs do not prejudice your patients' care
- act quickly to protect patients from risk if you have good reason to believe that you or a colleague may not be fit to practise
- avoid abusing your position as a doctor
- work with colleagues in the ways that best serve the patients' interests.

In all these matters you must never discriminate unfairly against your patients or colleagues. And you must always be prepared to justify your actions to them.

The guidance aims to promote the professional behaviours expected of medical students and help instil these behaviours in students. The guidance also aims to help medical schools reach decisions about a student's fitness to practise and in this way develop consistency in approaches to student fitness to practise. The GMC's Education Committee has a statutory duty (Medical Act 1983) to set and maintain the standards for undergraduate medical education. This committee has the power to visit universities to make sure that undergraduate teaching is consistent with the standards set out in the current edition of *Tomorrow's Doctors* (see Box 3.2). During these visits assessments are inspected to make sure that the standards expected at qualifying examinations are maintained and improved.

Box 3.2 *Tomorrow's Doctors:* main recommendations

- **Attitudes** and behaviour that are suitable for a doctor must be developed. Students must develop qualities that are appropriate to their future responsibilities to patients, colleagues and society in general.

- The **core curriculum** must set out the essential knowledge, skills, and attitudes students must have by the time they graduate.

- The core curriculum must be supported by a series of **student-selected components** that allow students to study, in depth, areas of particular interest to them.

- The core curriculum must be the responsibility of clinicians, basic scientists, and medical educationalists working together to **integrate** their contributions and achieve a common purpose.

- **Factual information** must be kept to the essential minimum that students need at this stage of medical education.

- **Learning** opportunities must help students explore knowledge, and evaluate and integrate (bring together) evidence critically. The curriculum must motivate students and help them develop the skills for self-directed learning.

- The **essential skills** that graduates need must be gained under supervision. Medical schools must assess students' competence in these skills.

- The curriculum must stress the importance of **communication skills** and the other essential skills of medical practice.

- The **health and safety of the public** must be an important part of the curriculum.

- Clinical education must reflect the **changing patterns of healthcare** and provide experience in a variety of clinical settings.

- **Teaching and learning systems** must take account of modern educational theory and research, and make use of modern technologies where evidence shows these are effective.

> **Box 3.2 *Tomorrow's Doctor:* main recommendations** *(continued)*
>
> ◆ **Schemes of assessment** must take account of best practice, support the curriculum, make sure that the intended curricular outcomes are assessed and reward performance appropriately.
>
> ◆ When designing a curriculum, putting it into practice and continually reviewing it, medical schools must set up effective **supervisory structures**, which use an appropriate range of expertise and knowledge.
>
> ◆ Selection, teaching, and assessment must **be free from unfair discrimination.**

The Education Committee makes recommendations to the Privy Council, the body that has powers to grant medical school status, about whether a university should:

◆ Be added to the list of universities that can award a UK medical degree (Section 8 of the Act).

◆ Be removed from the list of universities that can award a UK medical degree (Section 9 of the Act).

The first edition of *Tomorrow's Doctors* was published in 1993.[4] This signalled a significant change in the form of guidance to medical schools from the GMC. The emphasis moved from gaining knowledge to a learning process that includes the ability to evaluate data as well as to develop skills to interact with patients and colleagues. Medical schools across the UK welcomed this guidance and many introduced new, ground-breaking curricula. The GMC carried out a series of informal visits to medical schools to monitor their progress in putting the guidance into practice with a view to highlighting and sharing good practice as well as identifying areas causing difficulty or concern. A second round of informal visits was then carried out between 1998 and 2001. The GMC then reviewed progress, considering the strengths and weaknesses of its guidance. This review took account of developments in educational theory and research, and professional practice.

The second set of recommendations, published in 2003, replaced those in the first edition and identified the knowledge, skills, attitudes, and behaviour expected of new graduates. They:

◆ put the principles set out in *Good Medical Practice* at the centre of graduate education;

◆ make it clear what students will study and be assessed on during undergraduate education;

- make it necessary for all medical schools to set appropriate standards; and
- make necessary rigorous assessments that lead to the award of a primary medical qualification (PMQ).

These recommendations now provide the framework that UK medical schools use to design detailed curricula and schemes of assessment. They also set out the standards that are used to judge the quality of undergraduate teaching and assessments when the QABME teams visit medical schools and ask for written information.

The GMC Education Committee is now considering how *Tomorrow's Doctors* might be changed when a new edition is published in 2009. The current review of *Tomorrow's Doctors* builds on previous consultations undertaken by the GMC. It is considering if standards set out in the current edition are still relevant and appropriate and will again take account of developments in educational theory, research, and professional practice since the guidance was last published in 2003. The review is being organized in two phases. The first phase of the review is an informal information gathering exercise. Key issues are being sought from stakeholders including medical schools, students, QABME visitors, employers, patients, and the public. The outcomes of this process will form the development of revised draft guidance. The revised draft guidance will be published for consideration and feedback during a formal consultation period commencing in spring 2008. It is anticipated that the project will lead to a new, improved edition of *Tomorrow's Doctors* that will meet the changing context of the medical education environment and ensure undergraduate medical education continues to provide graduates with a strong foundation for future learning and practice.

The QABME processes are designed to:

- Make sure medical schools meet the outcomes in *Tomorrow's Doctors.*
- Identify examples of innovation and good practice.
- Identify concerns and help to resolve them.
- Identify changes schools need to make to comply with *Tomorrow's Doctors* and a timetable for their implementation.
- Promote equality and diversity in medical education.

The aims of the QABME programme are achieved through two core QABME processes: the Annual Return Process and the Visit Process. Continuous improvement of the QABME programme also takes place.

Each UK medical school must provide an annual return to the GMC that:

- Identifies significant changes to curricula, assessments or staffing.
- Highlights risks or issues of concern, proposed solutions and corrective actions taken.

- Identifies examples of innovation and good practice.
- Responds to issues of interest and debate in medical education, including promoting equality and valuing diversity.
- Identifies progress on any requirements or recommendations arising from the QABME visit process.

The GMC writes to each medical school towards the end of the calendar year to request the specific information required that year. School returns allow the GMC Education Committee to identify:

- Issues to explore with all medical schools.
- Examples of good practice that can be shared.
- Issues to be investigated with individual medical schools.

If the GMC then needs to investigate an issue, for example the introduction of a new curriculum or significant changes to the existing curriculum or facilities, the school may be requested to submit detailed information for analysis or may be selected for the QABME visit process.

The QABME visit process varies for established and new medical schools. For established schools, the GMC visits each medical school at least twice within every 10 years. Visits are undertaken on behalf of the GMC's Education Committee by a team of medical and educational professionals, medical students and lay members. The visiting teams are assigned to a school and are responsible for all stages of the visit process for their school.

The main stages of the visit process are:

- Stage 1: Collecting information (June–December)
- Stage 2: Confirming information (January–July)
- Stage 3: Integrating information and making judgements (June–August).

These time frames vary slightly to respond to individual school timetables. However, this three-stage process is designed to ensure that visiting teams collect information, explore information and observe examples of the teaching and learning process in a systematic way. Evidence is then triangulated and evaluated against the standards in *Tomorrow's Doctors*. Box 3.3 summarizes the range of activities that a visiting team may undertake. The visiting teams provide a report on their findings to the Undergraduate Board, which is a working group of the GMC's Education Committee. After consideration by the Education Committee the reports are published on the GMC website along with a response from each individual school. For each medical school listed you can access: the most recent quality assurance report – if quality assured; previous reports, if available; and the address of the medical school website.

Box 3.3 Range of activities undertaken by visiting team

+ Meetings of various members of the school
+ Observation of examination of clinical skills
+ Module and/or Phase Examination Board or other Board meeting observation
+ Site assessment: NHS Trusts and GP practices
+ Observation of clinical teaching
+ Discussions with GPs
+ Discussions with students, F1 doctors, and their educational supervisors
+ Discussions with teachers
+ Discussions with NHS and other service providers

(http://www.gmc-uk.org/education/undergraduate/undergraduate_qa/ medical_school_reports.asp).

The visit process for an established school is generally 18 months from notification of selection to the Education Committee's endorsement of the visiting team's report. The visit process may vary for established schools proposing major changes to curriculum, facilities, or supervisory structures. For example, if changes are limited to 1 or 2 years of the school's curriculum the visit process may be completed in the standard 18-month time frame. Alternatively, if extensive changes are planned across the curriculum the visit process may be repeated over a number of years as the changes are rolled out. Similarly, the visit process will vary for established medical schools wishing to change their degree awarding arrangements.

The process for monitoring the progress of newly established schools involves the same systematic three-stage process applied to established schools. New schools must pass the GMC's thorough assessments before they can award degrees. The GMC sets the standard that students must demonstrate to graduate but schools devise their own curriculum to enable students to meet the standards. The hypothesis is that a quality teaching environment will enable medical students to put into practice the principles that the GMC expect of doctors throughout their careers.

Quality assurance activities are carried out for each year for the duration of the first medical student intake's degree course, assessing the development and delivery. This process results in annual reports that enable the Education

Committee to gauge the progress of each school and compare progress across schools.

Four new medical schools have been established in England:

- Brighton and Sussex Medical School (Universities of Brighton and Sussex)
- Hull and York Medical School (Universities of Hull and York)
- Peninsula Medical School (Universities of Exeter and Plymouth)
- University of East Anglia Medical School

From June 2007, four medical schools in the UK were, for the first time, able to award their own primary medical qualifications. The schools have all completed the QABME process. The four schools include two new medical schools mentioned above: University of East Anglia Medical School and Peninsula Medical School. Two existing medical schools, Warwick Medical School and Cardiff Medical School can now also begin awarding degrees independently from their parent universities, having completed the GMC's Quality Assurance programme. This brings the total number of medical schools as recognized in the Medical Act from 23 to 27.

The Education Committee's recommendation to the Privy Council about awarding the status of medical school is informed by:

- the visiting team's findings on the first student intake's penultimate year, and
- plans for the students' final year of study.

The visiting team also monitors the implementation of the final year of the curriculum and assessments to ensure they are delivered as planned. Once a new school has been added to the list of universities that can award UK medical degrees it will be quality assured in the same way as established medical schools.

The GMC has built in a number of mechanisms to facilitate the continuous quality assurance of its processes. These include:

- annual evaluation of the programme
- a mandatory annual training programme for visitors
- informal and formal feedback processes for visited schools

The GMC believes that the views of schools help it to review and improve its processes. Schools are therefore requested to keep a log of issues with the process so concerns are identified and addressed in a consistent way. If the school identifies an urgent problem it is encouraged to contact the GMC staff member responsible for managing their visits. Non-urgent concerns are reported in the formal school feedback process at the end of the visit cycle.

We have used the QABME process of the GMC as an exemplar for quality assurance of undergraduate medical education. We recognize that similar models exist in other countries. In the Republic of Ireland, for example, the Council is also responsible for visiting the medical schools in Ireland at regular intervals and has in particular reviewed each school's core curriculum, foundation courses, integrated teaching and assessment procedures. The Council has made a number of recommendations on each visit, which then form the basis for subsequent visits (http://www.medicalcouncil.ie/education/default.asp).

Postgraduate medical education and training

The second section of the chapter focuses on how standards are set and monitored in postgraduate medical education and training in the UK by the Postgraduate Medical Education and Training Board (PMETB). It is important to note, however, that the GMC and the PMETB are jointly responsible for setting standards in the two-year foundation programme. The GMC sets the context and standards for foundation year one (F1) until the point of full registration and PMETB sets the standards for Postgraduate Education and Training including foundation year two (F2) following full registration with the GMC.

PMETB was established by the General and Specialist Medical Practice (Education and Training Qualifications) Order 2003,[5] thus signifying the advent of a single unified authority for postgraduate medical education and training. This new organization assumed its statutory powers as the UK competent authority on 30 September 2005 and subsumed the previous responsibilities of the Specialist Training Authority (STA) and the Joint Committee on Postgraduate Training for General Practice (JCPTGP). In addition, as a part of the 2003 order PMETB acts independently of government while being directly accountable to parliament and operating on an integrated basis across the four UK nations.

As an independent regulatory body, PMETB is responsible for ensuring that postgraduate medical education and training is of the highest possible standard, thus promoting the enhancement of the knowledge, skills, and attitudes of doctors, and the quality of healthcare provided for patients. PMETB carries out this remit through three main functions, i.e.

◆ *Setting and monitoring standards of postgraduate medical education and training,* including: curriculum approval and assessment; prospective approval of all training posts and programmes; quality assuring the management of postgraduate medical training; and setting the principles and standards for specialist recruitment and selection.

◆ *Certifying doctors for the GP and specialist registers*, including the assessment and award of the Certificate of Completion of Training (CCT) or the General Practice Certificate of Completion of Training (GPCCT) following the completion of training by trainee doctors. PMETB's responsibility also extends to the assessment of doctors who have not completed an approved UK training programme but who are considered in terms of experience as equivalent to the holder of a CCT or GPCCT.

◆ *Developing and promoting postgraduate medical education and training* through a variety of means, e.g. Deanery-wide inspection visits, trainer and trainee serveys.

The governance of PMETB is exercised through a Board consisting of 29 members, i.e. 17 medical, eight lay, and four representatives of the UK Departments of Health. In addition to the Board PMETB comprises two statutory committees, i.e.

◆ *Training Committee* with responsibility for developing standards for training; speciality curricula and specialist training entry. In addition, this committee is also responsible for promoting the quality and the quality assurance of education and training.

◆ *Assessment Committee* with responsibility for the assessment of those doctors who apply to the specialist and GP registers through the equivalence provisions or articles of the General and Specialist Medical Practice (Education, Training and Qualifications) order 2003; assessments undertaken by doctors during their training (including examination standards as

---

Box 3.4 Generic standards for Postgraduate Medical Education and Training

◆ Patient safety

◆ Quality assurance, review, and evaluation

◆ Equality, diversity, and opportunity

◆ Recruitment, selection, and appointment

◆ Delivery of curriculum, including assessment

◆ Support and development of trainees, trainers, and local faculty

◆ Management of education and training

◆ Educational resources and capacity

◆ Outcomes

evidence for entry to, progress through and exit from training; and certification at the completion of training).

In order to discharge its statutory function PMETB has an overall Chief Executive Officer and is structured around four directorates, i.e.: certification; policy and communication; quality; and finance and resources.

PMETB's generic standards for postgraduate medical education and training are clustered under nine separate domains that are listed in Box 3.4.

PMETB deanery-wide cross-speciality visits: a leader visitor's perspective

PMETB completed its first cycle of UK deanery-wide, cross-speciality visits in July 2007 and is now taking stock of how these visits should be further developed for the future. This section of the chapter recounts the author's (Neil Jackson) own experiences of participating in five PMETB Deanery visits, four as leader visitor and one as the Deanery Representative in the visiting team, supporting the leader visitor. Of the five visits, four were typical deanery-wide, cross-speciality visits and the fifth was a 'triggered' visit in a large foundation trust within the deanery boundary. The visits are summarized in Table 3.1.

For each deanery visit the leader visitor and visiting team work within the PMETB Quality Assurance Framework using the nine PMETB Domains (as detailed above) to assess the postgraduate medical education standards of the deanery and its educational network of Trusts and GP training practices.

Table 3.1 PMETB Deanery-wide visits 2006/2007.

Date	Deanery visit	Specialities
June 2006	West of Scotland (Leader Visitor)	Clinical Pharmacology and Therapeutics Geriatric Medicine Palliative Medicine Medical Microbiology and Virology General Practice
September 2006	South Yorkshire & South Humberside (Leader Visitor)	Chemical Pathology Clinical Genetics Histopathology
February 2007	Northern Ireland (Leader Visitor)	General Surgery
May 2007	Tri-Services (Deanery Representative supporting Leader Visitor)	Occupational Medicine Public Health
June 2007	South Yorkshire & South Humberside (Leader Visitor)	Paediatrics (Triggered Visit)

The role of the lead visitor

PMETB visits require detailed pre-visit preparation to promote team development and cohesion with firm leadership from the outset to ensure among other things that all team members contribute fully to the visit through their unique expertise. The leader visitor role also extends to ensuring that the visit programme is completed in a timely and efficient way; 'trouble shooting' where necessary; ensuring that evidence is appropriately gathered and triangulated throughout the visit and leading at the feedback session at the end of the visit.

For each of the visits listed above, five principles were adopted to underpin the visiting process, i.e.

+ Regulatory
+ Developmental
+ Dissemination of good practice
+ Peer review (of the Postgraduate Dean and Senior Deanery Team)
+ Testing the visit model

After completion of the visit the leader visitor must ensure that the visit report is drafted in good time (to meet required PMETB deadlines) and is agreed and signed off by all team members. The leader visitor also evaluates the performance of each team member during the visit and sends a report to PMETB. In addition, the team members evaluate the performance of the leader visitor and feed back to PMETB after the visit.

The structure of Postgraduate Medical Education and Training Board visiting teams

A typical PMETB visiting team for a Deanery-Wide cross-speciality visit might include the following members:

+ Leader visitor
+ Deanery representative
+ Specialist
+ Specialist
+ Specialist
+ GP
+ Lay visitor
+ Lay visitor
+ Trainee representative
+ PMETB observer

(NB: Two lay visitors contribute considerable 'non-medical' professional expertise to the visiting team and process.)

For a PMETB 'Triggered' visit a typical visiting team might be composed as follows:

+ Leader visitor
+ Specialist
+ Lay visitor
+ PMETB observer

What's a visit like?

Participating in a PMETB deanery visit is a high volume, high pressure activity and requires a sustained input of 2–3 days pre-visit preparation, 3–4 days for the visit itself and 1–2 days post-visit to finalize the report. Meanwhile, there is still the 'day-job' to do and all that goes with it!

Nevertheless, it is a privilege to be involved and can be exhilarating, interesting, and educational as well as hard work! It is also an opportunity for the cross-fertilization of ideas; for making new contacts; new friends and for renewing old acquaintances. There is also a considerable amount to be learned from the lay members of the visiting team. Evaluation and feedback are also two visit activities that present an interesting and complex challenge to any visiting team!

Models of good practice

All deaneries and their educational networks exhibit models of good practice and the following examples have been drawn from the deanery visits listed above, i.e.

+ Monthly clinical incident update (educational tool with no-blame culture).
+ Failure to provide appropriate trainee supervision = critical incident analysis within Trust.
+ Training video to demonstrate effective hand-over of patients.
+ Induction hand book/induction training package/electronic induction process.
+ High level of pastoral care for trainees.
+ Lay involvement in local quality control processes.
+ Development programme for postgraduate centre managers.
+ Deanery Information Strategy for General Practice.

Lessons learned from Postgraduate Medical Education and Training Board visits

Some interesting lessons have emerged from PMETB visits to deaneries and here are some examples (in no order of priority):

+ Visits are not for everyone! For a variety of reasons some members of visiting teams have found the challenge of one visit quite sufficient and have indicated that they do not wish to participate in others.

+ Pre-visit information has been refined to prevent visitor 'information overload'.

+ Visit programmes have been subject to 'fine tuning' following successive deanery visits, e.g. more time has been made available at the end of the visit to feedback individually to the Postgraduate Dean of the visited deanery.

+ Further work on PMETB domains is needed, e.g. outcomes (for greater clarity of the domain, including measurement and evaluation).

+ Visits are demanding for the visited as well as the visiting team!

+ The visit is a 'sampling process' and cannot cover everything!

+ There are benefits for all as a result of the visiting process.

+ The right balance between service provision and education and training in a Trust requires firm leadership from CEO/Board level downwards.

+ 'Big' issues are emerging from visits, e.g. induction (patient safety); educational supervisors (selection, support, and development).

+ The PMETB website is a useful learning tool! Visit reports, deanery responses, final PMETB decisions, and conditions of approval are posted on the PMETB website, and are there for all to see. All deaneries and their educational networks should be encouraged to visit the website to learn from the UK-wide visiting process in the quest to implement and enhance PMETB standards.

Postgraduate Medical Education and Training Board: Quality Assurance Framework

Having assumed its statutory responsibilities in September 2005 PMETB conducted a wide-ranging consultation between May and July 2007 to review its Quality Assurance Framework (QAF) for postgraduate medical education and training in the UK.[6] Various stakeholders were consulted, including those involved in the delivery of postgraduate education and training; patient groups and lay visitors; representatives of service, e.g. NHS, Independent

Health Sector, Strategic Health Authority (SHAs) and UK Government Department of Health.

As a result of the consultation process PMETB has developed and modified its QAF, and its main summary points are:

- *Deanery visits.* All 21 deaneries in the UK will receive a PMETB visit in the next 3 years as the second part of a 5-year cycle (2005–10) to focus on deanery quality management processes and the quality control aspects of their educational networks/providers. By the end of this 5-year cycle every deanery will thus have been visited at least twice.

- *Annual reports.* All deaneries will be required to submit annual reports to PMETB by way of a self-assessment against the generic standards for postgraduate medical education and training. The report will also need to include a reference to progress on continuous improvement in standards, and in particular the implementation of previous requirements as stipulated by PMETB following its last scrutiny of the deanery.

- *Response to concerns.* During the cycle PMETB will undertake random checks as appropriate to confirm the accuracy of information it has received. A range of methods will be adopted for this, including triggered visits where necessary.

- *National surveys.* Annual surveys of trainees and trainers will be carried out and the results published.

- *Curriculum review.* Specialist curriculum and assessment methodologies as previously approved by PMETB, may require development and modification in future and proposals for amendment will be reviewed as necessary by PMETB.

- *Action planning.* As part of their annual reports deaneries will have to declare their action plans for the benefit of members and organizations of their educational networks and to ensure continuous quality improvement.

Since the inception of PMETB one of the issues that has been subject to considerable debate and discussion is the definition of the terms Quality Assurance, Quality Control, and Quality Management. In its Quality Assurance Framework Consultation Report (September 2007) PMETB gives the following definition of these terms:

- *Quality Assurance.* 'This encompasses all the policies, standards, systems and processes directed to ensuring maintenance and enhancement of the quality of postgraduate medical education in the UK. PMETB will undertake planned and systematic activities to provide public and patient

confidence that postgraduate medical education satisfies given requirements for quality within the principles of better regulation.'

+ *Quality Control.* 'This relates to the arrangements (procedures, organization) within local education providers (health boards, NHS trusts,
independent sectors) that ensure postgraduate medical trainees receive
education and training that meets local, national and professional standards.'

+ *Quality Management.* 'This refers to the arrangements by which the postgraduate deanery discharges its responsibility for the standards and quality
of postgraduate medical education. It satisfies itself that local education
and training providers are meeting the PMETB standards through robust
reporting and monitoring mechanisms.'

Towards the end of 2007 PMETB published its new Quality Framework for
Postgraduate Medical Education and Training in the UK, which followed wide-
scale consultation, as detailed above.[7] PMETB is also developing an Operational
Guide and a series of informative booklets on 'The QF and what it means for
you' which are set to be published in 2008. PMETB has also stated it is intended
that the Operational Guide will be a 'live' web-based document covering the
practicalities of implementing the Quality Framework, whereas the booklets
will be designed with particular groups in mind, i.e.: patients; health services,
including employers; trainees; colleges/faculties, and deaneries.

Further information concerning PMETB and its Quality Standards for
postgraduate medical education and training can be obtained by visiting the
PMETB website: http://www.pmetb.org.uk/

References

1. General Medical Council. *Good medical practice.* London: GMC, 2001.
2. General Medical Council. *Medical students: professional behaviour and fitness to practise.*
   London: GMC, 2007.
3. General Medical Council. *Tomorrow's doctors.* London: GMC, 2003.
4. General Medical Council. *Tomorrow's doctors.* London: GMC, 1993.
5. General and Specialist Medical Practice (Education and Training Qualifications) Order
   2003.
6. PMETB Quality Assurance Framework: Consultation Report (September 2007).
7. The PMETB Quality Framework for Postgraduate Medical Education and Training in
   the UK (Autumn 2007).

Chapter 4

Patients' expectations

Angela Coulter

Introduction

What patients and the public expect from doctors is changing. It has always been expected that medical education will teach clinical knowledge and practical skills, as well as schooling students and trainees in a professional culture that emphasizes their responsibility to be trustworthy and act in the interests of their patients. In recent years, however, many people have come to expect more. Nowadays patients expect clinicians to respect their autonomy, to listen to them and inform them, to take account of their preferences, to involve them in treatment decisions, and to support their efforts in self-care. This includes taking action to prevent the occurrence or recurrence of disease, understanding the causes of illness and the treatment options, being involved in treatment decisions, monitoring symptoms and treatment effects, and learning to manage the symptoms of chronic disease. If they are to fulfil this role effectively, patients require help from clinicians who recognize and actively support their contribution and are willing to engage with them as healthcare partners.

Evidence from patient surveys and other research suggests that many doctors still adopt a dominant role in their encounters with patients rather than seeing them as active participants in their own healthcare. Although research evidence has long shown the complexity and negotiated nature of many doctor–patient relationships – especially in the case of chronic conditions – medical education has not always reflected this sufficiently, nor adequately prepared doctors for the more fully engaged patient of today. This chapter considers what needs to be done to ensure that medical education rises to this challenge.

What do patients and the public want?

The way people express their expectations of health services tends to vary according to whether they think of themselves primarily as users of the health service or as taxpayers, contributing to the costs of a service that they value and may need to use at any time in the future. Interestingly, surveys of patients (current or recent users) elicit more positive responses to questions about the state of the NHS than opinion polls among the general public. Public views are often influenced by media coverage that tends to focus on problems, whereas patients draw on their personal experience or that of their family and friends, which often leads them to give good reports on the care they received.

In 2003 the Department of Health in England undertook a major consultation on public priorities for the NHS. This gave a clear indication of the desire for a more active, engaged role on the part of patients. People want more choices, better information, and they expect to have a greater say in decisions about their health (Table 4.1).

Three-quarters of respondents to this survey put involvement in decisions at the top of their list of priorities, with half saying this aspect of care needed improvement. There was strong support also for the need to treat patients with respect, to listen to them, to offer them choices and to give them clear information – all of which are important attributes of patient-centred care.

Table 4.1 Important aspects of the NHS and the need for improvement, public survey, England 2003.[1]

	Proportion rating factor 'important'	Proportion saying 'needs improvement'
Involve patients in decisions about their condition or treatment	76%	51%
Treat patients with respect and dignity	59%	39%
Listen to the views and opinions of patients	47%	46%
Offer patients choice in the treatment they receive	46%	36%
Offer patients choice in the treatment date and time	42%	38%
Give clear information on what services are provided	38%	41%
Treat all people fairly	37%	25%
Offer patients choice in the services they can use	31%	29%
Offer patients choice of hospital	31%	26%
Offer patients choice of doctor	31%	25%
Focus on what patients want	24%	28%
Give clear information on the quality of services provided	21%	27%

A good doctor

What people expect of doctors tends to vary depending on whether one is talking about expectations of general practice or of hospital-based specialist care. Most people expect doctors to be clinically competent with a sound basis in scientific knowledge and technical expertise, but they also place considerable importance on communication skills and the doctor's personal commitment to their care.

General practice patients want to consult doctors who are good communicators, with sound, up-to-date clinical knowledge and skills, who are interested and sympathetic, involve them in decisions, give them sufficient time and attention, and provide advice on health promotion and self-care.[2] A systematic review of the literature on patients' priorities for general practice care, which examined 19 studies published between 1966 and 1995, found that the most important factors were:

◆ humaneness

◆ competence/accuracy

◆ patients' involvement in decisions

◆ time for care[3]

In the regular national patient surveys carried out in England most respondents give generally positive reports of the communication skills of GPs (Table 4.2).

However, certain aspects of communication are more problematic. When the focus shifts to involving patients in decisions about their care, sharing important information about side-effects, and copying referral letters to the patient, GP performance doesn't look so good (Table 4.3).

Only just over half of these primary care patients felt they had had sufficient involvement in decisions about prescribed medicines and a substantial minority felt they were given insufficient information about the possible side-effects.

Table 4.2 Patients' reports on GPs' communication skills. NHS primary care patient survey, England 2006.[4]

	n = 10 008
Had sufficient time to discuss health or medical problem with doctor	75%
Doctor listened carefully	82%
Doctor gave clear answers to questions	74%
Doctor clearly explained reasons for treatments/actions	76%
Had confidence and trust in doctor	76%
Treated with respect and dignity	92%

Table 4.3 Patients' reports on information and involvement in general practice. NHS primary care patient survey, England 2006.[4]

	n = 10 008
Had sufficient involvement in medication decisions	55%
Given sufficient information about medication side-effects	58%
Given a choice about where to be referred*	27%
Given copies of letters between GP and specialist*	25%

*Patients who had had a referral in the previous 12 months.

Less than a third of those who received a specialist referral said they were given a choice of where to be referred and only a quarter were given copies of referral letters. It would appear that general practice patients' expectations of involvement are not being met in many cases.

Hospital patients also have high expectations of doctors. Asked to list the most important aspects of a good quality inpatient stay, patients with recent experience of an inpatient stay identified the following top 10 priorities.[5]

1. The doctors know enough about my medical history and treatment.
2. The doctors can answer questions about my condition and treatment in a way that I can understand.
3. I have confidence and trust in the hospital staff who treat me.
4. The doctors wash or clean their hands between touching patients.
5. The nurses know enough about my medical history and treatment.
6. Before my operation or procedure I get a clear explanation of what will happen.
7. The risks and benefits of my operation or procedure are explained to me in a way that I can understand.
8. The nurses wash or clean their hands between touching patients.
9. The rooms and wards are clean.
10. The doctors and nurses are open with me about my treatment or condition.

Hospital patients want to be reassured that the doctors treating them have up-to-date medical knowledge and can communicate this effectively. They expect doctors to provide them with information about their treatment, to listen to them, to involve them in decisions, and to treat them humanely and with dignity. They also expect them to be conscientious about avoiding infection risks and to be open if mistakes are made.

Table 4.4 Patients' reports on hospital doctors' communication skills. NHS inpatient survey, England 2006.[6]

	n = 81 000
Given sufficient information about condition and treatment	79%
Given clear explanation of risks and benefits of operation or procedure	81%
Doctor gave clear answers to questions	68%
Family and friends had opportunity to talk to a doctor if they wanted to	84%
Given full information on likely impact of operation/procedure	56%
Given full information on how operation/procedure had gone	64%
Treated with respect and dignity	78%

Results from the national inpatient surveys show that communication between doctors and inpatients does usually achieve high standards (Table 4.4). The majority of patients were satisfied with hospital doctors' communication skills in the main, but hospital patients' expectations of involvement are often frustrated (Table 4.5).

These patient survey results suggest that there is a gap between what patients want and what they receive in respect of opportunities to participate in decisions about their care. Many patients are dissatisfied with this important aspect of doctor–patient communication.

A review of 134 observational studies found that most patients are happy to discuss their concerns, beliefs, experiences, and preferences, but health professionals do not always encourage them to do so.[8] Doctors often dominate discussion in the consultation, with patients relegated to a passive role. They tend to tell patients what they have decided, instead of informing them about the options and likely outcomes and asking them what they would prefer. There is evidence to suggest that practice patterns in the UK are worse in this respect than in other developed countries such as Australia, Canada, New Zealand, and the USA.[9]

Table 4.5 Patients in secondary care who had sufficient say in decisions about their care. NHS patient surveys, England 2004–6.[7]

Outpatients (2004)	70%
Emergency (2004)	64%
Coronary heart disease (2004)	61%
Inpatient (2006)	52%
Stroke (2004)	48%
Mental health (2006)	42%

Building partnerships with patients

It should be no surprise that patients nowadays expect to play a more active part in their care. The changes we see in patients' expectations are mirrored by changes in other aspects of everyday life. Consumerism is becoming a more powerful force – it will not go away. Paternalistic approaches are less readily tolerated and health professionals are likely to find that they have to devote more time to explaining and negotiating with patients than they might have had to 20 years ago.

This may appear challenging, but the rewards of a more equal partnership could be greater understanding, more shared responsibility, and more appropriate and effective healthcare. International evidence shows that involving patients in their care and treatment improves their health outcomes, their experience of the service, their knowledge and understanding of their health status, and their adherence to chosen treatment.[10]

In 2006 the GMC revised *Good Medical Practice,* its statement of the principles and values that underpin medical professionalism. The main difference between the new version and its predecessor was the addition of a section on working in partnership with patients. All doctors are now enjoined to:

+ Listen to patients and respond to their concerns and preferences.
+ Give patients the information they want or need in a way they can understand.
+ Respect patients' right to reach decisions with you about their treatment and care.
+ Support patients in caring for themselves to improve and maintain their health.

This requires a new relationship between clinicians and patients. Instead of the doctor being the primary decision-maker and care organizer, he or she is now expected to recognize and support the patient's role in promoting health and managing their own healthcare. Doctors have to learn to treat patients as important participants in the process of treating and managing disease. This involves understanding patients' role preferences, offering them appropriate information or guiding them to relevant information sources, and providing education and support in self-care, self-management, and shared decision-making.

Implications for medical education

While many doctors appreciate the need to treat patients as active players in theory, as the surveys show this is not always achieved in the real world of medical practice. Many trainees and experienced doctors feel ill-equipped to deal with the new demands.[11] Some feel threatened by informed, articulate patients and others are unsure how to engage with those who are less willing or able to ask questions and share their preferences. There is also some confusion among educators about how to respond to these needs.[12]

Much important work has been done to encourage understanding of the patient's perspective, especially in general practice training,[13,14] but there is still a tendency to encourage trainees to focus on the disease rather than the person, downplaying both the complexity of the doctor–patient encounter and the importance of patients' values, preferences and self-knowledge.[8,15] An overemphasis on the technical aspects of care negates the importance of the emotional and psychological responses to illness, which are a key part of patients' experience.

Fostering a culture of partnership between doctors and their patients requires doctors to develop a specific set of skills and attributes. In order to engage patients more fully, medical students and postgraduate trainees must learn about the theory and practice of developing health literacy, enabling shared decision-making, and supporting self-care, all of which demand excellent communication skills. Achieving this will require mastery of a new set of attitudes, knowledge, and competencies (see Box 4.1).

There is a great deal of good practice to draw on for teaching these competencies and some positive research evidence on the effectiveness of different approaches. For example, there is evidence that training in more patient-centred communication skills can lead to improvements in patients' experience.[8,16–20] Some key topics that ought to be regular features in medical curricula are described below.

Box 4.1 Competencies for patient partnership

- ◆ Understanding the patient's perspective, expressing empathy, and providing appropriate support.
- ◆ Guiding patients to appropriate sources of information on health and healthcare.
- ◆ Educating patients on how to protect their health and prevent occurrence or recurrence of disease.
- ◆ Eliciting and taking account of patients' preferences.
- ◆ Communicating information on risk and probability.
- ◆ Sharing treatment decisions.
- ◆ Providing support for self-care and self-management.
- ◆ Working in multidisciplinary teams.
- ◆ Managing time effectively.

Patients as educators

Despite a long tradition of involving patients in medical education, the potential teaching resource available through their more active involvement has not yet been fully exploited in all educational settings.[21] Educational activities have traditionally involved patients as relatively passive participants, for example, to illustrate symptoms or procedures, but there are clear benefits when patients are given a much more active role.[22] Direct contact with patients can help to develop students' and trainees' communication skills, professional attitudes, empathy, and clinical reasoning.[23,24]

When direct contact with patients cannot be arranged, other means of helping students and trainees to understand the patient's perspective can be useful. For example, the *British Medical Journal*'s series of articles written by patients describing their experiences, or the DIPEx website, which contains numerous video clips of patients telling their stories (http://www.dipex.org).

Providing information

Willingness to exchange information and share understanding of health problems and possible solutions are crucial elements in partnering with patients. Clinicians need to develop expertise in communicating health information in a comprehensible manner. This involves judging what information patients will find helpful, how much to give and the best way to give it, including the appropriate use of language. In order to do this effectively clinicians must learn how to encourage patients to tell them about their circumstances, beliefs, and experiences, and they must be very good listeners. They must also learn teaching skills in order to build health literacy (i.e. the ability to obtain, process, and understand health information) in their patients, and they must understand and take account of cultural differences.

Giving and receiving information from patients in the consultation is necessary but not sufficient. Many patients seek additional information, not necessarily because they don't trust what the doctor tells them, but because they want a deeper understanding than can be obtained in a single short consultation. Clinicians need to be able to guide their patients to reliable information sources and help them assess the quality of the information they find on the internet and elsewhere.

Risk communication

Most patients need expert help to understand risk and outcome probabilities and to deal with the uncertainties inherent in most treatment regimens. This requires skilled and sensitive communication tailored to the individual patient and delivered with empathy and understanding. Much work has been done to increase understanding of how people perceive risk, and how to present probabilities in a balanced and comprehensible manner.[25] For example, we know that it is better to use event rates (absolute risk) rather than relative risk, to use both positive and negative framing where possible, and to present different outcome probabilities using a common denominator and time frame. Graphical presentation can be helpful if well designed and computer-based packages allow clinicians to present personalized, rather than generalized figures on risk, which is much more helpful for patients.

Shared decision-making

The skills for involving patients in decisions need to be taught – they don't come naturally to most people. A substantial body of research has described the components of shared decision-making, outlining the theoretical concepts, observing the practice and measuring the effects.[26–28] Trainees need to learn how to share decisions, how to assess patients' reactions and modify the process accordingly, and how to handle any deviations from the norm. They also need to understand that outcomes are of importance to patients and how to find out what part they prefer to play in decisions about their treatment and care. Some patients want full information and expect to play a major part in decisions about treatment options, while others prefer the doctor to play the leading role. Determining the preferences of individual patients is not always straightforward.

Trainees need to observe the process of involving patients in decision-making as practised by skilled clinicians and they need opportunities to employ these skills with patients in real clinical settings. Their progress must be assessed by trained observers, including patients, and fed back to them.

Supporting self-care

In many cases patients, together with their family carers, expect to look after their own healthcare needs, so health professionals need to know how to access relevant self-care resources and how to help their patients make use of them. Detailed work has been carried out to describe and categorize the processes involved in supporting healthy lifestyles, promoting behaviour change, self-care of minor illnesses, recovery and rehabilitation after acute illness, and self-monitoring and self-management of chronic conditions. There is now a substantial evidence base telling us what works and what does not.[10] Medical education and training must enable doctors to support patients in the technical aspects of self-care or self-monitoring, as well as building patient confidence and self-assurance when doing so. Clinicians must also learn what can and cannot be left to patients and how to monitor and support patients who are providing care and treatment for themselves.

Teamwork and time management

Trainee doctors also need to learn how to deal with, and overcome, the many obstacles they are likely to face in trying to work in a more patient-centred manner. The partnership approach demands changes in the use of time as well as new skills. Where it is operating successfully, the key seems to be excellent multidisciplinary team-working. Clinical staff have re-examined and where necessary re-designed patient pathways to free up time to help patients absorb information, think through their options or learn new skills.[29] Different members of the clinical team work with patients in predetermined, well-coordinated ways. Medical students and trainees need to be prepared for this type of clinical process redesign. This might involve direct experience of different ways of organizing patient care, with students being encouraged to review different approaches critically from the viewpoint of the patient.

The scale of the challenge

The issues described above are complex. They go far beyond the basics that are commonly taught in undergraduate communication skills courses, which are too often repeated at the same basic level in postgraduate training. Underestimating the intellectual challenge required and the need for complex skill development can lead trainees to switch off the topic.

Engaging patients as partners requires demanding skills and attributes, yet apart from vocational training in general practice and some specialties (e.g. clinical genetics, psychiatry), postgraduate medical education has been slow to introduce teaching in advanced communication skills. The postgraduate curricula tend to have low aspirations in respect of these topics compared with the breadth and depth of the specialist medical knowledge and skills that trainees are expected to absorb. For example, most medical students receive some training in how to break bad news about prognosis, but they also need to know how to handle the consequences of medical errors and what and how to tell patients. Most medical schools teach students about the requirement for informed consent, but this needs to be followed up with training on how to communicate risk effectively to ensure that consent is truly 'informed'.

Role modelling is still an important component of education and training in medicine, but experienced role models who are expert in working in partnership with their patients may not always be available to trainees. There is a prevalent and somewhat complacent belief that most medical practice is already patient-centred, with only a small minority of doctors performing less than optimally. But, as we have seen, there is a substantial gap between what patients want in respect of involvement and what many experience.

Antipathy to the topic of interpersonal skills on the part of the medical establishment is often shared by medical students and trainees. Yet postgraduate deans often have to deal with trainees who have communication problems, which have their roots in a failure to understand and respect patients.[30] The dominance of the 'hard' sciences in medical education creates a lack of understanding of, and sympathy for, what are seen as 'soft' skills. This may be compounded by selection procedures that reward knowledge of basic science, but do not probe for empathy or interpersonal skills. The focus on interpersonal relations, which draws on the social sciences for its evidence base, is seen by some as not truly 'scientific', and hence not a high priority.

Building a new sense of professionalism that treats patients as true partners is not simple. Laudable aspirations will no longer suffice. The medical community must face up to the educational challenge of promoting effective patient partnership. This will require time, commitment, and additional resources, but everybody stands to gain from this. Many patients will welcome the chance to play an active role in their own healthcare, and many doctors will find it easier to respond to patient needs.

Promoting partnerships with patients is on the policy agenda; it is emphasized in professional guidance and codes; and it is beginning to appear explicitly in newly published medical curricula. It now needs to be taken to the next stage. This will involve developing practical methods for teaching and assessing the necessary skills and providing new and effective role models for best practice.

References

1. Leatherman S, Sutherland K. *Patient and public experiences in the NHS*. London: The Health Foundation, 2007.
2. Little P, Everitt H, Williamson I, *et al*. Preferences of patients for patient centred approach to consultation in primary care: observational study. *BMJ* 2001; **322**: 468–72.
3. Wensing M, Jung HP, Mainz J, Olesen F, Grol R. A systematic review of the literature on patient priorities for general practice care. Part 1: Description of the research domain. *Soc Sci Med* 1998; **47**(10): 1573–88.
4. Picker Institute Europe. *National survey of local health services 2006*. London: Department of Health, 2007.
5. Boyd J. *The 2006 inpatients importance study*. Oxford: Picker Institute Europe, 2007.
6. Healthcare Commission. *The views of hospital inpatients in England: key findings from the 2006 survey*. London: Healthcare Commission, 2007. http://www. healthcare-commission.org.uk/_db/_documents/Inpatient_survey_briefing_note pdf/ (accessed 26 October 2007).
7. Richards N, Coulter A. *Is the NHS becoming more patient-centred? Trends from the national surveys of NHS patients in England 2002–07*. Oxford: Picker Institute Europe, 2007.

8. Stevenson FA, Cox K, Britten N, Dundar Y. A systematic review of the research on communication between patients and health care professionals about medicines: the consequences for concordance. *Health Expect* 2004; 7(3): 235–45.

9. Coulter A. *Engaging patients in their healthcare: how is the UK doing relative to other countries?* Oxford: Picker Institute Europe, 2006.

10. Coulter A, Ellins J. *Patient-focused interventions: a review of the evidence.* London: The Health Foundation, 2006.

11. Smith R. Why are doctors so unhappy? *BMJ* 2001; **322**: 1073–4.

12. Gillespie R, Florin D, Gillam S. How is patient-centred care understood by the clinical, managerial and lay stakeholders responsible for promoting this agenda? *Health Expect* 2004; **7**: 142–8.

13. Tuckett D, Boulton M, Olson C, Williams A. *Meetings between experts.* London: Tavistock, 1985.

14. Pendleton D. *The consultation: an approach to learning and teaching.* Oxford: Oxford University Press, 1984.

15. Corke CF, Stow PJ, Green DT, Agar JW, Henry MJ. How doctors discuss major interventions with high risk patients: an observational study. *BMJ* 2005; **330**: 182–4.

16. Lewin SA, Skea ZC, Entwistle V, Zwarenstein M, Dick J. Interventions for providers to promote a patient centred approach in clinical consultations. *Cochrane Database of Systematic Reviews,* 2001, Issue 4. Art. No.: CD003267.

17. Griffin SJ, Kinmonth AL, Veltman MW, Gillard S, Grant J, Stewart M. Effect on health-related outcomes of interventions to alter the interaction between patients and practitioners: a systematic review of trials. *Ann Fam Med* 2004; **2**(6): 595–608.

18. Elwyn G, Edwards A, Hood K, *et al.* Achieving involvement: process outcomes from a cluster randomized trial of shared decision making skill development and use of risk communication aids in general practice. *Fam Pract* 2004; **21**(4): 337–46.

19. Fellowes D, Wilkinson S, Moore P. Communication skills training for health care professionals working with cancer patients, their families and/or carers. *Cochrane Database Syst Rev* 2004; CD003751(2).

20. Gysels M, Richardson A, Higginson IJ. Communication training for health professionals who care for patients with cancer: a systematic review of effectiveness. *Support Care Cancer* 2004; **12**(10): 692–700.

21. Wykurz G, Kelly D. Developing the role of patients as teachers: literature review. *BMJ* 2002; **325**(7368): 818–21.

22. Piachaud J. Teaching learning disability to undergraduate medical students. *Adv Psychiatric Treat* 2002; **11**: 334–41.

23. Spencer J, Blackmore D, Heard S, *et al.* Patient-orientated learning: a review of the role of the patient in the education of medical students. *Med Educ* 2000; **34**(851): 857.

24. Howe A, Anderson J. Involving patients in medical education. *BMJ* 2003; **327**(326): 328.

25. Thomson R, Edwards A, Grey J. Risk communication in the clinical consultation. *Clin Med* 2005; **5**(5): 465–9.

26. Charles C, Gafni A, Whelan T. Decision-making in the physician-patient encounter: revisiting the shared treatment decision-making model. *Soc Sci Med* 1999; **49**: 651–61.

27. Elwyn G, Edwards A, Gwyn R, Grol R. Towards a feasible model for shared decision making: focus group study with general practice registrars. *BMJ* 1999; **319**: 753–6.

28. Edwards A, Elwyn G, Wood F, Atwell C, Prior L, Houston H. Shared decision making and risk communication in practice: a qualitative study of GPs' experiences. *Br J Gen Pract* 2005; **55**(510): 6–13.

29. Wirrman E, Askham J. *Implementing patient decision aids in urology*. Oxford: Picker Institute Europe, 2006.

30. Hasman A, Coulter A, Askham J. *Education for partnership: developments in medical education*. Oxford: Picker Institute Europe, 2006.

Chapter 5

Predicting career destinations

Chris McManus and Michael J Goldacre

The most important asset of any healthcare system is its skilled workforce. Given the right workforce, sound knowledge-based decisions about all other aspects of resource provision for healthcare can follow. Doctors' individual clinical decisions, in sum, are a fundamental determinant of how healthcare budgets are spent. Medical practitioners take many years, and considerable cost, to train. It has been government policy in the UK – but inevitably a hard policy to implement with precision – to attempt both to minimize the under-provision of doctors and to minimize overprovision and involuntary medical unemployment. For all these reasons, it is critically important that those in medical education and training, in workforce planning, and in all aspects of healthcare provision, are well informed about doctors' career plans. Early career preferences reflect, at least in part, the learning and aspirations that medical students acquire at medical school. These are tempered by practical considerations and it is important to understand how doctors from different backgrounds, and perhaps particularly how men and women, differ in their career expectations. Knowledge about actual career progression, changes in choice, and eventual destinations is essential for the planning of postgraduate medical training and for the delivery of healthcare.

In the first part of this chapter we consider some basic principles, including psychology and personality, which influence career choice. In the second, we consider studies that identify what doctors say they want to do, as eventual careers, when they are newly qualified.

Principles of career choice

Medical careers, like all careers, are complex and difficult to predict, being influenced by a mix of factors that include fundamental interest in the specialty, aptitude for the specialty, temperament and personality, preferred styles of working, luck, opportunity, and practicalities. Indeed, it has been claimed that careers only make sense in retrospect; the journey travelled is clear, and explanations can be given for each turn along the way, but, for many individuals, the possibility of predicting in advance seems minimal.[1] For some doctors, their career trajectory can be likened to that of a ballistic missile, the target pre-programmed, and the destination reached direct, efficiently, and predictably.[2] However, for many doctors, careers are akin to the Brownian random walk of a microscopic particle, being continually buffeted by outside events as 'stuff happens'.

A good illustration of the problems of prediction and understanding is shown by Glin Bennet in his book *The wound and the doctor*,[3] where he describes his own very unusual career trajectory. For Bennet, 'there was never any plan', but instead 'at the major turning points I was guided by a vague sense of what was right and meaningful for me at the time'. Beginning as a surgeon, psychiatry was his eventual destination, his career moving between two of medicine's most dissimilar specialities. However, Bennet's career shows several features typical of many medical careers.

Bennet's initial inclination was 'a greater interest ... in the *practical* over the *theoretical*' (our emphases in italics). Then a key formative event pushed Bennet towards surgery, without which his surgical career may never have started: 'I had an opportunity to remove an appendix ... and that fired my enthusiasm for surgery and the technical challenges involved in performing operations'. Despite his practical interests, and having, 'performed practically all the operations in the surgical repertoire', Bennet realized, as a senior regis-trar, that 'learning operations and doing them for the first, second or third time is one thing. Repeating them endlessly was *not for me*'. Put simply, 'the prospect of repeating [these operations] for the rest of my working life was not appealing'.

The knight's move in Bennet's career progression occurred on a skiing holiday when he met a psychiatrist friend, and 'I knew in that instant that I, too, was going to take up psychiatry'. Although seemingly instantaneous and random, this meeting stimulated an appropriately prepared mind, and as Bennet said, 'must have activated a latent intention in myself'; 'the idea did not arise altogether out of the blue as I had long been interested in psychological ideas'.

Bennet's career emphasizes that, for some, their careers may be nigh on impossible to predict, but nevertheless can be seen as comprehensible and interpretable. The important paradox here was originally described in the nineteenth century by Adolphe Quetelet. Quetelet was impressed that while in an individual courtroom verdicts are difficult to predict, there is remarkable stability in the overall proportion of convictions (and he described how of 11 536 cases in French courts of assize between 1825 and 1830, 61.4% of cases resulted in a conviction, with remarkable constancy from year to year;[4] see also Senn[5] (p. 196 et seq)). Medical careers are similar. Despite much individual variation, medical careers *en masse* show surprising degrees of similarity, allowing workforce planners to make reasonable predictions, and occupational psychology to understand mechanisms and processes. As Quetelet said in 1835, 'The greater the number of individuals observed, the more do individual peculiarities ... become effaced ... [allowing] the general facts to predominate ...' (p. 172).[4]

A common error of medical educators is to assume that medical careers begin only as students enter medical school, are influenced only by medical school, and only medical education research informs. In reality, none is true for career choice. Medical school applicants are not a *tabula rasa*, but already have complex career attitudes, with clear specialty preferences and dislikes, long before they have entered the doors of a medical school. A more general look at occupational psychology is therefore necessary.

The structure of career preferences

An influential theory in occupational psychology is John Holland's hexagon model of career preferences.[6,7] A key insight is that people who are interested in one particular career also have other careers in mind that are attractive, and others that are not. A would-be biologist might be happy being an engineer or a museum curator, but may not consider accountancy or law as a career (and conversely, a would-be lawyer, might consider accountancy but not engineering or biology). From such preference data, Holland arranged careers into a hexagon (see Figure 5.1), in which RIASEC stands for Realistic, Investigative, Artistic, Social, Enterprising, and Conventional.

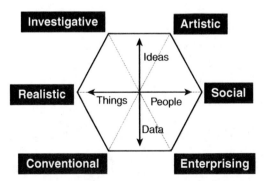

Fig. 5.1 Holland's RIASEC scheme for describing career preferences. Superimposed is Prediger's two-dimensional description of the hexagon in terms of ideas versus data and people versus things.

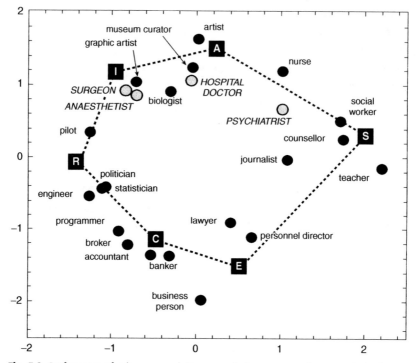

Fig. 5.2 Preferences of a large population sample for a range of careers, including four medical specialities (indicated with open circles and names in italic capitals). For further details see Petrides and McManus.[8]

Figure 5.2 shows the conventional RIASEC structure in the career interests of 1026 (non-medical) individuals.[8] This study also included four clinical specialities which cluster at the top, in the IA part of the hexagon, but with surgeon and anaesthetist towards I (and R) and psychiatrist between A and S. The precise structure of the Holland hexagon has been controversial (for an overview see Silvia[9]), but Prediger's description of two underlying dimensions, *Ideas versus Data*, and *People versus Things* (see Figure 5.1), is supported by our analysis.[8,10] To the public, medical careers are perceived mainly as concerned with ideas rather than data, but with medical specialities varying along the people–things dimension.

Although Holland's hexagon is often been applied to careers in general, much more rarely is it used to study specialities *within* careers (see Borges *et al.*[11]). Figure 5.3 analyses the specialty preferences of a large number of medical school applicants (and final year students show a similar picture). Holland's hexagon readily emerges from the clinical specialities, with surgeons being seen as the realists of medicine, physicians the investigators, psychiatrists

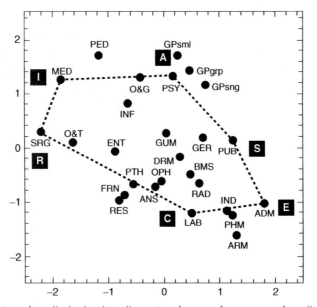

Fig. 5.3 Map of medical school applicants' preferences for a range of medical specialities. For further details see Petrides and McManus.[8] ADM, Administrative Medicine; ANS, Anaesthetics; ARM, Armed Forces; BMS, Basic Medical Sciences; DRM, Dermatology; ENT, Ear, Nose & Throat; FRN, Forensic; GER, Geriatrics; GPlrg, GP Large Group practice; GPsml, GP Small practice; GPsng, GP Single handed; GUM, Genito-urinary medicine; IND, Industrial Medicine; INF, Infectious diseases; LAB, Laboratory (Haematology, Clinical Chemistry, etc.); MED, Internal Medicine; O&G, Obstetrics & Gynaecology; O&T, Orthopaedics & Trauma; OPH, Ophthalmology; PED, Paediatrics; PHM, Pharmaceutical Medicine; PSY, Psychiatry; PTH, Pathology; PUB, Public Health; RAD, Radiology/Radiotherapy; RDL, Radiology; RDT, Radiotherapy; RES, Research; SRG, Surgery.

and GPs the artists, public health doctors as social, those in administrative medicine as enterprising and those in laboratory medicine as conventional, relative to other doctors.[8]

Although Figure 5.3 doesn't show it, just as 'a flea has smaller fleas ... and these have smaller still', so it seems probable that the principles of Holland's hexagon can also be found to apply within the subspecialities of psychiatry, paediatrics, obstetrics, and other broad areas of clinical practice. Obstetricians know that some obstetricians are realistic and practical, others are investigative, some are artistic, or social, or entrepreneurial or conventional, and subspecialities reflect this. Medicine is therefore a house with many rooms, allowing doctors to find congenial specialities or subspecialities for their needs. In Glin Bennet's case, despite his interest in 'the practical over the theoretical', he may have been at the A or S corner of surgery, a position that is relatively close to the R or I corner of psychiatry, making the jump from surgery to psychiatry less distant than it might seem. Certainly he describes his realism as a psychiatrist, when he found himself still interested in surgery, and 'became involved in consultations about psychological and social problems... in the surgical wards', and his surgical qualification, 'render me somehow more credible to my medical and surgical colleagues'.

Circumscription and compromise

Holland's hexagon is an idealized world of what one would *like* to do, not necessarily what one *can* do.

Linda Gottfredson has developed an influential theory of what she calls *circumscription* and *compromise* in career choice.[12–14] Gottfredson's early research considered career choice in adolescents, for whom careers differ primarily in perceived 'prestige level' (in effect the perceived academic achievement necessary) and the 'sextype rating' (the perceived appropriateness for a man or a woman; see Figure 5.4). Note here how the three medical specialities are all at the top of the prestige level, and surgery is seen as more

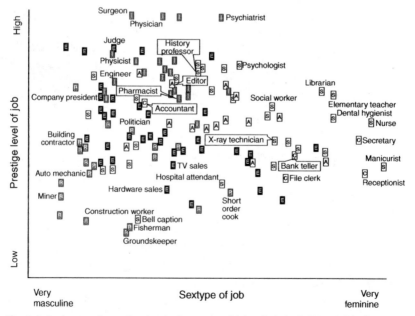

Fig. 5.4 Sextype and prestige level of a range of jobs. R, I, A, S, E, and C indicate Holland's RIASEC typing of the posts. Names of a selection of careers are indicated. Redrawn and adapted from Gottfredson.[12]

masculine than psychiatry. In an example, Gottfredson then considered how a 'hypothetical middle-class boy of average intelligence' may choose between careers. Vertical boundaries, shown in Figure 5.5, are set on the tolerable level of femininity (and might also be set for masculinity), and horizontal boundaries are set for the lower tolerable level of prestige, and the maximum tolerable level of effort. At that point the career space has been *circumscribed*, and only the careers remaining within the boundaries, the shaded area, are acceptable. An important feature of this model that is probably true of much career choice, is that most choices are *negative*. Students typically know better what they *don't* want to do, than what they *do*, so that specialities are successively rejected, perhaps paring away at maps such as that in Figure 5.3, until only a few remain. Of course sometimes there are exceptions to that rule, where individual idiosyncratic features result in positive, often very specific, career choices.[15]

The second component of Gottfredson's theory is far more practical, but is also essential. Even within a circumscribed set of possible careers, not all remaining careers are practicable, so *compromise* is necessary, perhaps due to a paucity of posts in particular specialities, in a geographical area, or which are compatible with family and other commitments. Compromise often means an

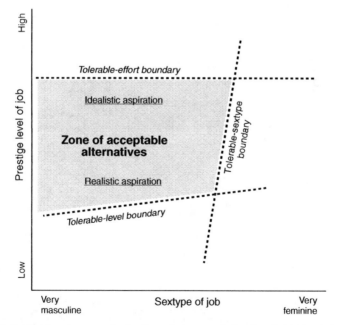

Fig. 5.5 Gottfredson's conceptualization of circumscription in relation to sextype and prestige level of a range of careers. Redrawn and adapted from Gottfredson.[12]

eventual specialty is not perfect but *satisfices* (Herbert Simon's neologism combining 'satisfy' and 'suffice').

Effects of medical school

Holland's hexagon and Gottfredson's circumscription and compromise are generic processes already in place before students enter medical school, perhaps influenced by personality and temperament.[16] Medical schools then further influence career choice, building on top of pre-existing preferences and interests. A brief overview will illustrate this for the single question of how students become interested in surgery, in medical school and in pre-registration house jobs. A powerful tool for analysing complex processes unfolding in time is structural equation modelling, which takes causal inter-relations into account and allows causality to be inferred from correlation. Figure 5.6 shows such a model for data from a large, national, longitudinal study of UK medical students.[17–19] Applicants to medical school in 1990 indicated their interest in a career in surgery, the same measure being repeated in their final year, PRHO year, and in 2002 when the students were then SpRs, SHOs, or in General Practice (see pale grey boxes across the bottom of Figure 5.6). The arrows linking these boxes show that interest in a surgical career is stable, each stage predicting subsequent interest, directly or indirectly.

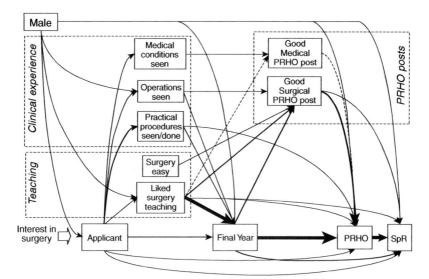

Fig. 5.6 Path model showing causal inter-relations of interest in surgery in medical school applicants, final year students, PRHOs, and SpR level doctors (including SHOs and GPs). Thickness of lines is proportional to strength of effect, and negative effects are shown as dashed lines. Source: IC McManus, unpublished analysis.

Other boxes show effects of background factors. Perceived quality of under-graduate surgical teaching is shown by the two boxes at lower left, a liking for surgery teaching strongly predicting interest in a surgical career (even after taking into account that surgically interested applicants are more likely to like surgery teaching). Similarly, students with greater experience of practical pro-cedures and operations (and students differ extensively[20]), are more likely to want to be surgeons. Having a surgical post that is perceived as good also increases interest in surgery, while a good medical PRHO post has the con-verse effect (and again, both effects are independent of an interest in surgery in the final year also predicting a better surgical PRHO post). Undergraduate surgical teaching, clinical experience, and house surgeon posts all therefore help determine an interest in surgery as a career. Similar effects of teaching are also found for careers in psychiatry.[21]

The model in Figure 5.6 also allows sex differences to be examined, which is of great interest as most surgeons in the UK continue to be male, despite a majority of medical students now being female. The influence of being male is shown by the top left-hand box in Figure 5.6. Not only are males more inter-ested in surgery when applying to medical school, but they like surgical teaching more, they see more surgical operations, and they find surgery pro-gressively more attractive in their final year, after PRHO posts, and as SpRs. The seemingly simple excess of male surgeons therefore results from complex interactions over time between sex, gender, career interests, and teaching and learning in medical schools and hospitals.

Medical career choices after qualification

The most comprehensive longstanding information about doctors' career choices in the UK comes from the Medical Careers Research Group (MCRG). This group has undertaken surveys, by postal questionnaire, of all graduates from all UK medical schools in selected years from 1974. It has surveyed the graduates towards the end of their first, third, and fifth years after qualification, and at longer time intervals after that. One of the important characteristics of the MCRG's study strategy is its prospective, longitudinal collection of information from the doctors. In relating eventual career destinations to early career choices, it can provide information about original choices that were gathered in the early years. It avoids any dependence on the doctors' memory of past decision-making and any possibility of recall bias.

Table 5.1 summarizes some of the MCRG's broad findings. A fundamental finding, if perhaps unsurprising, is that the great majority of newly qualified doctors intend to make a long-term career in medical practice. Only about 1% specifies, at the end of the first year after qualification, that they want

Table 5.1 Percentage of doctors in each year-of-qualification cohort who, at the end of the first year after qualifying, specified each career destination as their preference for their long-term career (and total numbers of doctors).

Specialty/choice*	1974/77	1980/83	1993/6	1999/2000	2002	All years, %	(All years, numbers)
General practice	33.2	40.9	22.7	25.3	22.7	29.7	(7314)
Hospital medical	21.3	15.4	23.1	20.9	22.1	20.2	(4989)
Surgical specialties	16.6	13.3	18.4	18.9	19.5	17.1	(4203)
Other clinical	27.2	27.7	32.8	31.0	34.0	30.0	(7444)
Not specified	1.1	2.2	1.8	2.4	1.0	1.8	(448)
Non-medical choices	0.6	0.5	1.2	1.5	0.7	0.9	(227)
Total	100	100	100	100	100	100	(24 625)

* The hospital medical specialties are those designated as such by the Department of Health (general medicine, cardiology, gastroenterology, etc.). Similarly, the surgical specialties are those so designated (general surgery, trauma and orthopaedics, cardiac surgery, etc.). Source: UK Medical Careers Research Group (UK McRG).

a non-medical career.[22,23] Only about another 2% felt unable to specify their preferred choice of eventual specialty. These percentages have shown no appreciable change across the cohorts.

General practice rose in popularity as a career choice between the 1970s and 1980s. Between 1983 and 1993 (when no national surveys were undertaken), the percentage of doctors who wanted a career in general practice was greatly reduced.[22,23] It is tempting to think that the perceived status of general practice in the UK waned between the 1980s and 1990s. In fact, even at the time when choice for general practice was particularly low, junior doctors none the less continued to hold general practice in high regard.[24] Specialist hospital practice, however, had become even more attractive to junior doctors.

As Table 5.1 shows, the hospital-based medical specialties and the surgical specialties grew in popularity between the 1980s and 1990s. Within the hospital specialties, there have been differing trends. For example, anaesthesia and radiology have grown a little in popularity;[25,26] obstetrics and gynaecology has become a little less popular in recent years, particularly among men;[27] and early career choices for psychiatry have remained remarkably constant at about 4% of all newly qualified doctors over many years.[28]

There are substantial differences between men and women in their career preferences,[22,23] as has already been seen for surgery. In the cohorts from 1974 to 1983, general practice was the preferred eventual career choice, as specified at the end of the first post-qualification year, of 45% of women and 34% of men. By the cohort of 2002, it had fallen to the first choice of 28% of women and only 15% of men. Relatively few women choose careers in the surgical specialties, although this is changing. In the cohorts from 1974 to 1983, surgery was the first choice of 20% of the men and only 5% of the women in year 1. In the cohort of 2002, it was the first choice of 31% of the men and 12% of the women. In the same cohort, obstetrics and gynaecology was the first choice of 3.4% of women and of a vanishingly small 0.7% of men. Historically, the proportion of women entering medicine has shown a large increase since the mid-1960s, an increase that has not always been reflected equally in different specialties, with women doctors perhaps to some extent compromising in their specialty choices, as opportunities became available.[29]

Certainty of choice

In addition to being questioned about their career choice, the doctors are invited to score their choice as definite, probable, or to signify that they are unsure about it. Considering the cohorts from 1974 to 1996 (whose experience will be described more fully below), at the end of the first year after qualifying 32% of doctors said that their career choice of specialty was definite, 52% said probable, and 17% were not really sure. Towards the end of year 3, 50% were definite, 41% probable, and 9% not really sure. Specialties with high levels of certainty in year 1 included general practice (90% definite or probable, 43% definite), surgery (respectively 90% and 31%), and psychiatry (89% and 37%). Specialties with lower than average levels in year 1 included the hospital medical specialties (70% said definite or probable, 13% definite) and radiology (respectively, 79% and 18%). Women were consistently less definite about their choices than men, which may indicate that women tend to feel less confident than men about the compatibility of career choices with their role in family life. It also follows that pressure to reduce the time after qualification at which doctors make final career choices may be a more important reduction in flexibility for women than for men.

Early career choices and eventual career destinations

In Table 5.2, the early specialty choices of the cohorts who qualified between 1974 and 1996 are compared with their specialty destinations later in

Table 5.2 Percentage of doctors who initially chose each broad specialty group, and eventually practised in it long term*: choice made at year 1, 3, and 5 after qualification.

Specialty group†	Year 1	Year 3	Year 5
General practice	78	84	90
Hospital medicine	42	63	82
Paediatrics	47	64	79
Surgery	57	76	88
Obstetrics and gynaecology	46	71	82
Accident and emergency	22	51	70
Anaesthetics	60	76	87
Radiology	39	79	89
Pathology	58	74	88
Psychiatry	68	83	89

*Based on the qualification cohorts of 1974, 1977, 1983, and 1993 at 10 years after qualification, and the 1996 cohort at 7 years. Source: UK MCRG.

†The hospital medical specialties are those designated as such by the Department of Health (general medicine, cardiology, gastroenterology, etc.). In this and subsequent tables, an early choice for any specialty within the broad group, and a destination in the same specialty or another specialty within the same group, is counted as a 'match' of choice and destination. Similarly, the surgical specialties are those so designated (general surgery, trauma and orthopaedics, cardiac surgery, etc.), and a choice and destination within the broad group is counted as a 'match'.

their careers. The table shows, for example, that 78% of the doctors who said in year 1 that they would like a career in general practice, and 84% of those who gave such a choice in year 3, eventually worked as general practitioners. Sixty eight per cent of those who said that they would like a career in psychiatry in year 1, and 83% of those in year 3, eventually practised in the specialty. There were lower levels of agreement between early choice and eventual destinations for the hospital medical specialties, accident and emergency, obstetrics and gynaecology, pathology, and radiology. Within the broad specialty grouping of surgery, there were particularly high levels of agreement between early choice and eventual careers for oral and maxillofacial surgery (many were qualified dentists when they entered medical school) and for ophthalmology.

The doctors' early levels or certainty (or lack of it) about their early career choices were also highly predictive of their future pathways. For example, of those who expressed a preference for general practice in year 1, it was the eventual career destination for 84% of those who were definite in their choice, for 75% who said that their choice was probable, and for only 60% who were not really sure. General practice was the branch of medicine with the highest level of agreement between early choice, and between each level of certainty of choice, and eventual destination.

Early career choices for all specialties were highly predictive of eventual career destinations. Consider, for example, a specialty such as pathology in which early career choices are less predictive of eventual destinations than in most specialties (Table 5.2). Even for pathology, 58% of the doctors who said that it was their first choice of career in year 1, and 77% of those who said that their year 1 choice was definite, eventually had a career in pathology. As a comparison, to demonstrate how far from random their career trajectories are, about 4% of UK medical graduates enter career posts in pathology.

It is none the less clear that, like Glin Bennet, many doctors do switch choice in the early post-qualification years. Indeed, of 1735 doctors in the MCRG database who initially chose surgery as a career, 16 (0.9%), like Bennet, eventually became psychiatrists, while two (0.5%) of the 381 doctors who initially chose psychiatry followed the reverse path and eventually became surgeons. Early career choices represent aspiration, hope, and, no doubt, determination. For some, opportunities and aspiration may not coincide; and, for others, aspirations may in any case change. Another way of studying the relationship between early career choice and eventual destination, analytically, is to start with the doctors' eventual career destination and to look back at their original choices. Table 5.4 shows that, for example, 66% of career general practitioners, and 91% of surgeons, had decided on their long-term specialty career in their first year after qualification. Half or fewer of all career anaesthetists, patholo-gists, or radiologists had chosen their specialty in their first year. It is evident that career choices have firmed up considerably by the end of year 3: 97% of surgeons, and the great majority of doctors in other specialties, had made up their minds by the end of year 3. None the less, some still subsequently switched. Differences between early choice as aspiration (Tables 5.2 and 5.3), and early choice on the pathway to what doctors actually do subsequently (Table 5.4), no doubt reflect a mix of stability and change in choice and the sheer practicality of changing choice. For example, Table 5.4 shows that anyone not on track to becoming a surgeon in year 3 (perhaps even in year 1) is very unlikely to become a surgeon. At least in the past, much more flexibility has been exercised, and has been possible, in switching in the early years to general practice, anaesthetics, pathology, or radiology (all of which are numer-ically large specialties). It is possible, but beyond the scope of this chapter, to document the profiles of career changes between specialties in detail.[30] Understanding the profile of career changes that are common is important in ensuring that appropriate flexibility is planned into postgraduate training programmes.

Table 5.3 Percentage of doctors who initially chose each broad specialty group, and eventually practised in it long term:* choice made at year 1, 3, and 5 after qualification – all who said that their choice was definite (D), probably (P), or that they were not really sure (NS).

Specialty group	Year 1			Year 3			Year 5		
	D	P	NS	D	P	NS	D	P	NS
General practice	84	75	60	90	80	56	94	81	64
Hospital medicine	59	45	30	75	64	50	90	78	50
Paediatrics	69	45	28	77	63	29	88	74	44
Surgery	68	55	25	83	72	45	92	76	69
Obstetrics and gynaecology	59	49	15	83	60	37	87	72	38
Accident and emergency	42	25	8	72	54	10	83	57	33
Anaesthetics	74	58	46	83	69	61	92	81	68
Radiology	50	38	31	89	70	46	94	79	33
Pathology	77	56	26	87	66	33	90	78	39
Psychiatry	78	66	47	87	82	53	93	87	59

* Based on the qualification cohorts of 1974, 1977, 1983, and 1993 at 10 years after qualification, and the 1996 cohort at 7 years. Source: UK MCRG.

Table 5.4 Percentage of all doctors, who practised in each specialty in the long term, who had chosen the specialty as their first choice of career in year 1, 3, and 5 after qualification.

Specialty group	Year 1	Year 3	Year 5
General practice	66	84	93
Hospital medicine	71	79	89
Paediatrics	64	78	87
Surgery	91	97	97
Obstetrics and gynaecology	67	82	87
Accident and emergency	15	50	73
Anaesthetics	50	81	89
Radiology	23	61	89
Pathology	47	75	87
Psychiatry	55	75	90

* Based on the qualification cohorts of 1974, 1977, 1983, and 1993 at 10 years after qualification, and the 1996 cohort at 7 years. Source: UK MCRG.

There is a mismatch between early career choices of UK doctors and the specialty profile of career posts in the UK.[23] For example, currently a higher percentage of young doctors want careers in the hospital medical specialties, and in surgery, than the percentage distribution of posts in these specialties in career grades. In making their early choices, too few choose general practice, psychiatry, radiology, and pathology. The UK has been a net importer of doctors for decades. The fact that so many UK-qualified doctors have been able to follow their preferred choice of specialty probably results, at least in part, from the fact that overseas-qualified doctors have staffed some of the less popular specialties without displacing UK-qualified doctors from training grades in the more popular specialties. This may change.

Medical school, graduate status at entry to medical school, ethnicity, location of home, and training

There are some significant differences between medical schools in the specialty choices made by their qualifiers.[31] For example, a smaller percentage of qualifiers from Oxford and Cambridge than from other schools seek careers in general practice. Graduate entrants to medical school are a little more likely than non-graduate entrants to choose an eventual career in general practice, but the differences between graduate and non-graduate entrants in career choices are small.[32] Ethnicity of UK-qualified doctors – at least at the level of white and non-white – has very little influence on career choice.[33]

Location of home and of place of training influences location of eventual practice. For example, of the qualifiers in the years studied between 1974 and 1993, 38% went to medical school in their home region, 42% obtained their eventual post in the same region as their medical school, and 38% eventually practised in the same region as their family home at the time when they entered medical school.[33] It is common for doctors to want to stay reasonably close to their family roots and location of training.

Leaving UK medicine

The MCRG routinely asks doctors whether, apart from short breaks abroad, they intend to practice medicine in the UK 'for the foreseeable future'. About 75% say 'yes-definitely' or 'yes-probably' when asked in year 1. Of these, 91% eventually practised medicine in the UK. Of those who were undecided in year 1, the figure was 78%; and, of those who said they probably or definitely would not, 63% eventually did.[35]

Doctors who say that they may not continue practising medicine in the UK are far more likely to say that they would practise medicine abroad than would give up medicine.[35] This is amply borne out by what doctors actually do: for young doctors, practising overseas, notably in Australasia and North America, is far more common than quitting medicine.[36]

The future

Studies that cover long time-scales to compare early intentions and eventual destinations draw heavily, inevitably, on data from cohorts that qualified years ago. There have been major policy changes in the UK in recent years to shorten postgraduate training, and to structure it more tightly, with the aim of providing quicker and more certain pathways to career grade status.[37–39] It can be anticipated that career pathways in the future, and the timing of career decisions, will differ from those of the past. Some doctors are certain, in their early postgraduate years, about their eventual choice of specialty. Early entry to run-through training in their specialty of choice should benefit many (providing that they have sufficient breadth of generalist postgraduate training, too, as appropriate to practise in their chosen specialty). It is also clear that a substantial minority of doctors would welcome the retention of some flexibility in the early postgraduate years, so that they can experience work in a number of different specialty areas before making their final choice.

Conclusions

Although a fair amount is known about medical careers in the aggregate, there is still relatively little knowledge about the intellectual processes whereby individual doctors end up in particular specialities. The problem of prediction is in fact even larger than it seems, because most research we have described, particularly the longitudinal studies, is based on graduates of UK medical schools. For the future, there is a major gap in knowledge about doctors' career choices and destinations in the UK that needs to be filled: little is known about the career preferences of overseas-qualified doctors in the UK. In the decade from 1987 to 1996, the General Medical Council reported new registrations of doctors that averaged 3691 UK-qualified doctors per year (almost all qualified in the previous year) and 3832 overseas-qualified doctors per year. In 1997–2006, the most recent decade for which figures are complete, it reported an annual average of 4422 UK-qualified doctors and 6709 overseas-qualified doctors. UK-qualified doctors are currently a minority of all newly registered doctors. Little is known systematically about the careers of doctors who received their basic medical training outside the UK and who are now registered to practise in the UK, and research is urgently needed.

Acknowledgements

The surveys undertaken by the Medical Careers Research Group are funded by the English Department of Health's Policy Research Programme. Chris McManus's longitudinal studies of doctors are currently funded by the London Deanery. The views expressed in this chapter are those of the authors and not necessarily those of the funding bodies.

References

1. McManus IC. Medical careers: stories of a life. *Med Educ* 1997; **31** (Suppl. 1): 31–5.

2. Handfield-Jones RS, Mann KV, Challis ME, *et al.* Linking assessment to learning: a new route to quality assurance in medical practice. *Med Educ* 2002; **36**: 949–58.

3. Bennet G. *The wound and the doctor: healing, technology and power in modern medicine.* London: Secker and Warburg, 1987.

4. Stigler SM. *The history of statistics: the measurement of uncertainty before 1900.* Cambridge, MA: Harvard University Press, 1986.

5. Senn S. *Dicing with death: chance, risk and health.* Cambridge: Cambridge University Press, 2003.

6. Holland JL. *Making vocational choices: a theory of careers.* New York: Prentice Hall, 1973.

7. Holland JL. *Making vocational choices: a theory of vocational personalities and work environments.* Lutz, FL: Psychological Assessment Resources, 1997.

8. Petrides KV, McManus IC. Mapping medical careers: questionnaire assessment of career preferences in medical school applicants and final year students. *BMC Med Educ* 2004; **4**,18.

9. Silvia PJ. *Exploring the psychology of interest.* New York: Oxford University Press, 2006.

10. Prediger DJ. Holland's hexagon is alive and well – though somewhat out of shape: response to Tinsley. *JVB* 2000; **56**: 197–204.

11. Borges NJ, Savickas ML, Jones BJ. Holland's theory applied to medical specialty choice. *J Career Assessment* 2004; **12**: 188–206.

12. Gottfredson LS. Circumscription and compromise: a developmental theory of occupational aspirations. *J Counsel Psychol* 1981; **28**: 545–79.

13. Gottfredson LS. Gottfredson's theory of circumscription, compromise, and self-creation. In *Career choice and development* (Ed. Brown D). San Francisco, CA: Jossey-Bass, 2002.

14. Gottfredson LS. Using Gottfredson's theory of circumscription and compromise in career guidance and counseling. In *Career development and counseling: putting theory and research to work* (Eds Brown SD, Lent RW). New York: Wiley, 2005, pp. 71–100.

15. Crimlisk H, McManus IC. The effect of personal illness experience on career preference in medical students. *Med Educ* 1987; **21**: 464–7.

16. Borges JL, Savickas ML. Personality and medical specialty choice: a literature review and integration. *J Career Assessment* 2002; **10**: 362–80.

17. McManus IC, Richards P, Winder BC, Sproston KA, Styles V. Medical school applicants from ethnic minorities: identifying if and when they are disadvantaged. *BMJ* 1995; **310**: 496–500.

18. McManus IC, Richards P, Winder BC. Intercalated degrees, learning styles, and career preferences: prospective longitudinal study of UK medical students. *BMJ* 1999; **319**: 542–6.

19. McManus IC, Keeling A, Paice E. Stress, burnout and doctors' attitudes to work are determined by personality and learning style: a twelve year longitudinal study of UK medical graduates. *BMC Med* 2004; **2**: 29.

20. McManus IC, Richards P, Winder BC, Sproston KA. Clinical experience, performance in final examinations, and learning style in medical students: prospective study. *BMJ* 1998; **316**: 345–50.

21. McParland M, Noble LM, Livingston G, McManus IC. The effect of a psychiatric attachment on students' attitudes to and intention to pursue psychiatry as a career. *Med Educ* 2003; **37**: 447–54.

22. Lambert TW, Goldacre MJ, Edwards C, Parkhouse J. Career preferences of doctors who qualified in the United Kingdom in 1993 compared with those of doctors qualifying in 1974, 1977, 1980 and 1983. *BMJ* 1996; **313**: 19–24.

23. Lambert TW, Goldacre MJ, Turner G. Career choices of the United Kingdom medical graduates of 2002: questionnaire survey. *Med Educ* 2006; **40**: 514–21.

24. Lambert TW, Evans J, Goldacre MJ. Recruitment of UK-trained doctors into general practice: findings from national cohort studies. *Br J Gen Pract* 2002; **52**: 364–72.

25. Turner G, Goldacre MJ, Lambert TW, Sear J. Career choices for anaesthesia: national surveys of graduates of 1974–2002 from UK medical schools. *Br J Anaesth* 2005; **95**: 332–8.

26. Turner G, Lambert TW, Goldacre M. Career choices for radiology: national surveys of graduates of 1974–2002 from UK medical schools. *Clin Radiol* 2006; **61**: 1047–54.

27. Turner G, Lambert TW, Goldacre MJ, Barlow D. Career choices for obstetrics and gynaecology: national surveys of graduates of 1974–2002 from UK medical schools. *Br J Obstet Gynaecol* 2006; **113**: 350–6.

28. Goldacre MJ, Turner G, Fazel S, Lambert TW. Career choices for psychiatry: national surveys of graduates of 1974–2000 from UK medical schools. *Br J Psychiatry* 2005; **186**: 158–64.

29. McManus IC, Sproston KA. Women in hospital medicine: glass ceiling, preference, prejudice or cohort effect? *J Epidemiol Community Health* 2000; **54**: 10–16.

30. Goldacre MJ, Lambert TW. Stability and change in career choices of junior doctors: postal questionnaire surveys of the United Kingdom qualifiers of 1993. *Med Educ* 2000; **34**: 700–7.

31. Goldacre MJ, Turner G, Lambert TW. Variation by medical school in career choices of UK graduates of 1999 and 2000. *Med Educ* 2004; **38**: 249–58.

32. Goldacre MJ, Davidson JM, Lambert TW. Career preferences of graduate and non-graduate entrants to medical schools in the United Kingdom. *Med Educ* 2007; **41**: 349–61.

33. Goldacre MJ, Davidson JM, Lambert TW. Country of training and ethnic origin of UK doctors: database and survey studies. *BMJ* 2004; **329**; 597–600. http://bmj.com/cgi/doi/10.1136/bmj.38202.364271.BE

34. Parkhouse J, Lambert TW. Home, training and work: mobility of British doctors. *Med Educ* 1997; **31**: 399–407.

35. Lambert TW, Goldacre MJ, Parkhouse J. Intentions of newly qualified doctors to practise in the United Kingdom. *BMJ* 1997; **314**: 1591–2.

36. Moss P, Lambert TW, Goldacre MJ, Lee P. Reasons for considering leaving UK medicine: questionnaire study of junior doctors' comments. *BMJ* 2004; **329**: 1263–5.

37. Working Group on Specialist Medical Training. *Hospital doctors: training for the future.* London: UK Department of Health, 1993.

38. Department of Health. *Modernising medical careers – the response of the four UK health ministers to the consultation on Unfinished Business: proposals for reform of the senior house officer grade.* London: Department of Health, 2003.

39. Tooke J. *Aspiring to excellence: findings and recommendations of the independent inquiry into modernising medical careers.* London: MMC Inquiry, 2007. http://www.mmcinquiry.org.uk/

Chapter 6

Extending learning into the community

Val Wass

Introduction

Medical education is gradually moving away from the tradition of hospital-based, disease-focused training. 'Gradual' is the key word as the pace of change has been relatively slow. Until recently the community remained a distant place where, if one failed to meet the training expectations of a hospital career, one might 'end up' working. A deep cultural educational divide existed between secondary and primary care with a strong assumption that clinical skills could only be learnt in the former. Over the past 40 years this has been challenged with some success.

In the UK a significant milestone occurred in 1972 when the recommendation that vocational training for general practice should include a year of supervision in primary care *per se* was accepted.[1] In the undergraduate arena the need for medical students to experience community care has also gradually evolved. In the UK strong support from the General Medical Council (GMC) has been of paramount importance. *Tomorrow's Doctors*,[2] first published in 1993, clearly highlighted the need for more education in the community. Its implementation has been ensured through GMC quality assurance procedures. Similar challenges to include community services in the delivery of undergraduate medical education have occurred in North America.[3,4] Modernising Medical Careers in the UK has now offered a further significant advance. Primary care attachments during Foundation training[5] have allowed all young doctors, regardless of their career aspirations, to experience work in primary care. The extension of education into the community is on the move. Yet there is much still to be understood and overcome if all the opportunities available for learning in the community are to be effectively harnessed. For clinical learning to truly embed in the community a better understanding of both the forces driving the change and the barriers to be overcome is essential.

There has been a culture of arguably artificial divide within medical education for too long. For clinical education to extend effectively into the community true integration of learning is essential. These 'divides' must be bridged. The Flexnerian model of undergraduate teaching[6] delivered medical student education as 2 years of dedicated basic medical science knowledge followed by 3 years of hospital-based clinical training. Although welcome at the time the advantages of early patient contact to set scientific knowledge in a practical context has been increasingly recognized. The new medical schools have taken a very positive approach to early learning in the community.[7] Yet in the more traditional schools, despite an overt commitment to education in the community,[8] a hidden teaching hospital anti-curriculum can still exist.[9] This culture of separation has been unwittingly established not only at the community versus hospital or primary versus secondary care level. An undergraduate–postgraduate divide also sits uncomfortably in the arena. Tensions of responsibility between universities and deaneries and thus funding streams for education exist. This is currently under discussion as recommendations from the Tooke report[10] are reviewed. The debate continues on the point at which university and GMC quality assurance ends and deanery and the governance of the Postgraduate Medical Education Training Board (PMETB) assume responsibility. This is set against the reality of a continuum of education within the National Health Service (NHS). To ensure effective extension of learning into the community and appropriate resourcing these divisions of care and responsibility need to be addressed.

As the publication of this book highlights, we are at a crucial point of change in clinical training. Extending education into the community has two important facets. It has the potential to bring all the contexts in which healthcare is being delivered together. This would ensure trainees both achieve the full benefits of experiential learning and develop a comprehensive understanding of patients' holistic experiences of their illness and their journey through the NHS. At the same time the changes we are seeing in methods of training and assessment, as outlined in other chapters, must be addressed. Community learning must rest seamlessly alongside hospital education and meet the standards for quality assurance set by the GMC and PMETB.

This chapter will review the forces driving the change to extend education into the community and the difficulties to be overcome. The implications of training in the community for (1) students and trainees, (2) tutors, and (3) patients with evidence of its efficacy will then be outlined before analysing implications and ways forward for the future.

The driving forces for change

Changing healthcare

Healthcare in the UK is changing radically. Provision within the NHS has become increasingly dispersed by new government initiatives both to move specialist care into the community and to create alternative providers fostering explicit choice for patients. The concept of a well defined interface between community and hospital care for planning and resourcing experiential learning is rapidly losing clarity. Healthcare is fragmenting arguably to the extent that the primary -secondary care divide between 'generalism' and 'specialism' no longer exists. In future hospital specialists and general practitioners are likely to work side by side in the community. What are the challenges we now face?

More diverse pathways of access to acute care

Patients' experiences have become increasingly disjointed and complex as access pathways to acute healthcare change. Internationally duty hour reforms in hospital have impacted on education.[11] In the UK with the loss of 24-hour GP responsibility for cover and the introduction of various schemes for out of hours services new structures for training must be considered if trainees are to gain sufficient experience and understanding of acute care.[12] Walk-in centres attract a certain group of patients and offer different educational opportunities for those learning about healthcare.[13] Accident and emergency attachments are experiencing a change in referral patterns. Unless appropriately supported by a community-orientated physician this again risks a distorted view of the impact of acute minor illness on patients. The ability to follow the progression and/or resolution of these problems offered through continuity of care in general practice may be lost.

Creation of tiered referral systems

A similar risk occurs with the learning of diagnostic skills. The introduction of enhanced services within primary care and community second tier referral centres increasingly deflects common disorders from the hospital arena. Important diagnostic decisions, requiring specialist expertise, are now being made in new territory lying between traditional primary and secondary care as we know it. The process of using investigation to move from an undifferentiated diagnosis to a definitive one will not necessarily now be observed in the hospital outpatient clinic. The creation of GPs with a specialist interest can deskill their GP colleagues and thus equally threaten comprehensive education in primary care attachments.[14]

Movement of chronic disease management into the community

Much of common chronic disease management, e.g. diabetes, asthma, and cardiovascular care, occurs increasingly outside hospitals. The range of community services is also extending beyond practices as GP's and community nurses with a specialist interest are commissioned to extend services into community centres. This is creating an additional level of care between the GP surgery and the hospital. Herein lies a double-edged sword. If trained with insufficient experience of these community services, students, and postgraduate trainees see only the very serious complications referred to secondary care. These represent the tip of the 'care' iceberg. Without experience of chronic disease management at the community 'coal face' their understanding of the problems faced by patients becomes increasingly distorted. Fragmentation of services carries a significant risk of failure to understand the essentials of health promotion and prevention.

Streamlining of hospital services

Patients spend increasingly less time in hospital and the number of beds has decreased. Over the past 20 years the average length of stay has fallen from 12 to 7 days.[15] This rapid patient turnover has clear implications for hospital training. The introduction of intermediate care services to accelerate discharge of the elderly may further increase patient turnover. This represents another arena where trainees may miss learning about rehabilitation of the elderly unless community learning is appropriately organized. Similarly with the increasing use of day surgery and community centres or private providers for these services, experience of common conditions such as hernias, cataracts breast diagnostic services, etc. may also be missed.

Changing medical education

Education is undergoing change too. The current fragmentation of healthcare is by no means unique to the UK. It is internationally recognized that continuity is a fundamental principle of high-quality medical education.[16] The need for continuity between undergraduate and postgraduate curricula has also been firmly argued.[17] Many of these new educational issues, which hold key importance for the development of community learning, are addressed in more detail in other chapters. To summarize briefly the following changes must be considered.

The undergraduate curriculum

We await a new version of *Tomorrow's Doctors*.[2] However, its fundamental philosophy will undoubtedly continue. Both the move from a disease-based curriculum to embrace a more holistic community-based approach to healthcare and the encouragement of more self-directed mature learning to foster continuous professional development should remain. High technology hospital medicine will inevitably continue to progress and rightly so. Care must be taken to ensure an appropriate balance is available to enable future doctors to make appropriate career choices earlier than has been necessary in the past. Experience in the community is essential to this. It remains to be seen to what extent the GMC address the important changes in healthcare we are experiencing.

Outcomes based training curricula

Training curricula are increasingly based on outcomes and observed demonstration of competence. Both the 2-year Foundation Programme[5] and new Royal College training curricula, designed to meet the Postgraduate Medical Education Training Board (PMETB) principles and standards for competence,[18] illustrate this. The emphasis on competence is increasingly shifting the role of the teacher to one of observation and assessment of skills in the work place. If experience in the community is not appropriately constructed then both integration of 'knowledge' with 'practice' and the pursuit of a tick box 'can do' mentality are risked. This arguably detracts from excellence as a performance goal.[19] The focus on competency has resource implications for community tutors too. Sufficient teaching time must be protected for these tasks. Tutors need to be trained to perform the assessments and give appropriate feedback. Increasingly it is apparent that to cover the GP curriculum vocational training in primary care needs a greater community focus. Fortunately this is under review in the Tooke report.[10]

Professionalism

The Royal College of Physicians Working Party, tasked with redefining professionalism for the twenty-first century, highlighted the need to aim for 'excellence' not 'competence'; standards higher than ones of 'mere capability'.[20] Many of the report's recommendations are compatible with learning in the community. Opportunities to increase experience through patient contact, to develop management skills, to work interprofessionally and to build appropriate multiprofessional team working skills lie well within the scope of community healthcare delivery. The report emphasizes that doctors must not only learn to *lead* well. They must also develop the flexibility needed to *follow* other health professionals where appropriate and to communicate across a range of cultural diversity. GP trainers can act as excellent role models through one to one attachments in the community and are trained to give feedback on professional behaviour. These skills should be fostered not lost in community education.

These current changes in both healthcare and education can be harnessed to extend learning into the community. Careful attention must first be paid to the implications:

Implications for the extension of community-based learning into the community

The impact on students and trainees

Since the General Medical Council first highlighted the need for a more community-based undergraduate medical education[21] strong evidence has increasingly accrued that it is an effective means of learning core medical skills. The Department of Health London Initiative Zone Educational Incentives (LIZEI) in the 1990s enabled London Medical Schools to develop and evaluate primary care driven undergraduate educational initiatives in the community. These demonstrated that GPs: (1) could teach clinical skills as well as their hospital colleagues;[22] (2) were motivated by teaching medical students;[23] and (3) gave students a wealth of experience of common and chronic diseases in contrast to the acute experiences of the hospital.[24] Nigel Oswald extended the model analysing the experiences of a small student cohort of Cambridge students on a continuous 15-month attachment in general practice. Following patient pathways from primary into secondary care provided sufficient clinical exposure to specialist care for the students to develop core clinical skills and perform at the same level as their hospital educated colleagues.[25] Admittedly this was a selective student group with appropriate resourcing. However, the principle that students can learn core skills from patients in the community has been established.

Examination performance continues to confirm that students learn equally well in primary care[22,25,26] and that a rural setting is as good as an urban one.[27] Furthermore, students themselves are capable of directing their own learning. They can use the broad spectrum of opportunity to fill in gaps in their knowledge and skills.[28] These deficiencies are widening due to increasing specialization within hospital firms, high patient turnover, and the move of chronic disease management into the community. Internationally the need to extend education into the community accords with the UK experience. Reports from the USA,[29] Australia,[30] and Europe[31] all reach similar conclusions. General Practitioners are keen to involve their healthcare teams in teaching and this can enhance their professional self-image.[32]

Increasingly, UK medical schools have built on this evidence developing curricula that focus on 'the patient' rather than 'the disease'. New schools offer a high proportion of experience (up to 35%) in primary care to ensure regular patient contact from the moment of arrival on the course;[7] a contentious change for those embedded in traditional teaching hospital tertiary care delivery. There is a view that new medical schools risk 'training social workers not doctors'. This traditionalist view may impact on students.

A hidden curriculum[9,33] favouring specialist training and undermining community attachments can have a powerful influence.[34] Inevitably the quality of the placements also affects the student experience. High-quality attachments motivate students and can alter career choice favourably towards primary care.[33,34] Negative experiences on the other hand are difficult to reverse.[9] With increasing pressure on placements and fragmentation of delivery, the importance of the GP tutor as a role model – the one to one teaching they offer and the professional values intrinsic to it – must be acknowledged. Every effort should be made to sustain this as learning extends into the community.

Similarly pilot schemes exploring early attachments originally as pre registration house officers[35] and more recently as part of the Foundation programme pilots[36] confirm that young doctors benefit from a period of time working in general practice regardless of their proposed career pathway. Anecdotally, as it is too early for full evaluation, the 4-month attachment also provides valuable learning in Foundation years. It would be regrettable if this was lost in the reorganization of specialist training. The community opens new learning opportunities to doctors in training that should be viewed as symbiotic with experience in hospital.[37] Both are needed. Emerging evidence suggests the balance of the learning environments is important to the development of professional identity and career selection.[38] Appropriate experience of work in the community and hospital post registration appears to offer valuable learning for those in training. Thus the experiences of the Foundation programme should not be lost in reorganization. It is not a case of substitution but one of achieving the correct balance between community and hospital.[39]

Implications for patients

Patients are equally crucial stakeholders in community learning. They have been as open to engagement in teaching students in general practice as they have in hospital.[40] A true sense of altruism and personal gain remains. This must be fostered given the range of educational experience interviewing patients in both the surgery and in their homes can offer.[41] Not only are the patient-centred values of primary care effectively modelled to students.[42] Patients perceive their role as that of a teacher[43] who can inform and influence students.

There are some caveats. Consent, confidentiality and access to notes must be transparently agreed to reassure both patients and students.[44] Some patients report difficulty in talking about personal issues in front of students[45] and increasingly consent for a student to observe an intimate examination is refused.[46] This affects students who need reassurance that patients have consented to their presence. Male students can feel significantly disadvantaged in reaching competency in Obstetrics and Gynaecology. However, there is accruing evidence that both students and patients value their teaching experiences within primary care.[47] The quality of the placement is crucial.[9,48]

Implications for community tutors

There is strong evidence that GPs and their patients contribute significantly to community education. It is estimated that more than a half of all GPs teach; over a third for universities. Increasingly teaching is becoming intrinsic to the role of the community physician. Securing adequate protected time to teach, remuneration, and lack of facilities has caused frustrations for a long time.[49] Increasing expansion of medical school intakes, alongside the introduction of the Foundation programme in General Practice, have exacerbated these problems. Ideally facilities for training students and Foundation doctors should match deanery standards set for vocational training. Expansion of community teaching has outstripped the resources needed for this. Capacity is limited by available space, particularly for students to interview patients. This is increasingly found to be limiting a practice's commitment to teaching. Remuneration for teaching is poor and fails to cover locum costs or compete with alternative income sources. Compared with the hospitals, community teaching receives a relatively lower proportion of the Service Increment for Teaching (SIFT). Siddiky estimates that on average 9% of the UK undergraduate curriculum is now taught in the community remunerated by only 5% of the teaching income.[50] Given that it is crucial that community educators maintain their educator role[51] what are the implications for the future?

As healthcare changes, education and the resources supporting it must change too. Failure to address this will deny those in training access to patients and appropriate role models. This requires strategies that acknowledge the findings described above.

The future

Future change must be supported by evidence. Education will almost certainly continue to extend into the community at all levels of service provision. Much of the evidence accrued over the last 10 years as cited in this chapter investigates the primary–secondary care interface. However, as with so much of educational research, the evaluation lies mostly at the level of satisfaction.[52] If we are to realign education with healthcare then robust evidence is needed to support proposals for change, explore any added value of learning in the range of community services offered and identify any impact on patient care.[53] One study in East London demonstrated a relationship between practice involvement in teaching and higher scores on a range of performance and organizational quality indicators.[54] We need research at a level that addresses learning outcomes, behavioural change, and healthcare performance.[52] In the meantime to keep abreast of change in healthcare and ensure appropriate educational use of the extended resources the following key areas need to be addressed.

The curriculum

As healthcare disperses across a range of providers, the continuity and context of the available learning opportunities must be explicit within the curriculum.[16] The need for more integration[55] and stronger undergraduate–postgraduate links[56] has already been argued. Without doubt the relative dispersal of healthcare requires a fundamental rethink of medical education. If we accept that we learn experientially from patients (and I suspect few would dispute this) then more direct integration of educational opportunities and processes with clearly defined learning outcomes is essential. Linking the range of experiences offered within and without hospital with educational goals mapped against the curriculum is essential. Attachment either to a hospital firm or primary care practice is no longer going to suffice if all the intermediate community tiers of the healthcare system are to be harnessed and integrated for learning. We need models for both tracking student activities and evaluating their learning experiences.[57]

The patient 'journey'

Students can be successfully encouraged to direct their own learning and follow 'patient journeys' both between primary and secondary care placements[30] and in rural settings.[25] As healthcare moves beyond the relatively 'simple' primary – secondary divide, frameworks on which to build this experience are needed if students are to develop a holistic approach to care and understand the progression and/or resolution of illness. One model might be to develop Health Education Zones where a central teaching hospital and attached district general hospitals link with their local primary care and mental health trusts and community intermediate care services. The development of an integrated community learning environments within these zones to embrace undergraduate and postgraduate training and multiprofessional learning would require integration of deanery and university resources.[58] If appropriately resourced students could follow patients within their community locality.

Community tutors

The professional commitment of a doctor to teach must also be nurtured.[59] This is increasingly highlighted within training curricula.[60] As we move to competency and workplace-based teaching and assessment, the apprenticeship learning resources within practices could be harnessed, for example, to share teaching responsibilities and spread workload for GP tutors. For example, the registrar might observe the Foundation trainee who in turn teaches the year 5 medical student. Thus those teaching revisit their own previous learning and enhance their teaching portfolio while those being taught have the advantage of the immediacy of a young role model. The multiprofessional resource of the practice must also be used to full advantage embracing the skills of other health professionals.[61] Change is essential if the one-to-one teaching offered by primary care is to be maintained.[62] It is encouraging that innovations are beginning to emerge[63,64] as creative use of existence resources is essential.

Financial resources

Provided appropriate resourcing is available, portfolio GPs appear keen to teach centrally in hospitals as problem-based learning tutors, mentors, and assessors. Joint GP–consultant-led firms have proved successful in opening the eyes of both consultants and GPs to life on the other side of the traditional 'fence'. The major challenge as healthcare changes lies in the resources. Secondary care Service Increment for Teaching (SIFT) resources must follow the patients into the community. Politically these monies have become embedded in hospital service. Identifying and moving resources for reimbursing community tutors is undoubtedly the greatest challenge we face in extending community training to reflect twenty-first century healthcare.

The extension of education into the community is essential if those in training are to experience the actualities of modern healthcare. This is reflected throughout the world with increasing recognition that integration and flexibility are of paramount importance as we move to modify educational opportunities to embrace both changing service delivery and modern approaches to medical education. Clear strategies to develop curricula and resource change are essential to achieve this. Reflection across the content of this book provides an ideal opportunity to start to develop the links and ideas necessary to keep abreast change. We must ensure the resources available in the community for learning are harnessed to the best advantage of trainees, patients, and their tutors.

References

1. Royal Commission on Medical Education 1965–8 (Todd Report). London: HMSO (Cmnd 3569), 1968.

2. General Medical Council. *Tomorrow's Doctors*. London: GMC, 1993. http://www.gmc-uk.org/.

3. Seifer SD. Service-learning: community-campus partnerships for health professions education. *Acad Med* 1998; **73**: 273–7.

4. Hennen B. Demonstrating social accountability in medical education. *Can Med Assoc J* 1997; **156**: 365–7.

5. Modernising Medical Careers: The Foundation Programme. http://www.mmc.nhs.uk/pages/foundation.

6. Flexner A. *Medical education in the United States and Canada*. Bethesda, MD: Science and Health Publications, 1910.

7. Howe A, Campion P, Searle J, Smith H. New perspectives – approaches to medical education at four new UK medical schools. *BMJ* 2004; **329**: 327–32.

8. O'Neill PA. Problem-based learning alongside clinical experience: reform of the Manchester curriculum. *Educ Health* 1998; **11**: 37–48.

9. Firth A, Wass V. Medical students' perceptions of Primary Care: The influence of tutors, peers, and the curriculum. *Educ Primary Care* 2007; **18**: 364–72.

10. Tooke Report. 2008. http://www.mmcinquiry.org.uk/.

11. Woodrow S, Segouin C, Armbruster J, Hamstra S, Hodges B. Duty hours reforms in the United States, France, and Canada: Is it time to refocus our attention on education? *Acad Med* 2006; **81**: 1045–51.

12. Jones R. Should general practitioners resume 24 hour responsibility for their patients? *BMJ* 2007; **335**: 696.

13. Salisbury S, Munro J. Walk-in centres in primary care: a review of the international literature. *Br J Gen Pract* 2003; **53**, 53–9.

14. Wilkinson D, Dick M-LB, Askew DA. General practitioners with special interests: risk of a good thing becoming bad? *Med J Aust* 2005; **183**: 84–6.

15. Black D, Pearson M. Average length of stay, delayed discharge, and hospital congestion. *BMJ* 2002; **325**: 610–11.

16. Hirsh DA, Ogur B, Thibault GE, Cox M. 'Continuity' as an organizing principle for clinical education reform. *New Engl J Med* 2007; **356**: 858–65.

17. Jones R, Oswald N. A continuous curriculum for general practice? Proposals for undergraduate-postgraduate collaboration. *Br J Gen Pract* 2001; **463**: 135–7.

18. PMETB. Principles of good medical education and training. http://www.pmetb.org.uk/media/pdf/o/b/PMETB-GMC_ _(2005).pdf.

19. Hodges B. Medical education and the maintenance of incompetence. *Med Teach* 2007; **28**: 690–6.

20. Royal College of Physicians. *Doctor in society: medical professionalism in a changing world*. London: RCP, 2005. http://www.rcplondon.ac.uk/pubs/books/docinsoc.

21. General Medical Council. *Tomorrow's Doctors*. London: GMC, 2003. http://www.gmc-uk.org/education/undergraduate/undergraduate_policy/tomorrows_doctors.asp.

22. Murray E, Jolly B, Modell M. Can students learn clinical method in general practice? A randomised crossover trial based on objective structured clinical examinations. *BMJ* 1997; **315**: 920–3.

23. Hartley SH, MacFarlane F, Gantley M, Murray E. Influence on general practitioners of teaching undergraduates: qualitative study of London general practitioner teachers. *BMJ* 1999; **319**: 168–71.

24. Bryant P, Hartley S, Coppola W, Berlin A, Modell M, Murray E. Clinical exposure during clinical method attachments in general practice. *Med Educ* 2003; **37**: 790–3.

25. Oswald N, Alderson T, Jones S. Evaluating primary care as a base for medical education: the report of the Cambridge Community-based Clinical Course. *Med Educ* 2001; **35**: 782–8.

26. Worley P, Esterman A, Prideaux D. Cohort study of examination performance of undergraduate medical students in community settings. *BMJ* 2004; **328**: 207–9.

27. Waters B, Hughes J, Forbes K, Wilkinson D. Comparative academic performance of medical students in rural and urban clinical settings *Med Educ* 2006; **40**: 117–20.

28. Smith P, Morrison J. Clinical clerkships: students can construct their own learning. *Med Educ* 2006; **40**: 884–92.

29. Peters AS, Schnaidt K, Seward SJ, Rubin RM, Feins A, Fletcher RH. Teaching Care Management in a Longitudinal Primary Care Clerkship. *Teach Learn Med* 2005; **17**: 322–7.

30. Worley P, Prideaux D, Strasser R, March R, Worley E. What do medical students actually do on clinical rotations? *Med Teach* 2004; **26**: 594–8.

31. Haffling A-C, Håkansson A, Hagander B. Early patient contact in primary care: a new challenge. *Med Educ* 2001; **35**: 901–8.

32. Howe A. Teaching – practice: a qualitative factor analysis of community based teaching. *Med Educ* 2003; **34**, 648–55.

33. Henderson E, Berlin A, Fuller J. Attitude of medical students towards general practice and general practitioners. *Br J Gen Pract* 2002; **52**: 359–63.

34. Howe A, Ives G. Does community based experience alter career preference? New evidence from a prospective longitudinal cohort study of undergraduate medical students. *Med Educ* 2001; **35**: 391–7.

35. Williams C, Cantillon P, Cochrane M. Pre-registration rotations into general practice: the concerns of pre-registration house officers and the views of hospital consultants. *Med Educ* 2000; **34**: 716–20.

36. Beard J, Strachan A, Davies H *et al.* Developing an education and assessment framework for the Foundation Programme. *Med Educ* 2005; **39**: 841–51.

37. Worley P, Prideaux D,Strasser R, Magarey A, March R. Empirical evidence for symbiotic medical educational comparative analysis of community and tertiary-based programmers. *Med Educ* 2006; **40**: 109–16.

38. Cross V, Hicks C, Parle J, Field S. Perceptions of the learning environment in higher specialist training of doctors: implications for recruitment and retention. *Med Educ* 2006; **40**: 121–8.

39. Morrison J. Learning in teaching hospitals and the community: time to get the balance right. *Med Educ* 2006; **40**: 92–3.

40. Thistlethwaite JE, Jordan JJ. Patient-centred consultations: a comparison of students' experience and understanding in two clinical environments. *Med Educ* 1999; **33**: 678–85.

41. Howe A, Anderson J. Involving patients in medical education *BMJ* 2003; **327**: 326–8.

42. Howe A. Patient-centred medicine through student-centred teaching: a student perspective on the key impacts of community-based learning in undergraduate medical education. *Med Educ* 2001; **35**: 666–72.

43. Stacy R, Spencer J. Patients as teachers: a qualitative study of patients' views on their role in a community based undergraduate project. *Med Educ* 1999; **33**: 688–94.

44. O'Flynn N, Spencer J, Jones R. Consent and confidentiality in teaching in general practice: survey of patients' views on presence of students. *BMJ* 1997; **315**: 1142–5.

45. O'Flynn N, Spencer J, Jones R. Does teaching during a general practice consultation affect patient care? *Br J Gen Pract* 1997; **49**: 7–9.

46. O'Flynn N, Rymer J. Women's attitudes to the sex of medical students in a gynaecology clinic: cross sectional survey *BMJ* 2002; **325**: 683–4.

47. Lucas B, Pearson D. Learning medicine in primary care: medical students' perceptions of final year placements. *Educ Prim Care* 2005; **16**: 440–9.

48. Silverstone Z, Whitehouse C, Willis S, McArdle P, Jones A, O'Neill PA. Students' conceptual model of a good community attachment. *Med Educ* 2001; **35**: 946–56.

49. Mathers J, Parry J, Lewis S, Greenfield S. What impact will an increased number of teaching general practices have on patients, doctors and medical students? *Med Educ* 2004; **38**: 1219–28.

50. Siddiky A. Teaching in General Practice. *Br J Gen Pract* 2004; **54**: 640.

51. Prideaux D, Alexander H, Bower A *et al.* Clinical teaching: maintaining an educational role for doctors in the new health care environment *Med Educ* 2000; **34**: 820–6.

52. Kirkpatrick D. Levels of evaluation. http://www.science.ulster.ac.uk/caa/presentation/kirkpatrick/index.htm.

53. Gray RW, Carter YH, Hull SA, Sheldon MG, Ball C. Characteristics of general practices involved in undergraduate medical teaching. *Br J Gen Pract* 2001; **51**: 371–4.

54. Pearson B, Lucas B. Learning medicine in primary care: what is the added value? *Educ Prim Care* 2005; **16**: 424–31.

55. Worley P, Silagy C, Prideaux, Newble D, Jones A. The parallel rural community curriculum: an integrated clinical curriculum based in rural general practice. *Med Educ* 2000; **34**: 558–65.

56. Jones R, Oswald N. A continuous curriculum for general practice? Proposals for undergraduate–postgraduate collaboration. *Br J Gen Pract* 2001; **51**: 135–8.

57. Dornan T, Boshuizen H, King N, Scherpbier A. Experience-based learning: a model linking the processes and outcomes of medical students' workplace learning. *Med Educ* 2007; **41**: 84–91.

58. Mckinlay D, Lewis B. Working together across the undergraduate–postgraduate divide in the North West. *Educ Prim Care* **16**: 729–31.

59. General Medical Council UK. *Good Medical Practice*. London: GMC, 2006. http://www.gmc-uk.org/guidance/good_medical_practice/index.asp.

60. Royal College of General Practitioners Curriculum for Vocational Training. http://www.rcgp-curriculum.org.uk/.

61. Howe A, Billingham K, Croft D. Can nurses teach tomorrow's doctors? A nursing perspective on involvement in community-based medical education. *Med Teach* 2000; **22**: 576–81.

62. Charlton R, Prince R, Bhattacharya A, Reid D. One-to-one teaching in primary care. *Educ Prim Care* 2006; **17**: 518–20.

63. Edwards J, Goulding S, Leach J. The general practice foundation placement: innovations for added value. *Educ Prim Care* 2007; **18**: 443–9.

64. Lake J, Bell J. How do educational supervisors view innovative training posts? An evaluation of the Portsmouth experience. *Educ Prim Care* 2007; **18**: 588–92.

Chapter 7

Peer-assisted learning

Peter Cantillon and Liam Glynn

Introduction

'To teach is to learn twice' (Joubert, 1754–1824) is an aphorism that is much quoted in educational literature. It is particularly apt in the context of peer learning. Peer-assisted learning (PAL) has been described as: 'people from similar social groupings who are not professional teachers helping each other to learn, and learning themselves, by teaching'.[1] Peer learners (and peer teachers) share similar social status and are not content experts in the subject matter that is being taught. The definition of PAL was later refined to the 'development of knowledge and skills through active help and support among status equals or matched companions'.[2] In this definition PAL is viewed as an active learning process in which learners cooperate as equals to achieve knowledge and skill learning goals.

PAL is not a recent educational invention. In fact peer teaching has been traced back to the time of Aristotle when he used student leaders (or archons) to disseminate his ideas among his followers. More recently PAL was evident in descriptions of nineteenth century primary school education when teachers, overwhelmed by large student numbers used senior children to teach younger children. One of the earliest descriptions of PAL in third-level education was by Marcel Goldschmid at McGill University in Montreal in 1970. He used PAL approaches to address the largely passive learning evident in his large undergraduate classes of 200 or more students. He initiated peer-lead discussion groups in which students engaged with course content, addressed misconceptions, and produced educational product. He found that PAL made significant differences to the quality of student learning and improved their appreciation of the courses he was teaching.[3]

Theory of peer-assisted learning

PAL is strongly rooted in educational theory. The cognitive tradition, which concerns itself with how new knowledge is acquired, stored, and reproduced, explains the effects and the effectiveness of PAL in terms of the benefits for the student teacher. Gartner *et al.*[4] outlined a number of cognitive benefits that accrue from being a peer tutor or teacher. The act of preparing for teaching student colleagues requires a review of prior knowledge that helps the peer teacher to develop a deeper and more flexible grasp of fundamental principles. More importantly the peer teacher must also reorganize the material to make it understandable for others. In other words the PAL teacher has to convert book knowledge into a form that can be readily understood and absorbed by peer learners. Thus peer teachers not only develop deeper knowledge of the subject matter, but they also develop knowledge of how to teach and explain difficult concepts.

Whitman and Fife[5] found that when students learn material for their own needs they seem to learn it differently than when they learn it for the purpose of teaching others. Benware and Deci[6] showed that students who were randomly assigned to learn a topic with the purpose of teaching, performed better in a subsequent test of knowledge and understanding than students who learned it for the purpose of passing a test. While involvement in PAL has clear benefits for peer teachers it also has benefits for learners.

There is a large literature that demonstrates the benefits of learning in collaborative settings. Vygotsky[7] one of the early proponents of collaborative learning, described a theory of learning through social interaction based on what he termed the 'zone of proximal development.' The zone represents the difference between what a learner can achieve independently and what he/she can achieve with the support of a more experienced person. The involvement of a person with deeper or better knowledge enables a less competent person to carry out a task or solve a problem that would be impossible if learning independently. In PAL the role of the more experienced person is not necessarily played by the peer teacher who is not a content expert. Rather, the combined prior knowledge of the group provides the stimulus and support to bring each learner further than they would have travelled individually.

Most forms of PAL involve collaborative learning. A particular characteristic of peer-assisted 'collaborative' learning is the peer tutor's intuitive understanding of the misconceptions and knowledge gaps of the learners. PAL tutors are well placed to provide assistance that is pitched at the right level and delivered appropriately to support peer learners navigate the subject matter.

Whitman and Fife[5] shows how PAL increases both the peer teachers' and learners' motivation to learn. PAL has also been shown to increase the self-esteem of peer teachers. Peer teachers became more confident not only about the subject matter but also about their ability to explain concepts and identify misconceptions and others. Peer teachers are also more likely to develop better self-awareness, an essential prerequisite for self-directed learning.[2]

Categories of peer learning

The concept of PAL is interesting to consider in the context of teacher hegemony. Traditionally education is founded on the intellectual authority of the teacher and the subservience of the learner. The authority in PAL is shared between the peer tutor and the learners. The authority gap between tutor and learner is minimal and this changes the learning environment fundamentally. Goldschmid and Goldschmid[3] published the first extensive review of PAL in education. In it they identified five different peer teaching models:

1. The teaching assistant model in which high performing students are asked to help other students to grasp essential concepts and prepare for assessments.

2. The peer tutor model in which a more experienced student is paired with a less experienced student. The purpose of such a pairing is to provide content guidance and academic support.

3. The peer counsellor model in which more senior students provide mentorship to more junior students in the areas of study habits and strategies for improving performance.

4. The peer partnership model in which students meet to discuss course content and critique each others written work (i.e. very similar to informal student study groups).

5. The peer workgroup model in which student are assigned to collaborative groups to achieve a common set of goals, e.g. a project, a presentation, etc.

Whitman and Fife[5] grouped the five Goldschmid PAL models into either 'near-peer' or 'co-peer' categories as follows (see Table 7.1).

A *near-peer* model of PAL means that the peer tutor is ahead of the peer learners in terms of seniority, experience or academic achievement. Examples of 'near peer' PAL include:

1. A third year medical student facilitating a first year student group.

2. A high achieving student is asked to support students who are struggling with the course content.

Table 7.1 Peer teaching models.

Near-peer	Peer teaching assistants
	Peer tutors
	Peer counsellors
Co-peer	Peer partnerships
	Peer work groups

Co-peer models of PAL represent a partnership in which learners of equivalent experience or seniority learn from and with each other. 'Co-peer' groups are often established to carry out a project-based tasks or form naturally among students to prepare for assessments.

Falchikov[8] provided a more up to date definition in which he described three categories of peer tutoring that can apply in a single institution. The categories represent a refinement of the near-peer and co-peer categories outlined above. The Falchikov categories include:

1. Same level peer tutoring with equal status (this is where learners have equal status in terms of experience and attainment levels).

2. Same level peer tutoring with unequal status (this is where learners may be selected for the role of tutor on the basis of superior academic achievement over other students).

3. Cross level peer tutoring (this describes PAL where more senior students peer tutor more junior students (e.g. third year student peer tutor first year students).

When thinking about introducing PAL in a new setting it is important to decide whether the peer learners and tutors should have equal (co-peer) or unequal (near peer) status. Critical factors include the learning goals (can the students achieve the goals with or without 'near peer' guidance?); the nature of the learning task, the required peer teacher role (tutor or facilitator) and the feasibility of establishing PAL within the curricular structure.

The benefits of peer-assisted learning

PAL has been shown to have benefits for peer tutors, peer learners, and for the design and delivery of courses. From a course director's perspective PAL can reduce workload by devolving teaching responsibility. While PAL should never be viewed as 'teaching on the cheap' it does represent an effective form of active learning in which the students take a far greater responsibility for the delivery of course material.

PAL represents an inexpensive way to organize small group education in situations where there are relatively high staff–student ratios. It also enhances student socialization that is an important part of third-level education. Student-led small group learning has been shown to stimulate better sharing of individual perspectives, leading to deeper understanding and enhanced personal development.[2] Interestingly students who regularly volunteer to act as peer teachers are more likely to pursue academic careers.[5]

Given the relative informality of PAL, students feel more comfortable discussing personal viewpoints and performance issues with peers compared with teachers. The PAL learning environment is perceived as less threatening, and students feel freer to express doubts, misconceptions and erroneous thinking. It has also been shown that near-peer tutors are often better at explaining concepts to junior colleagues than more experienced teachers. Near peer tutors are 'consciously competent' and are therefore more aware of the subject matter that presents conceptual challenges for student colleagues. PAL enhances the student teacher's self-esteem and represents an important addition to their curriculum vitae.

There is good evidence to show that PAL leads to learning outcomes that are at least equivalent to those achieved with more traditional teacher led forms of education. A recent systematic review of PAL effectiveness[9] showed that the academic performance of students who received peer tutoring when compared with students in a more traditional programme, was significantly better. Santee and Garavalia[9] also found that studies that compared the academic performance of students who learned using PAL as opposed to faculty directed tutoring did at least as well in terms of assessment outcomes.

The drawbacks of peer-assisted learning

It is difficult to locate literature that describes the disadvantages or difficulties associated with organizing PAL, yet it is important to be aware of the implications of introducing PAL into a course or institution.

PAL represents an organizational challenge. Students who are not trained as teachers are being asked to supervise or facilitate the learning of others. There may also be considerable faculty opposition to such an innovation given the many prejudices about students in the health professions. If PAL is to be successful it needs to be organized appropriately and peer tutors need to be trained for what they do. They should acquire a clear understanding of their brief, the learning objectives, and the purposes of their involvement. It is likely that they will also need written guidance in the form of a handbook or guide to remind them of what they should be doing.

The introduction of PAL may lead to considerable variance in the learning outcomes achieved between different PAL groups. If, for example, peer-assisted tutors vary in their ability to stimulate group engagement with the learning task, large differences in learning achievement may result. Is such variance tolerable? What means are there to ensure that the variance between groups is minimized? There is also a concern that students who attend PAL may not take it seriously. In fact one of the key outcomes that should be measured for PAL intervention is attendance. If sessions are poorly or not attended are they worth continuing with?

One of the areas of PAL that is poorly described in the literature is the management of the relationship between senior teachers and PAL tutors. How can teachers manage the process of PAL appropriately while being sufficiently distant from it to allow it to progress creatively? Clearly it would be inadvisable to micro-manage PAL and yet how distant should teachers remain from the process? How should they measure the outcomes and assess the success of the initiative? Many senior teachers do not want to devote the time to establishing PAL networks or sign up to it half-heartedly.

If these concerns are to be addressed any new PAL initiative needs to be carefully piloted, evaluated, and reported. Teachers need to be convinced that PAL at the very least leads to equivalent learning outcomes compared with traditionally teaching formats. It also needs to be clearly demonstrated that the costs of establishing PAL (timetabling, training peer teachers, evaluating PAL) do not overwhelm the institution's ability to cope.

Senior teachers who direct PAL programmes need to establish a means of supervision that is on the one hand sufficiently close to ensure consistent instructional quality between groups yet distant enough to avoid stifling creativity. Teachers should also carefully consider what content is appropriate to be learned in a PAL environment. For example, it may be relatively easy to use PAL for learning about material that is largely factual; however, it may be more difficult to train PAL teachers to facilitate peer learners to navigate complex or abstract content. PAL tutors who have only recently familiarized themselves with a topic may lack the versatility to explain abstract concepts using different examples and analogies.

Summary

PAL is increasingly recognized within medical education as a valuable educational approach that can deliver effective learning at a lower cost than traditional approaches. PAL has been shown to improve assessment performance,[10,11] lower student stress and enhance learner satisfaction through the establishment of a reciprocal social support system.[12] Researchers have shown that pairing junior and senior undergraduate students provides psychological support and aids professional and personal development.[13] Peers teachers can take on many roles, including role models, monitors, counsellors, and assessors. However, the most commonly cited form of PAL in the literature is that of peer *tutoring*, where more senior students help more junior learners in specific educational tasks. PAL can been used to deliver a wide variety of teaching from factual knowledge[11] to communication[14] and clinical examination skills.[15]

In addition, PAL can have a powerful influence on the development of professional 'attitudes'. PAL tutors are often viewed as very influential role models by peer learners.[16] However, the effectiveness of peer tutoring depends very much on effective planning. We will now describe a number of essential steps for the implementation of PAL.

Making peer-assisted learning happen

Step 1. Securing faculty and student 'buy-in'

The survival of any educational initiative will often depend on faculty support. PAL will not prosper if it is regarded as an *add-on* or as an educational eccentricity. Rather it must be formally timetabled, assessed, and evaluated. For this to happen teacher colleagues must agree to and support its implementation (Box 7.1 summarizes the main 'selling' points). It is also important that the students should be aware that PAL is an endorsed and valued part of their learning programme otherwise they may devalue its significance and fail to attend.

Step 2. Structure and content

PAL is often praised for it's versatility,[1] yet there are obvious perils in placing students in tutor roles. They are neither content experts, nor qualified teachers.

Box 7.1 Key points when explaining peer-assisted learning to colleagues/faculty

1. Frees faculty time and makes small group teaching for large classes possible.

2. PAL is very versatile and can be used to develop student knowledge, skills, *and* attitudes.

3. PAL has been shown to encourage deep learning and disseminates teaching skills among the student body.

4. PAL has been shown to improve examination scores, student satisfaction, and student's ability to self-direct their own learning.

5. For any new PAL initiative training will be provided for course directors and peer teachers. Peer teachers will be supported through monitoring and regular feedback on performance.

6. New PAL initiatives will be thoroughly evaluated and quality assured. The results of any evaluation will be fed back to course directors and teaching staff.

Thus the student tutor role should emphasize facilitation rather than of formal teaching.[17] The ideal setting for PAL to flourish is small group learning, where the student tutor facilitates discussion and reflection among peer learners and, if appropriate, corrects misconceptions and provides explanations of difficult concepts.

The Falchikov[8] classification of peer tutoring described above is useful to consider when deciding whether the peer learners and tutors should be 'same' or 'cross' level and should have equal or unequal status. This will be decided by a combination of factors, including: learning goals (Do the students need 'cross' level guidance to achieve the learning goals?); the nature of the learning task (Does the task require a collaborative effort from 'same' level peers or the advice, experience and direction of a more senior student?); the required peer teacher role (tutor or facilitator); and the feasibility of establishing PAL within the curricular structure (Are the 'cross' level peers available at the same time?).

Step 3. Participants

Learner selection

Student participation in a PAL initiative may be compulsory, optional, or selective (e.g. targeted at weaker students). Where 'same' level peer tutoring in taking place, it may be advantageous to mix low and high achievers as low achievers have been shown to make greater learning gains in mixed-ability groups.[18] It is also worth considering alternating the learner and tutor roles in 'same' level PAL groups, as it has been shown that students who act as both the agents and recipients of peer tutoring will make greater learning gains than those who participate in fixed recipient roles.[19]

Tutor selection

Some PAL programmes, particularly in the USA, base cross level peer tutor selection on academic performance. However, there is good evidence that weaker students may be just as appropriate as peer tutors. The benefits of working as a PAL tutor have been described in primary, secondary,[20] and tertiary education.[21,22] In fact the results of studies among children, suggest that acting as a peer tutor may be a particularly useful method for enhancing the academic performance of low-achieving children.[20] In addition, weaker students acting as peer tutors may be better at identifying concerns and problems of peer learners. The 'peer' effects in learning are multiple, complex, and often occur simultaneously and in a reciprocal fashion,[9] and should therefore not be denied to students with poorer academic performance.

Training

Training is an essential element of effective PAL programmes.[2] The key role of the peer tutor is usually facilitation, and training should therefore focus on the development of facilitation skills. These sessions should ideally be led by a content expert and an expert in healthcare education using a combination of direct instruction, modelling, and supervised practice activities, such as role-play. These can be used to teach behaviours such as giving setting appropriate learning goals, using questions to prompt critical thinking as well as how to provide effective feedback.[2] Training peer teachers represents the largest task in PAL programmes for course directors and senior teachers. Teach the teacher workshops in which several peer tutors can be developed simultaneously are more efficient. Training needs to be followed up with observation of peer teachers as they work and peer teacher reflections on their teaching role.

Step 4. Establishing a safe learning environment

Safe learning environments are vital in order to engage students in purposeful learning experiences, encourage constructive interactions among tutors and students and enable students to control their own learning effectively. This will only happen to its fullest extent if PAL is student-led and the explicit involvement of teaching staff is kept to a minimum. However, the use of PAL can also lead to a decline in the *quality* of student learning, such that it becomes more focused on assessment and less on understanding course material.[23] Training peer tutors to recognize and avert the natural student tendency to focus on the assessment requirements has been shown to alleviate this trend.[24]

Step 5. Feedback and evaluation

PAL requires careful design and appropriate evaluation. This is particularly important when PAL is a new initiative and the doubters are gathering like vultures on a carcass. Classically, evaluation is divided into outcome and process evaluations. In terms of evaluating outcomes the most revealing is a direct comparison of assessment outcomes between PAL and non-PAL groups of learners. However, it may be difficult to create valid comparisons and lower level outcome evaluations may be more appropriate such as student attendance, continuous assessment results, independent reviewer judgements of student work, qualitative interviews with participants to examine positive and negative aspect of the PAL environment and process.

A more common and perhaps easier form of evaluation is so-called 'process' evaluation. Process evaluation examines the experiences and operation of the PAL intervention. This is usually done using some form of evaluation tool such as a post hoc questionnaire or interview. Process evaluation can also be done by recording PAL events and reviewing the process with external experts. PAL process is often evaluated by external reviewers who 'sit in' on PAL sessions as non-participant (or participant) observers. Obviously, this can inhibit the free and forthcoming student expression inherent in PAL so it should be kept to a minimum. However, it has the advantage of being able to provide timely and specific feedback to peer tutors which they often desire. Where deficits are identified, tutors can be offered the opportunity to re-train. The results of any process or outcome evaluation need to be disseminated widely among the proponents and detractors of a new PAL scheme. The results should lead to a discussion of relative merits and difficulties associated with PAL.

Conclusions

The benefits of PAL are well established with positive effects on the quality of student learning, assessment performance, and student satisfaction. PAL can also help hard-pressed institutions to offer greater access to small group learning formats in a climate of steadily increasing class sizes. It is imperative, however, to consider the real challenges of introducing PAL (summarized in Box 7.2) before commencing such an initiative. As with much educational delivery, the success of PAL will rest largely on the organizational issues of tutor training, proper timetabling and set-up as well as adequate feedback and evaluation. However, given the well established benefits for both students and faculty, PAL is an educational innovation that should be actively considered by all medical education providers.

Box 7.2 Making peer-assisted learning happen

Step 1. Securing faculty and student 'buy-in'

- Secure agreement and support from teaching colleagues.
- Ensure PAL is enshrined in curricular timetables.
- Build in robust process and outcomes evaluation of PAL.
- Ensure that PAL is perceived by students as being 'valued' by faculty.

Step 2. Structure and content

- Select the course content that is suitable for a PAL approach.
- Decide whether 'same level' or 'cross' level peer teaching is required.

Box 7.2 Making peer-assisted learning happen *(continued)*

Step 3. Participants

- Choose between compulsory, optional or selective student participation.
- Decide whether 'mixed-ability' or 'same-ability' groups are required.
- Choose whether peer teachers and peer learners should have fixed or alternating teacher/learner roles.
- If using a 'cross-level' peer teaching approach decide whether peer teachers should be based on seniority or academic performance.
- Plan appropriate training for peer tutors.

Step 4. Establishing a safe learning environment

- Ensure that PAL student-led.
- Ensure that faculty role is viewed as external and supportive.
- Ensure that peer teacher training includes group facilitation skills.

Step 5. Feedback and evaluation

- Monitor and provide feedback on tutor performance.
- Provide re-training to tutors if required.
- Perform an outcome evaluation using assessment performance, attendance records, etc.
- Carry out a process evaluation using post hoc questionnaires, non-participant observation, student interviews, etc.
- Disseminate evaluation results widely to faculty.

References

1. Topping KJ. The effectiveness of peer tutoring in further and higher education: A typology and review of the literature. *Higher Educ* 1996; **32**(3): 321–45.
2. Topping KJ, Ehly S. *Peer-assisted learning*. Mahwah, NJ: Laurence Erlbaum Associates Inc., 1998.
3. Goldschmid B, Goldschmid M. Peer teaching in higher education; a review. *Higher Educ* 1976; **5**: 9–33.
4. Gartner A, Kohler M, Riessman F. *Children teach children: Learning by teaching.* New York, Harper Row, 1971.

5. Whitman NA, Fife JD (Eds). *Peer teaching: to teach is to learn twice.* ASHE-ERIC Higher Education Report No. 4. Washington DC: Office of Educational Research and Improvement, 1988.

6. Benware CA, Deci EL. Quality of learning with an active versus passive motivational set. *Am Educ Res J* 1984; **21**: 755–65.

7. Vygotsky LS. *Mind in society: the development of higher psychological processes.* Cambridge, MA: Harvard University Press, 1978.

8. Falchikov N. *Learning together. peer tutoring in higher education.* London, UK: Routledge Falmer, 2001.

9. Santee J, Garavalia L. Peer tutoring programs in health professions schools. *Am J Pharm Educ* 2006; **70**: 1–10.

10. Ebbert MR, Morgan PM, Harris LB. A comprehensive student peer-teaching programme. *Acad Med* 1999; **74**: 583–4.

11. Trevino PM, Eiland DC. Evaluation of basic science, peer tutorial programme for first- and second-year medical students. *J Med Educ* 1980; **55**: 952–3.

12. Fantuzzo JW, Dimeff LA, Fox SL. Reciprocal peer tutoring: a multimodal assessment of effectiveness with college students. *Teach Psychol* 1989; **16**(3): 133–5.

13. Escovitz ES. Using senior students as clinical skills teaching assistants. *Acad Med* 1990; **65**: 733–4.

14. Glynn L, MacFarlane A, Kelly M, Cantillon P, Murphy A. Helping each other to learn – a process evaluation of peer assisted learning. *BMC Med Educ* 2006; **6**: 18.

15. Field M, Burke J, Lloyd D, McAllister D. Peer-assisted learning in clinical examination. *Lancet* 2004; **363**: 490–1.

16. Parr JM, Townsend MAR. Envoirnments, processes and mechanisms in peer learning. *Int J Educ Res* 2002; **37**: 403–23.

17. Wallace J. Student as mentor and role model to support effective learning. In *Mentoring – the new panacea?* (Ed. Stephenson J). Norfolk, UK: Peter Francis, 1997; pp. 78–92.

18. Tudge J, Rocoff, B. *Peer influences on cognitive development.* Hillsdale, NJ: Laurence Erlbaum Associates Inc., 1989.

19. Rosen S, Powell ER, Schubot DB, Rollins P. Peer tutroing outcomes as influenced by the equity and type of role assignment. *J Educ Psychol* 1978; **69**: 244–52.

20. Allen VL, Feldman RS. Learning through tutoring: Low-achieving children as tutors. *J Exp Educ* 1973; **42**: 1–5.

21. Annis LF. The processes and effects of peer tutoring. *Hum Learn* 1983; **2**: 39–47.

22. Bargh JA, Schul Y. On the cognitive benefits of teaching. *J Educ Psychol* 1980; **72**(5): 593–604.

23. Ashwin P. Peer support: relations between the context, process and outcomes for students who are supported. *Instructional Sci* 2003; **31**: 159–73.

24. Packham G, Miller C. Peer-Assisted Student Support: a new approach to learning. *J Further Higher Educ* 2000; **24**: 55–65.

Chapter 8

Assessment in medical education and training 1

Val Wass and Cees van der Vleuten

Introduction

Education is increasingly regarded as a life-long continuum. The same principle applies to assessment. This book argues for a more mature, peer-assisted, formative style of learning (Chapters 7 and 14) robust standards for education and professionalism (Chapters 1 and 2), flexible formative training to address continuing professional development (Chapter 11), and increased patient and peer involvement (Chapter 4). If these concepts are to be embraced then, as education becomes more multifaceted, so should test methodology. Assessment must evolve to match the training curriculum.

The concept of artificially staging examinations at pre-fixed points in training can now be confidently challenged.[1] The pitfalls of traditional end point examinations are increasingly recognized.[2] The move towards objective standardized assessment can foster rote learning at a superficial reductionist level rather than self-directed adult learning styles.[3] The restrictions of high stakes, large-scale test methodology, and limited resources may inadvertently fail both to mirror desired education goals and measure qualities relevant to actual performance.[4] Learners progress at different rates. Traditional methods have not necessarily identified candidates' true levels of expertise[5] or provided sufficient formative feedback for remedial help where appropriate. As the culture of training changes then so must the culture of testing. To align with the issues highlighted in other chapters assessment in medical education and training needs to move forward.

The move internationally towards competency based curricula for clinical training[6-8] has significant implications for assessment. We define competency as 'the ability to handle a complex professional task by integrating the relevant cognitive, psychomotor and affective skills'. It is immediately apparent that the old model of testing against single competencies categorized under 'knowledge', 'skills', or 'attitudes' fails to achieve the integration now required to achieve competency.[9] A more integrated approach is essential.

The changes introduced by Modernising Medical Careers in the UK have begun to stimulate a new assessment culture. The Foundation programme[10] aims to provide more support for a doctor's transition from undergraduate to postgraduate training. It is formative, portfolio based, and uses a variety of assessment tools centred on performance in the workplace. This is radically different from summative methods traditionally used in medical schools. Similarly, the assessment principles (Box 8.1) introduced by the Postgraduate Medical Education Training Board (PMETB)[11] have encouraged UK Royal Colleges to review their specialist training curricula. They aim to provide supportive, formative, reflective, and transparent assessments that foster an educational continuum. The goal is to ensure doctors emerge from training with clear frameworks for keeping up to date and continuing their professional development. Assessment is intrinsic to driving these educational changes and ensuring that competencies are tested as integrated not isolated skills.

At the same time there is concern that if assessment becomes too focused on the demonstration of competence alone, it will become too trivial.[4] We risk the development of a tick box 'can do' mentality. The Royal College of Physician's report on Medical Professionalism highlights the need for professional excellence not just the 'capacity to do something'.[12] It concludes that, for the twenty-first century, professionalism requires a higher standard than mere capability. The need to develop longitudinal programmes of assessment to accommodate this range of needs is becoming clear.[13]

Box 8.1 Summary of PMETB principles for assessment[11]

1. Methods must reflect the assessment's intended purpose/content
2. Reference assessment content to Good Medical Practice
3. Ensure methods used to set standards are in the public domain
4. Involve lay members in the assessment process
5. Have mechanisms for giving students feedback on performance
6. Use appropriate criteria for examiner training
7. Use standardized documentation that is available nationally
8. Be sufficiently resourced

Miller's model of competence assessment[14] has provided an invaluable framework over the past 15 years for clinical competency testing. Matching existing test methodologies with 'the triangle' has increasingly highlighted the lack of methodology to robustly assess performance (the tip of the triangle) and the need to adjust test methodology as expertise develops. The model now needs reconsideration. Some have suggested inversion of the triangle.[15] We propose a three-dimensional approach to the Miller model. It must now evolve to emphasize the importance of measuring 'domain independent' skills not necessarily specific to the domain of medicine but essential facets of professional behaviour. Progression to expertise and excellence is also intrinsic to this model. Professional judgement is essential to place the doctor on the appropriate point on the novice to expert scale.[16] Increasingly programmes must be designed to offer more flexibility, more formative feedback, longitudinal assessment that adapts testing to expertise and involves all stakeholders in setting standards and quality assurance. This is the new culture.[17,18]

This chapter aims to provide a framework in which to place the basic principles underpinning the design of a longitudinal assessment programme for training. We offer a broad evidence-based overview of available methods and their quality assurance to ensure programmes are 'fit for purpose'. The structure offered supports the subsequent chapter, which outlines in more detail how assessment is keeping abreast of the challenges presented by changes in education.

Designing assessment programmes

We have formulated a 10-principle model to guide readers through the challenges of assessment programme design and quality assurance (Table 8.1). There is a large literature on clinical assessment. We highlight references we view as most accessible and practical to support the principles laid out.

Principle 1: Define the purpose

Clarity and transparency of purpose from the start are essential. Use assessment to 'mirror' and 'drive' the educational outcomes of the training programme.

Assessment drives learning. Ideally this should not be the case. The curriculum should be designed to motivate learning. Assessment should follow to ascertain that the required learning has occurred. In actuality at all levels of education, whether undergraduate[9,20] or postgraduate,[21] trainees feel

Table 8.1 Ten principle steps for the design and quality assurance of an assessment programme.

	Principle	Step
1	Define the purpose of the test	Clarity and transparency of purpose from the start are essential. Use assessment to 'mirror' and 'drive' the educational outcomes of the training programme
2	Select the overarching competency structure	Define the learning outcomes you aim to assess over the training period. At which level: knowledge, competence, or performance?
3	Define the longitudinal novice to expert pathway	The programme design should include longitudinal assessment elements and acknowledge the development of expertise across training. At what level on the novice to expert scale are you testing?
4	Design a blueprint	Map the competencies being tested against the curriculum: blueprint to ensure the design is comprehensive and reflects the philosophy of the curriculum
5	Balance formative and summative feedback	A balance is essential between formative and summative assessment. We need more evidence on how to achieve this within assessment programmes
6	Choose appropriate tools	Apply the 'Utility equation' (see text) to determine which tests to use and when
7	Involve stakeholders	Ensure stakeholders (trainers, trainees, managers, patients) are actively involved in the designing and evaluating the programme
8	Aggregation/triangulation	Judgements of overall performance must be based on aggregated multiple sources of information and triangulation of findings
9	Programme evaluation	There must be systematic attention to feedback, both quantitative and qualitative
10	Quality assurance (of test design and administration)	The assessment programme must be continuously monitored and adjusted to ensure constructive alignment with the curriculum and its impact on learning.

Modified from Baartman.[19]

overloaded by work. They focus on and prioritize those aspects of the course that are tested not the overall curriculum.

To overcome this, the assessment programme must be designed to mirror and drive the educational intent. The balance is a fine one. Pragmatically, it is the most appropriate engine to which to harness the curriculum. Yet one can be too enthusiastic. Creating too many burdensome time-consuming assessment 'hurdles' can detract from the educational opportunities of the curriculum itself.[18] The assessment must have clarity of purpose and be designed to encourage learning. Careful planning is essential. In reality the first decision lies in agreeing how to maximize educational achievement. This cannot be an afterthought. Those designing the assessment must be very clear on their direction of travel and make their purpose transparent to those being assessed.

Principle 2: Select the overarching competency structure

> Define the learning outcomes you aim to assess over the training period. At which level: knowledge, competence, or performance?

As highlighted above Miller's pyramid (Figure 8.1) provides an important framework for establishing the aim of an assessment.[14] It conceptualizes the essential facets of clinical competence. The base represents the knowledge components of competence: 'knows' (basic facts) followed by 'knows how' (applied knowledge). The progression to 'knows how' highlights that there is more to clinical competency than knowledge alone. 'Shows how' represents a behavioural rather than a cognitive function, i.e. it is 'hands on' and not 'in the head'. Assessment at this level requires the ability to demonstrate a clinical competency in a simulated environment.

The ultimate goal for a valid assessment of clinical aptitude is to test *performance*, i.e. what the doctor actually *does* in the workplace. Over the last four decades assessment research has focused on developing valid ways of assessing the summit of the pyramid, i.e. a doctor's actual performance.[15,22] Assessment design must develop to address the values and behaviours intrinsic to modern medical professionalism.[11] Our modification of the triangle (Figure 8.1) to include 'domain-independent skills' aims to emphasize the importance of this third dimension. As highlighted in the Royal College of Physicians Report[12]

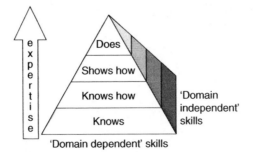

Fig. 8.1 Modification of Miller's triangle.[14]

these aspects of care, such as leadership and management skills, are becoming increasingly important. The competencies developed by the Royal College of Physicians and Surgeons of Canada illustrate this well.[8] Methodology for measuring this third dimension remains challenging.[23]

Principle 3: Define the novice to expert pathway

The programme design should include longitudinal assessment elements and acknowledge the development of expertise across training. At what level on the novice to expert scale are you testing?

Any assessment design must accommodate the progression from novice through competency to expertise. It must be clear against what level the student is being assessed. First year students may require a foundation of basic factual knowledge. In contrast at the trainee level the ability to synthesize and evaluate knowledge should be measured. It is important this is acknowledged and tested appropriately. Frameworks have been suggested for mapping this progression for clinical competency.[24,25] Work remains to be done in incorporating models of professional development in expertise into assessment methodology and determining the level of performance to be expected at different points in training. For example, written assessment methods have been developed that evaluate the distance or concordance of examinees' clinical scripts with domain experts.[26]

When designing an assessment package, conceptual clarity is essential to identify the level of expertise anticipated at that point in training. It is not uncommon to find questions in postgraduate examinations assessing basic factual knowledge at undergraduate level rather than the applied knowledge more reflective of the candidate's postgraduate experience. Similarly fragmented OSCEs assessing isolated skills with analytical scoring methods may be appropriate in early undergraduate training. Later in training integrative OSCEs are needed to assess integrated skills, including the professional quality of the performance. These need the holistic judgements of experts and for appropriate standards to be set.[27] The question 'Is the test appropriate for this level of training?' must always be asked.

Principle 4: Design a blueprint

Map the competencies being tested against the curriculum: blueprint to ensure the design is comprehensive and reflects the philosophy of the curriculum.

Once the purpose of the assessment is agreed, test content must be carefully planned against the intended learning outcomes, a process known as 'blue printing'.[28] In the UK both the General Medical Council (GMC) and PMETB, who quality assure undergraduate[29] and postgraduate[11] assessments respectively, recommend mapping the curriculum against the GMC recommendations for Good Medical Practice.[30] In the past blueprinting has been difficult for postgraduate collegiate examinations, where curriculum content remained more broadly defined.[31] To address these difficulties and the requirements of PMETB, colleges are now revising their curricula developing clear learning outcomes. An example from the Royal College of General Practitioners can be found on the PMETB website.[32]

The integral design (blueprint) must include:

1. *A conceptual framework.* A structure against which to plan the content of the assessment programme is essential. Good Medical Practice provides a useful one.[30] The design of the blueprint can be used to reflect the educational goals (principle one). Thus Good Medial Practice emphasizes the importance of covering our three-dimensional model to include domain dependent and independent skills.

2. *Adequate sampling.* Blueprinting must also ensure that the contextual content of the curriculum is covered. Content needs careful mapping within the framework to ensure students are comprehensively and fairly assessed. Probably the most important evidence to emerge from recent assessment literature is the realization that competencies are context bound and not generalizable.[9] Professionals do not perform consistently from task to task.[33] This applies as equally to professional behaviours[23] and communication skills as it does to practical skills. Two important lessons have emerged. First, wide sampling of content is essential.[13,28] This was the main catalyst for the development of Objective Structured Clinical Examinations[34] and the demise of testing on a single long case.[35] However, in recent years the emergence of more psychometric analysis of traditional methods, such as long cases[36] and orals,[37] has demonstrated that all assessment tools can be used to assess reliably provided sufficient contexts are covered. The second lesson, i.e. that all methods are relevant provided the test is long enough to sample adequately,[9] has been key to the move to programmes and packages.[13] We have been released from the stringencies of examinations.

Sampling broadly to cover the full range of the curriculum is of paramount importance if fair and reliable assessments are to be guaranteed.[38] The blueprint collates learning outcomes with the levels of competency (principle 2) and expertise to be measured (principle 3). Contextual domains can be plotted within the framework to check that sampling is adequate.

The blueprint at the same time provides a chart to ensure that appropriate assessment tools are chosen.[32] Many medical curricula define learning outcomes in terms of knowledge, skills, and attitudes. These cannot be validly assessed using a single test format. All assessments must ensure the test being used is appropriate to the outcome being tested. To assess clinical competence validly, we are moving from a battery of different examinations to an assessment package where performance in the workplace can be included alongside high stakes examinations, such as multiple choice tests.[13] Given the complexity of clinical competency itself, it is hardly surprising that single examinations in isolation fail to be valid.

Principle 5: Balance formative with summative feedback

A balance is essential between formative and summative assessment. We need more evidence on how to achieve this within assessment programmes.

To promote deeper learning, assessment should be 'formative'. Trainees must learn from tests and receive feedback to build on their knowledge and skills. If they do not meet the standard, there should be further opportunities to try again until the competency is ultimately achieved. Feedback should encourage trainees to identify their strengths and weaknesses and map their progress. Weak students should be identified and given remedial help. This is the explicit focus of assessment in the Foundation Programme[10] and intrinsic to the developing new culture for assessment.[17]

At the same time, with an increasing focus on examples of doctors' underperformance[39] and public demand for assurance that doctors are competent to practise, assessment must, at times, have a 'summative' function. Tests of clinical competence are necessary to make end-point decisions on whether a doctor can be certified as 'fit to practise'. Such tests generally take a 'snapshot' of ability at a defined moment. This is clearly important at fixed points in the longitudinal trajectory of training: registration as a doctor, certification of completion of training and revalidation for medical regulation. The candidate has a fixed time frame and number of attempts in which to succeed. The two forms of assessment are stark in contrast (Box 8.2). Both are necessary. However, longitudinal assessment programmes have the distinct advantage of offering ample opportunities for formative feedback and avoiding highly resourced examinations barren of significant educational outcomes. By building a portfolio of information on trainees across the assessment blueprint using formative

Box 8.2 Formative versus summative assessment

Formative assessment

- Breaks learning into manageable modules
- Allow repeated attempts to master the content of each module
- Is not perceived as threatening (low stakes)

Summative assessment

- Is an end-point examination
- Can block intended career progression (high stakes)
- Is perceived as threatening

assessments, we hope to blur the divide and reduce the need for tools which are only summative.

This raises a challenge for all involved in medical education. Many argue a test cannot be simultaneously formative and summative. Yet if assessment focuses only on certification and exclusion, the all important influence on the learning process will be lost. Superficial learning, aimed purely at passing the test can result. The PMETB principles[11] emphasize the importance of giving students feedback on all assessments encouraging reflection and deeper learning. The challenge is to connect formative and summative assessment. Preferably every assessment should be embedded within the training programme[40] providing feedback to the learning while at the same time providing ample information to be aggregated into a trustworthy decision.[1] All those designing and delivering high stakes tests should explore ways of doing this and make their intentions transparent to candidates. There is little doubt this is a real challenge. Outcomes to date are optimistic. A recent literature review on portfolios found no evidence that the summative nature of the portfolio hampered or detracted from the formative value.[41] This is clearly a key area for evaluation and research.

Principle 6: Select appropriate assessment tools

The Utility Equation
Utility = Reliability × Validity × Feasibility × Acceptability × Educational Impact[40]
Apply the 'Utility equation' to determine which tests to use and when.

The practicalities of delivering assessments cannot be ignored. No tool is perfect. Choice is generally a compromise. Using the integral design (blueprint), appropriate tools can be selected to reflect the philosophy of the training programme. The 'utility equation' provides guidance for matching test method to the competency being assessed in the context of the blueprint.[42] It aims to counterbalance the selection of assessment methods and deliver a comprehensive, robust, and educationally transparent assessment package.

The equation acknowledges that the choice of tool and aspirations for high validity and reliability are constrained by the restraints of feasibility, e.g. resources to deliver the tests and acceptability to the candidates, e.g. level of examination fee. No test can score uniformly high on all five factors. Some trade-off is inevitable to ensure that the purpose of the assessment is achieved. The next step is to select the most appropriate assessment method for each learning outcome to ensure the educational goals (principle 1) and levels of competency and expertise (principles 2 and 3) are achieved at the required level of feedback (principle 5). The blueprint design (principle 4) is absolutely fundamental to this.[32] Assessment methods should only be selected when all these five steps are in place.

How do you choose which assessment methods to meet the intents of the programme design?

Two key concepts, validity and reliability, are essential when selecting, evaluating and interpreting assessments:

- *Validity*: Was the assessment valid? Did it measure what it was intended to measure?
- *Reliability*: What is the quality of the results? Are they consistent and reproducible?

It is important to remember that validity is a conceptual term that should be approached as a hypothesis and cannot be expressed as a simple coefficient.[43,44] It is evaluated against the various facets of clinical competency: In the past these facets have been defined separately[45] acknowledging that appraising the validity of a test requires multiple sources of evidence (Table 8.2).

We have added consequential validity.[46] This is not a traditional facet of validity. However, as we define the first principle of designing an assessment package as the need to consider the educational impact of the programme, it seems a fair criterion. 'Does the test produce the desired educational outcome?' is we believe a key question to ask. We highlight this as another area of assessment requiring more longitudinal research.

Table 8.2 Traditional facets of validity.

Type of validity	Test facet being measured	Questions being asked
Face validity	Compatibility with the curriculum's educational philosophy	What is the test's face value? Does it match up with the educational intentions?
Content validity	The content of the curriculum	Does the test include a representative sample of the subject matter?
Construct validity	The ability to differentiate between groups with known difference in ability (beginners versus experts)	Does the test differentiate at the level of ability expected of candidates at that stage in training?
Predictive validity	The ability to predict an outcome in the future, e.g. professional success after graduation	Does the test predict future performance and level of competency?
Consequential validity	The educational consequence of the test	Does the test produce the desired educational outcome?

It is now argued that validity is a unitary concept that requires these multiple sources of evidence to evaluate and interpret the outcomes of an assessment.[43] Intrinsic to the validity of any assessment is analysis of the scores to quantify their reproducibility. An assessment cannot be viewed as valid unless it is reliable.

Two aspects of reliability must be considered, i.e. (1) *inter-rater reliability*, which correlates the consistency of rating of performance across different examiners, and (2) *inter-case reliability*, which quantifies the consistency of performance of the candidate across the cases. The latter gives a measure of the extent context specificity has been addressed by the assessment blueprint to ensure candidate performance is accurately rank ordered. It is a quantifiable measure that can be expressed as a coefficient either using Classical Test theory[47] or Generalizability theory.[48,49] A perfectly reproducible test would have a coefficient of 1.0, i.e. 100% of candidates would achieve the same rank order on re-testing. In reality, tests are affected by many sources of potential error such as examiner judgements, cases used, candidate nervousness, and test conditions. High stakes test generally aim for a reliability coefficient of greater than 0.8.

Relying on the reliability coefficient *per se* is now accepted as potentially misleading. Ranking is essentially a norm referenced process affected by the spread of ability of the candidates. A more acceptable alternative to assure reliability of the pass/fail cut off is to adjust for variances in ability between cohorts. The standard deviation of the scores and the reliability of the test are used to estimate the standard error of measurement on the original scoring scale. This can be applied to decisions of the pass/fail cut-off level.[50]

Sufficient testing time is essential in order to achieve adequate inter-case reliability. As described above, it is becoming increasingly clear that whatever the test format, ensuring adequate breadth of content sampling, is critical to the reliability of the test.[9,13] Increasing the number of judges over different cases improves reliability but to a lesser extent.[38,51] Examiners make judgements rapidly[52] though and a range of assessors is also important. We stress the importance of the planning framework for workplace-based assessments of performance to ensure sampling across different contexts is monitored and content specificity addressed.

A guide to selection of tools: How do you select the most appropriate assessment methods?

Assessing the apex of Miller's pyramid, 'the does', is the international goal of the twenty-first century for all involved in clinical competency testing. The ensuing chapter will describe in detail practical aspects of applying these principles to undergraduate and postgraduate assessments in both primary and secondary care. Here we aim to provide a brief overview appraising currently available assessment tools in the light of the above principles of assessment programme design.

The assessment of 'knows' and 'knows how'

Many examinations both undergraduate and postgraduate focus on the pyramid base: 'knows' (the straight factual recall of knowledge) and to a lesser extent on the 'knows how' (the application of knowledge to problem solving and decision making).

Tests of factual recall can take a variety of formats. Multiple choice formats are universally the most widely used. Although time consuming to set, these tests have high reliability; a large number of items can be tested and marked within a relatively short time frame. A variety of question formats exist. Increasingly true/false MCQ formats are being replaced by single best answer and extended matching questions using short and long menus of options.[53,54] Some argue that only 'trivial' knowledge can be tested. By giving options, candidates are cued to respond and the active generation of knowledge is avoided. Although reliable, criticism of the validity of the MCQ has stimulated much research into alternative options.

Essays and orals as tests of knowledge have lost popularity over the years. This relates partly to reliability and partly to feasibility. It is difficult to produce highly reliable assessments using either tool because of problems in standard-izing questions,[37,51] inconsistency in marking[55] and lack of sufficient testing time to address context specificity. Undue pressure is placed on the examiner resource. Reliability can be achieved using short answer written formats[56] and also through more standardized orals[38] but both are resource intensive. Despite this, orals have remained popular in the UK, and other European countries on the grounds of validity. Many argue that the ability to recall and synthesize information can best be judged in the face to face encounter. Thus it is not surprising that more structured oral interactions have been introduced into workplace-based assessments as 'case base discussions' between the trainee and trainer in some postgraduate assessment programmes.[10,32,39]

The 'key feature' test developed in Canada avoids cueing by allowing short written 'uncued' answers to clinical scenarios and limiting the assessment of each scenario to key issues only.[57,58] This enables a large number of scenarios to be covered within a feasible time limit. Using the MCQ format attempts at focusing the content within the question formats using clinical scenarios or scientific extracts for critical appraisal are proving successful.[59] Computer simulations can replace the written or verbal scenarios and, hopefully, with the development of multimedia, can be used to raise the level of clinical testing.[60,61] The dynamic and complex situations created in the past have been complicated and require enormous resources rarely available at university or deanery level. A focus on producing short simulations that can test at an appropriate applied knowledge level continues to challenge those developing this test format.

The assessment of 'shows how' and 'does'

We are experiencing a stimulating change in approach to assessment. Originally when the need to address context specificity became apparent North America was quick to abandon traditional clinical examinations favouring the knowledge tests described above as they were reliable and legally defensible. Now the trend is being reversed.

Traditional assessments: long and short cases and orals

These traditional methods stood to be challenged on the grounds of both authenticity and unreliability. Long cases were often unobserved. Thus this method, relying on the candidate's presentation, represented an assessment of 'knows how' rather than 'shows how'. Generally, only one long case and three or four short cases were used and context specificity was not adequately addressed. Attempts have been made to improve the long case format; the Objective Structured Long Examination Record (OSLER)[62] and the Leicester Assessment Package.[63] Observation improves the validity of the long case.[64]

Decreasing the length of time available to assess a case and allowing more cases to be assessed within a given testing time may also be an option.

Although unlikely to ever reach feasibility for high stakes testing, a better understanding of the psychometrics of these methods has reopened them to modification for use in the workplace. The 'Mini CEX' format,[65] introduced in the USA, is essentially a modification of an observed long case in the clinical setting. The method takes 'snapshots' of the integrated assessment by focusing on one of a range of predetermined areas, e.g. observation of history taking, the physical examination or the management of the case but not the entire process. As few as 10 cases may be enough for a reliable judgement of clinical competency to be made.[66]

However, a strong case has been made for seeking new psychometric approaches. Cronbach himself was reviewing his theories before he died.[67] Pleas have been made from both sides of the Atlantic for new methodology to chart and combine judgements made during training and form a reliable judgement of the trainee's aptitude;[68,69] another area for much needed research!

The Objective Structured Clinical Examination (OSCE)

As a potential solution to the problems of adequate sampling and standardization of cases, the OSCE[70] has gained increasing popularity on both sides of the Atlantic. Candidates rotate through a series of stations based on clinical skills applied in a range of contexts. The structured assessment, which provides wide sampling of cases, each with an independent examiner, improves reliability but this examination format is expensive, labour intensive, and a challenge to feasibility. Validity may be lost at the expense of reliability as complex skills, requiring an integrated professional judgement, become fragmented by the relatively short station length (generally 5–10 minutes).[3] Communication skills and attitudinal behaviours can be simultaneously assessed. Interestingly these skills are also proving to be context specific and to have low generalizability across clinical contexts.[71–73] OSCEs are also proving less objective than originally supposed. Scoring against a check-list of items is not ideal.[74] The global performance may reflect more than the sum of the parts.[3] Global ratings are increasingly used but neither offer a true 'gold standard' of judging performance.[75,76] Rater training is required to ensure consistency and care has to be taken not to discriminate.[77]

The use of standardized patients versus real patients remains an area of interest. Simulations are becoming the norm as it proves increasingly difficult to use real patients.[78,79] Extensive training to ensure reproducibility and consistency of scenarios is required.[80] Increasingly more intricate instruments are being developed to develop more integrated assessments of procedural skills.[81]

Given the high reliabilities required of the North American licensing tests, the high costs of training can be justified but, perhaps, at the cost of validity. Performance on an OSCE is arguably not the same as performance in real life.[82]

The assessment of 'does'

The real challenge lies in the assessment of actual performance in practice, i.e. the tip of the pyramid. Increasing attention is being placed on this in the postgraduate assessment arena.[10] Revalidation of a clinician's fitness to practise and the identification of poorly performing doctors are increasingly areas of public concern.

Any attempt at assessment of performance has to balance the issues of validity and reliability. Interestingly modifications of the more traditional methods are now coming to the fore. Assessments of clinical competencies in the Foundation programme are workplace based and incorporate adaptation of the observed long case (mini CEX), direct observation of procedures (DOPs) and an 'oral' type assessment 'case based discussion'.[10] In a sense there is a swing away from the OSCE back to more traditional methods modified to address the issue that led to their demise, i.e. context specificity.

Similarly most knowledge tests can be improved to test at the 'knows how' rather than 'knows' level, but it remains difficult to assess synthesis and evaluation. Workplace-based assessments, e.g. audit projects and portfolios, may well prove the answer to assessing a trainee's ability to apply knowledge at this level. Broadly defined as a tool for gathering evidence and a vehicle for reflective practice, a wider understanding is developing of the portfolio's potential use in assessment. What it adds in validity to formative assessment needs to be weighed against its reliability for use in summative purposes.[83] A recent literature review suggests these difficulties may not be insuperable.[41] The Learning portfolio for the Foundation programme provides an interesting example[10] and we need more evidence of its efficacy as an assessment tool.

Whether these methods can ever achieve more than medium stakes reliability given the difficulties of standardizing content and training assessors remains to be seen. With adequate sampling across contexts, assessors and methods workplace assessment should be able to realize adequate reliability. Other biases, such as score inflation due to the formative nature of the assessment might be a concern.[84]

In choosing methods compromise is inevitable. Decisions need to be carefully weighed in relation to both the purpose and context of the assessment and to the assessment programme as a whole. One may, for example, choose a method with lower reliability to emphasize the effect on learning or perhaps even because stakeholders believe it's acceptable. This may be defensible if the method chosen is only a small part of a total assessment programme. Other tests, more rigorous in terms of reliability, should also be included. The overall programme may contain any method, whether traditional or modern depending on its function but should meet the quality criteria. It should be noted also that more criteria exist in addition to those mentioned in the utility formula.[85]

Principle 7: Involve stakeholders

> Ensure stakeholders (trainers, trainees, managers, patients) are actively involved in the designing, setting standards, and evaluating the assessment programme.

PMETB principles (Box 8.1) state categorically that lay members must be involved in the assessment process. This is can be informative to the process and crucial to setting standards.

How you decide on who should pass or fail: standard setting

Inferences about examinee performance are critical to any test of competence. When assessment is used for summative purposes, the pass/fail level of a test must be agreed. Well defined and transparent procedures need to be set in place to do this.[86] The move to criterion referencing to set standards offers an ideal opportunity for stakeholders outside the speciality to be involved.

Criterion referencing

Comparison of performance to peers, i.e. **norm referencing** can be used in examination procedures where a specified number of candidates are required to pass. Performance is described relative to the positions of other candidates and it is agreed that a fixed percentage fail, e.g. all candidates one standard deviation below the mean. Thus the variation in difficulty of the test is compensated for. However, variations in ability of the cohort sitting the test are not taken into account. If the group is above average in ability, those who might have passed in a poorer cohort will fail. This is clearly unacceptable for clinical competency licensing tests, which aim to ensure that candidates are safe to practise.

A clear standard, below which the doctor would not be considered 'fit to practise' needs to be defined. Such standards are set by **criterion referencing,** where the minimum standard acceptable has to be decided. The reverse problem now faces the assessor. Although differences in candidate ability are accounted for, variation in test difficulty becomes the key issue. Standards should be set for each test, item by item. Various methods have been developed to do this; 'Angoff', 'Ebel', 'Hofstee', 'Contrasting method'.[87–89] These can be time consuming but essential and enable a group of stakeholders (not just examiners) in the assessment to participate.

More recently methodology has been introduced using the examiner cohort itself to set the standard. Examiners, after assessing the candidate, indicate which students they judge to be borderline. The mean mark across all examiners (and there is invariably a range) is taken as the pass/fail cut-off.[90] The robustness of this method across different cohort of examiners remains to be seen.[91] Recently, this borderline method has been extended to more reliable regression techniques that are very suitable for application in OSCEs.[92] The choice of method will depend on available resources, the consequences of misclassifying passing and failing examinees and decisions on how stakeholders can be involved.

Principle 8: Aggregation/triangulation of results/judgements

> Decisions in achieving the training standard for the programme are based on the triangulation of aggregated information across multiple sources of information/methods of assessment/moments of assessment.

Triangulation

The complexity of measuring professional performance is now acknowledged.[13] As assessment design develops the need to combine assessments of performance in the workplace alongside high stakes competency has been increasingly recognized and needs a new psychometric approach.[68] It is important to develop an assessment programme to build up evidence of performance in the workplace and avoid reliance on examinations alone. Triangulation of observed contextualized performance tasks of 'does' must be assessed alongside high stakes competency based tests of 'shows how'. The GMC's performance procedures, where workplace assessments are triangulated with a knowledge test and an OSCE provides such a model.[39] However, as highlighted above, we have yet to be sure whether workplace-based assessment alone can ever achieve more than medium stakes reliability; a challenge that faces us all as we move into assessment programme design.

Principle 9: Feedback and judgement

> Trainers and assessors need to have the requisite skills for feedback and judgement. These are not innate skills.

The contrasting roles of assessors involved in formative and summative processes have to be acknowledged. Tasks range from educational supervision to summative judgements of fitness to progress in high stakes examinations. Whatever their role, all assessors must have the requisite skills, understand the process, and be trained to make sound judgements against the criteria being assessed at the required standard of expertise. This is not without significant pitfalls.[52] Work from the Royal College of General Practice emphasizes the importance of selecting and training assessors.[93] Just as it cannot be assumed that any professional competent in their work can necessarily teach, the same applies to assessment. Not all teachers can make clear judgements or rank order performance consistently. Selection and training of assessors is essential to ensure they: (1) have the skills; (2) understand the process of the assessment; and (3) can address issues of equal opportunity.[93,94]

Principle 10: Quality control

> The programme must include quality control on test design and test administration. The assessment programme should continuously be monitored and adjusted through evaluation of its constructive alignment and effect on learning.

Test construction is a tedious process. One may become a good item writer but one never becomes perfect. Many of our in-house tests are of poor quality.[95] Test material should be reviewed with experts on committees in advance of test administration and statistics included in all post-administration reviews. This has a dramatic impact on the original test material[96] and significantly raises the quality of the assessment.[97]

The assessment programme as a whole must be closely monitored. Periodic reviews and evaluation of the programme, both psychometrically and educationally, are essential to quality assurance. Even the best planned methodology may ultimately be reduced to a trivial exercise if not delivered appropriately in real practice. A dynamic process of continuous reform, parallel to an appropriate curriculum assurance system, is absolutely essential.

Conclusions

Assessment at the apex of Miller's pyramid, 'the does', is the international challenge of the twenty-first century for all involved in clinical competence testing. In outlining a framework for developing programmes to do this, we have inevitably simultaneously highlighted areas of uncertainty and concern open to further research. We need to understand much more about the outcomes of assessment. Tensions continue between methodologies that support trainees formatively and those needed for licensing purposes to assure the public the same trainees, on exiting from speciality training, are 'fit for purpose'. We argue a package of methods is most appropriate; workplace-based assessment combined with high stakes examinations is currently being developed in most college postgraduate qualifications.

Further research into the utility of workplace-based assessment and the use of portfolio assessment is essential. In addition we need to understand more on the assessment of attitudinal behaviours and how these inform the development of medical professionalism. Finally, we must increase our understanding of the design, implementation, and maintenance of assessment programmes as a whole. Many challenges face us. We trust this current review provides a useful outline from which to proceed.

References

1. van der Vleuten CPM. Validity of final examinations in undergraduate medical training. *BMJ* 2000; **321**: 1217–19.

2. van der Vleuten CPM, Norman GR, de Graaff E. Pitfalls in the pursuit of objectivity: issues of reliability. *Med Educ* 1991; **25**: 110–18.

3. Talbot M. Monkey see, monkey do: a critique of the competency model in graduate medical education. *Med Educ* 2004; **38**: 587–92.

4. Hodges B. Medical education and the maintenance of incompetence. *Med Teacher* 2006; **28**: 690–6.

5. Hodges B, Regehr G, McNaughton N, Tiberius R, Hanson M. OSCE checklists do not capture increasing levels of expertise. *Acad Med* 1999; **74**: 1129–34.

6. Weigel T, Mulder M, Collins K. The concept of competence in the development of vocational education and training in selected EU member states. *J Vocat Educ Training* 2007; **59**: 51–64.

7. Accreditation Council for Graduate Medical Education (AGCME) Common Program Requirements: General Competencies (2007). http://www.acgme.org/outcome/comp/GeneralCompetenciesStandards21307.pdf.

8. CanMEDs Framework (2005). http://rcpsc.medical.org/canmeds/bestpractices/framework_e.pdf.

9. Wass V, van der Vleuten CPM, Shatzer J, Jones R. Assessment of clinical competence. *Lancet* 2001; **357**: 945–9.

10. Modernising Medical Careers (2008). http://www.foundationprogramme.nhs.uk/pages/home/training-and-assessment.

11. Southgate L, Grant J (2004). Principles for an assessment system for postgraduate training. Postgraduate Medical Training Board. http://www.pmetb.org.uk/fileadmin/user/QA/Assessment/Principles_for_an_assessment_system_v3.pdf.

12. Doctors in Society: Medical Professionalism in a Changing World (2005). http://www.rcplondon.ac.uk/pubs/books/docinsoc/.

13. van der Vleuten CPM, Schuwirth LWT. Assessing professional competence: from methods to programmes. *Med Educ* 2005; **39**: 309–17.

14. Miller GE. The assessment of clinical skills/competence/performance. *Acad Med* 1990; **65**: S63–7.

15. Rethans J, Norcini J, Baron-Maldonado M, *et al.* The relationship between competence and performance: implications for assessing practice performance. *Med Educ* 2002; **36**: 901–9.

16. Coles C. Developing professional judgement. *J Contin Educ Health Prof* 2002; **22**: 3–10.

17. Birenbaum M, Breuer K, Cascallar E, *et al.* Position paper. A learning integrated assessment system. *Educ Res Rev* 2006; **1**: 61–7.

18. Swanwick T, Chana N. Workplace assessment for licensing in general practice. *BJGP* 2005; **55**: 461–7.

19. Baartman L. 'Assessing the assessment'. Development and use of quality criteria for competence assessment programmes. PhD thesis, Utrecht University, 2008.

20. Frederiksen N. The real test bias. Influences of testing on teaching and learning. *Am Psychol* 1984; **39**: 193–202.

21. Dixon H. Candidates' views of the MRCGP examination and its effects upon approaches to learning: a questionnaire study in the Northern Deanery. *Educ Prim Care* 2003; **14**: 146–57.

22. Schurwith L, Southgate L, Page G, *et al.* When enough is enough: a conceptual basis for fair and defensible practice performance assessment. *Med Educ* 2002; **36**: 925–30.

23. Stern D. *Measuring medical professionalism.* Oxford University Press, 2005.

24. Eraut M. *Developing professional knowledge and competence.* London: Falmer Press, 1994.

25. Dreyfus HL, Dreyfus SE. *The power of human intuition and expertise in the era of the computer.* New York: Free Press, 1986.

26. Charlin B, van der Vleuten CPM. Standardized assessment of reasoning in contexts of uncertainty: the script concordance approach. *Eval Health Prof* 2004; **2**: 304–19.

27. Norcini J. Setting standards on educational tests. *Med Educ* 2003; **37**: 464–9.

28. Dauphinee D, Fabb W, Jolly B, Langsley D, Wealthall S, Procopis P. Determining the content of certifying examinations. In *The certification and recertification of Doctors: Issues in the assessment of clinical competence* (Eds Newble D, Jolly B, Wakeford R). Cambridge University Press, 1994; pp. 92–104.

29. The General Medical Council Education Committee. *Tomorrow's doctors: recommendations on undergraduate medical education.* London: GMC, 2005. http://www.gmc-uk.org/education/undergraduate/undergraduate_policy/tomorrows_doctors.asp.

30. The General Medical Council. *Good Medical Practice.* London: GMC, 2007. www.gmc-uk.org/guidance/good_medical_practice/index.asp.

31. Hays RB, van der Vleuten CPM, Fabb WE, Spike NA. Longitudinal reliability of the Royal Australian College of General Practitioners Certification Examination. *Med Educ* 1995; **29**: 317–21.

32. Rughani A. Assessment blueprint of General Practice (2007). http://www.pmetb.org.uk/index.php?id=968.

33. Swanson DB, Norman GR, Linn RL. Performance-based assessment: lessons learnt from the health professions. *Educ Res* 1995; **24**: 5–11.

34. Newble D. Techniques for measuring clinical competence; objective structured clinical examinations. *Med Educ* 2004; **38**: 199–203.

35. Wass V, Jones R, Vleuten van der C. Standardised or real patients to test clinical competence? The long case revisited. *Med Educ* 2001; **35**: 321–5.

36. Wass V, van der Vleuten CPM. The Long case. *Med Educ* 2004; **38**: 1176–80.

37. Wass V, Wakeford R, Neighbour R, van der Vleuten CPM. Achieving acceptable reliability in oral examinations: An analysis of the Royal College of General Practitioner's Membership Examination's oral component. *Med Educ* 2003; **37**: 126–31.

38. Newble D, Dawson B, Dauphinee D, *et al.* Guidelines for assessing clinical competence. *Teach Learn Med* 1994; **6**: 213–20.

39. Southgate L, Cox J, David T, Hatch D, Howes A, Johnson N. The General Medical Council's Performance Procedures: peer review of performance in the workplace. *Med Educ* 2001; **35**: 9–19.

40. Wilson M, Sloane K. From principles to practice: An embedded assessment system. *Appl Measurement Educ* 2000; **13**: 181–208.

41. Driessen E, Tartwijk J van, van der Vleuten CPM, Wass V. Portfolios in medical education: why do they meet with mixed success? A systematic review. *Med Educ* 2007; **41**: 1224–33.

42. van der Vleuten CPM. The assessment of professional competence: developments, research and practical implications. *Adv Health Sci Educ* 1996; **1**: 41–67.

43. Downing SM. Validity: on the meaningful interpretation of assessment data. *Med Educ* 2003; **37**: 830–7.

44. Messick S. Validity. In *Educational measurement*, 3rd edn (Ed. Linn RL). New York: American Council on Education Macmillan, 1989; pp. 13–104.

45. Crossley J, Humphris G, Jolly B. Assessing health professionals. *Med Educ* 2002; **36**: 800–4.

46. Messick S. The interplay of evidence and consequences in the validation of performance assessments. *Educ Res* 1995; **23**: 13–23.

47. Cronbach LJ. Coefficient alpha and internal structure of tests. *Psychometrika* 2004; **16**: 297–334.

48. Brennan, RL. *Elements of generalisability theory*. Iowa, USA: American College Testing Program, 1983.

49. Shavelson RJ, Webb NM. *Generalisability theory: a primer*. Newbury Park, CA: Sage Publications, 1991.

50. Norcini JJ. Standards and reliability in evaluation: when rules of thumb don't apply. *Acad Med* 1999; **74**: 1088–90.

51. Swanson DB. A measurement framework for performance based tests. In *Further developments in assessing clinical competence* (Eds Hart IR, Harden RM). Montreal: Can-Heal, 1987; pp. 13–45.

52. Williams RG, Klamen DK, McGaghie WC. Cognitive, social and environmental sources of bias in clinical performance ratings. *Teach Learn Med* 2003; **15**: 270–92.

53. Case SM, Swanson DB. Extended Matching Items: a practical alternative to free response questions. *Teach Learn Med* 1993; **5**: 107–15.

54. Case SM, Swanson DB. *Constructing written test questions for the basic and clinical sciences*. Philadelphia, PA: National Board of Examiners.

55. Frijns PHAM, van der Vleuten CPM, Verwijnen GM, Van Leeuwen YD. The effect of structure in scoring methods on the reproducibility of tests using open ended questions. In *Teaching and assessing clinical competence* (Bender W, Hiemstra RJ, Scherbier AJJA, Zwierstra RP). Groningth: Boekwerk, 1990; pp. 466–71.

56. Munro N, Denney ML, Rughani A, Foulkes J, Wilson A, Tate P. Ensuring reliability in UK written tests of general practice; the MRCGP examination 1998–2003. *Med Teach* 2005; **27**: 37–45.

57. Page G, Bordage G, Allen T. Developing key-feature problems and examinations to assess clinical decision-making skills. *Acad Med* 1995; **70**: 194–201.

58. Farmer EA, Page G. A practical guide to assessing decision making skills using the key features approach. *Med Educ* 2005; **39**: 1188–94.

59. Cantillon P, Irish B, Sales D. Using computers for assessment in medicine *BMJ* 2004; **329**: 606–9.

60. Schuwirth LWT, van der Vleuten CPM. The use of clinical simulations in assessment. *Med Educ* 2003; **37** (Suppl. 1): 65–71.

61. Guagnano MT, Merlitti D, Manigrasso MR, Pace-Palitti V, Sensi S. New medical licensing examination using computer-based case simulations and standardized patients. *Acad Med* 2002; **77**: 87–90.

62. Gleeson F. The effect of immediate feedback on clinical skills using the OSLER. In *Proceedings of the sixth Ottawa conference of medical education* (Eds Rothman AI, Cohen R). Toronto: University of Toronto Bookstore Custom Publishing, 1994; pp. 412–15.

63. Fraser R, Mckinley R, Mulholland H. Consultation competence in general practice: establishing the face validity of prioritised criteria in the Leicester assessment package. *Br J Gen Pract* 1994; **44**: 109–13.

64. Wass V, Jolly B. Does observation add to the validity of the long case? *Med Educ* 2001; **35**: 729–34.

65. Norcini JJ, Blank LL, Duffy FD, Fortuna GS. The mini-CEX a method for assessing clinical skills. *Ann Intern Med* 2003; **138**: 476–81.

66. Durning S J, Cation LJ, Markert RJ, Pangaro LN. Assessing the reliability and validity of the Mini-Clinical Evaluation Exercise for Internal Medicine residency training. *Acad. Med* 2002; **77**: 900–4.

67. Cronbach LJ, Shavelson KJ. My current thoughts on Cronbach alpha and successor procedures. *Educ Psychol Meas* 2004; **64**: 391–418.

68. Schuwirth L, van der Vleuten CPM. A plea for new psychometric models in educational assessment. *Med Educ* 2006; **40**: 296–300.

69. Kuper A, Reeves S, Albert M, Hodges B. Assessment do we need to broaden horizons? *Med Educ* 2007; **41**: 1121–3.

70. Harden RM, Gleeson, FA. ASME Medical Educational Booklet No. 8 Assessment of medical competence using an objective structured clinical examination (OSCE). *J Med Educ* 1979; **13**: 41–54.

71. Shatzer JH, Wardrop JL, Williams RC, Hatch TF. The generalizability of performance of different station length standardised patient cases. *Teach Learn Med* 1994; **6**: 54–8.

72. Colliver JA, Willis MS, Robbs RS, Cohen DS, Swartz MH. Assessment of empathy in a standardized-patient examination. *Teach Learn Med* 1998; **10**: 8–11.

73. Colliver JA, Verhulst SJ, Williams RG, Norcini JJ. Reliability of performance on standardised patient cases: a comparison of consistency measures based on generalizability theory. *Teach Learn Med* 1989; **1**: 31–7.

74. Reznick RK, Regehr G, Yee G, Rothman A, Blackmore D, Dauphinee D. Process-rating forms versus task-specific checklists in an OSCE for medical licensure. *Acad Med* 1998; **73**: S97–9.

75. Regehr G, MacRae H, Reznick R, Szalay D (1998). Comparing the psychometric properties of checklists and global rating scales for assessing performance on an OSCE-format examination. *Acad Med* 1998; **73**: 993–7.

76. Swartz MH, Colliver JA, Bardes CL, Charon R, Fried ED, Moroff S. Global ratings of videotaped performance versus global ratings of actions recorded on checklists: a criterion for performance assessment with standardized patients. *Acad Med* 1999; **74**: 1028–32.

77. Wass V, Roberts C, Hoogenboom R, Jones R, van der Vleuten C. Effect of ethnicity on performance in a final objective structured clinical examination: qualitative and quantitative study. *BMJ* 2003; **326**: 800–3.

78. Howley LD. Performance assessment in medical education. Where we've been and where we're going. *Eval Health Prof* 2004; **27**: 285–303.

79. Sayer M, Bowman D, Evans D, Wessier A, Wood D. Use of patients in professional medical examinations: current UK practice and the ethico-legal implications for medical education. *BMJ* 2002; **324**: 404–7.

80. van der Vleuten CPM, Swanson DB. Assessment of clinical skills with standardised patients: state of the art. *Teach Learn Med* 1990; **2**: 58–76.

81. Kneebone R, Nestel D, Yadollahi F, Brown R, Nolan C, Durack J. Assessing procedural skills in context: exploring the feasibility of an Integrated Procedural Performance Instrument (IPPI). *Med Educ* 2006; **40**: 1105–14.

82. Ram P, van der Vleuten CPM, Rethans JJ, Schouten B, Hobma S, Grol R. Assessment in general practice: the predictive value of written-knowledge tests and a multiple-station examination for actual medical performance in daily practice. *Med Educ* 1999; **33**: 197–203.

83. Driessen EW, Tartwijk van J, Overeem K, Vermunt JD, van der Vleuten CPM. Conditions for successful reflective use of portfolios in undergraduate *Med Educ* 2005; **39**: 1221–9.

84. Govaerts MJ, Vleuten CP M van der, Schuwirth L.W, Muijtjens AM. Broadening perspectives on clinical performance assessment: rethinking the nature of in-training assessment. *Adv Health Sci Educ Theory Pract* 2007; **12**: 239–60.

85. Baartman LKJ, Bastiaens TJ, Kirschner PA, van der Vleuten CPM (2006). The wheel of competency assessment: presenting quality criteria for competency assessment programmes. *Studies in Educational Evaluation* 2006; **32**: 153–77.

86. Developing and maintaining an assessment system – a PMETB guide to good practice (2006). http://www.pmetb.org.uk/fileadmin/user/QA/Assessment/Assessment_system_guidance_0107.pdf.

87. Cusimano MD. Standard setting in medical education. *Acad Med* 1996; **71**: S112–20.

88. Norcini J. Setting standards on educational tests. *Med Educ* 2003; **37**: 464–9.

89. Champlain de A. Ensuring the competent are truly competent: An overview of common methods and procedures used to set standards on High Stakes Examinations. *J Vet Med Educ* 2004; **31**: 62–6.

90. Wilkinson TJ, Newble DI, Frampton CM. Standard setting in an objective structured clinical examination: use of global ratings of borderline performance to determine the passing score. *Med Educ* 2001; **35**: 1043–9.

91. Downing SM, Lieska GN, Raible MD. Establishing passing standards for classroom achievement tests in medical education: a comparative study of four methods. *Acad Med* 2003; **78**: S85–7.

92. Kramer A, Muijtjens A, Jansen K, Dusman H, Tan L, van der Vleuten CPM. Comparison of a rational and an empirical standard setting procedure for an OSCE. Objective structured clinical examinations. *Med Educ* 2003; **37**: 132–9.

93. Wakeford R, Southgate L, Wass V. Improving oral examinations: selection, training and monitoring of examiners for the MRCGP. *BMJ* 1995; **311**: 931–5.

94. Roberts C, Sarangi S, Southgate L, Wakeford R, Wass V. Examinations – equal opportunities, ethnicity, and fairness in the MRCGP. *BMJ* 2000; **320**: 370–4.

95. Jozefowicz RF, Koeppen BM, Case SM, Galbraith R, Swanson DB, Glew RH. The quality of in-house medical school examinations. *Acad Med* 2002; **77**: 156–61.

96. Verhoeven BH, Verwijnen GM, Scherpbier AJJA, Schuwirth LWT, van der Vleuten CPM. Quality assurance in test construction: the approach of a multidisciplinary central test committee. *Educ Health* 1999; **12**: 49–60.

97. Wallach PM, Crespo LM, Holtzman KZ, Galbraith RM, Swanson DB. Use of a committee review process to improve the quality of course examinations. *Adv Health Sci Educ Theory Pract* 2006; **11**: 61–8.

Chapter 9

Assessment in medical education and training 2

Gareth Holsgrove and Helena Davies

Introduction

Until comparatively recently, assessment in UK medical education and training consisted almost exclusively of formal, high-stakes examinations. Little, if any, assessment was undertaken outside the examination hall, and the only outcome of which the candidate was usually aware was whether or not they appeared on the pass list. This situation only began to change significantly during the 1990s as new undergraduate curricula were introduced that followed the principles set out in *Tomorrow's doctors*.[1] These principles led to a number of changes that were without doubt educationally beneficial, and as a result are likely to have improved patient care. The content and delivery of the curriculum improved – in many instances, very substantially – and new and more appropriate assessment methods came into widespread use. Furthermore, assessment came to be used more creatively to monitor and guide progress and plan educational programmes, rather than just to determine who passed or failed.

This chapter is concerned with changes in assessment that have come about, in part as a result of the *Tomorrow's doctors* curricula. It focuses on contemporary best practice in assessment, both in the workplace and the examination hall. We also take the opportunity to look towards potential developments in assessment in medical education and training over the next few years because we see the major changes that are currently underway continuing with two particular priorities – the quality of postgraduate medical examinations and the design of assessment programmes based on a utility model.

We shall not dwell on the theoretical aspects of assessment, which are covered elsewhere, and extremely well, by many authors, including Streiner and Norman,[2] Wood,[3] and Downing and Haladyna.[4] Nor shall we describe specific methods in detail, as this, too, has been done both by the present authors[5] and many others.[6–9] Instead, we shall consider the practical implications of assessment in both undergraduate and postgraduate medical education.

Principles and standards of assessment

In respect of educational innovation and making improvements, UK post-graduate medical training has generally tended to lag behind its undergraduate counterpart. There are exceptions to this broad statement, of course. For example, postgraduate training for general practice has been in the educational vanguard for many years and continues to be so. Nevertheless, the general picture is not only that postgraduate medical training was educationally less sound than at undergraduate level, but that the great influence of the medical royal colleges could be perceived as an obstacle to developments in assessment in the undergraduate curriculum. For example, some medical schools were unwilling to replace out-dated examination methods such as multiple true/false questions with more appropriate formats because, it was argued, 'The Membership examinations use them, and we must prepare our students by using the same methods'.

For many years, the methods and standards in undergraduate medical education have been governed by the parent university and, even though they are all ultimately approved by the General Medical Council (GMC), there are substantial differences between medical schools. These include differences in the structure, content, and delivery of the curriculum, and the methods of assessment.

Similarly, in postgraduate medical education until recently each medical royal college was almost completely autonomous in determining the content and conduct of their examinations, in setting the pass mark, and in handling appeals.

This is not to argue against differences between medical schools, or that the important educational role of the royal colleges should be reduced. On the contrary, the different approaches to organizing and delivering the curriculum should help potential medical students to select the most appropriate schools to apply to. Also, there is currently enormous scope for the educational roles of the royal colleges to be developed and some are responding very effectively to this opportunity. However, there is still a need for more consistency in standards and principles for both curricula and assessment, as well as in strengthening accountability and quality assurance. This is already happening rapidly in postgraduate medical education, and is coming about through two main developments.

The first is that medical education is now established as a recognized specialty – indeed, it has been claimed to be the fastest-growing specialty in medicine. As well as highly regarded professional organizations such as the Association for the Study of Medical Education (ASME), the Association for

Medical Education in Europe (AMEE), and the newly formed Academy of Medical Educators, there is now a substantial body of high quality literature in medical and dental education, mainly through journals such as *Medical Education*, *Medical Teacher*, *Advances in Health Sciences Education*, *Academic Medicine*, and *Teaching and Learning in Medicine*. Among the major contributors to this literature are the team at Maastricht (particularly Lambert Schuwirth and Cees van der Vleuten), Brian Jolly, John Norcini, Val Wass, and others. Unusually, perhaps, in education, both innovative thinking and consistency in key messages are evident in contemporary publications in this area.

The second development that is driving improvements in postgraduate medical education in the UK is the work of the Postgraduate Medical Education and Training Board (PMETB). This is now the statutory body for quality and standards in postgraduate medical education. After a rather hesitant start, which resulted in it going live 1 year later than originally intended, at the time of writing (late 2007) PMETB has completed the first round of approval of the postgraduate curricula and assessment programmes (PMETB calls them assessment systems) for the UK medical specialties and subspecialties. This approval process was based on two key documents that have done much to place postgraduate medical education in its current position where, in some respects, it is now ahead of many undergraduate programmes. These two documents are the *Principles for an assessment system for postgraduate training*[10] and *Standards for curricula*.[11] All postgraduate medical curricula are now fully compliant with the PMETB curriculum standards, and all their associated assessments all comply, at this stage, with the assessment principles 1, 2, and 5. These require that the assessment system must be fit for a range of purposes (principle 1); that assessments are referenced to curricula, which in their turn, are referenced to *Good Medical Practice*[12] (principle 2); and that assessment must provide relevant feedback (principle 5). Full compliance with all nine principles must be achieved by 2010, and further details are given in the section below on 'Looking to the future'. Furthermore, many curricula are likely to require reapproval over the next few years because the GMC published a new edition of *Good Medical Practice* in November 2006.[13] The 2006 edition has a different structure and content to its predecessor, and several of the approved curricula are based on the earlier (2001) version and will therefore need to be updated. PMETB plans to consider both curricula and assessment systems together in the next round of the approval process to ensure that both elements are clearly recognized as integrated components of the overall curriculum, and that the entire curriculum, including assessments, are fully compliant with the *Standards* and *Principles* by 2010.

The purpose of assessment

The first of PMETB's principles for assessment[10] requires that assessments must be fit for a range of purposes, and that these must be clearly stated. PMETB also requires that the methods for setting standards (which would generally be what we think of as the pass mark) are transparent and in the public domain[10] (principle 4). The standard setting process is also likely to involve consideration of the purpose of assessments. For example, a prelude to two common methods of standard setting for formal examinations – Angoff's and Ebel's methods (see, for example, reference 14 for further details) – requires the panel of examiners to agree on the purpose of the examination. At first sight, this appears to be such an obvious point that it can be taken as read – indeed, it is almost an insult to ask! However, experience has shown that opinions among examiners often vary quite substantially, even when considering the same examination. They usually agree that one purpose is to identify which candidates meet the required standard to pass and those that do not. Often, they agree that the examination determines to a great extent what the candidates learn. However, a multitude of other purposes can also be proposed. These might vary from those of no educational value whatsoever – making a profit for the examining body is a common one – to those with only a vague or presumed educational implication, such as raising or maintaining the status of the awarding body or the qualification it awards. These two purposes can, of course, work together if the examination is an essential one for professional development; leads to a qualification that is highly regarded in the profession; is expensive to take; and has a low proportion of candidates who pass. Readers might be able to think of an example of such an examination, for they are not unknown in medicine.

Contemporary best practice is that the purpose of examinations must not only be agreed, but also made known to the examiners, candidates, other stakeholders, and any other interested individual. It is also good practice to publish details of how the pass mark is decided, and this will soon be a mandatory PMETB requirement. Therefore, the practice commonly adopted in the past, where a pass mark was arbitrarily predetermined – and often set down in the examination regulations – would no longer be defensible. A proper method of standard setting will be required, and the purpose of the assessments must be clearly defined.

Following the *Tomorrow's doctors* reforms, formal examinations have still remained a major feature of undergraduate medical student life, but now they are increasingly supplemented by formative assessments – that is, assessments that provide feedback on progress and attainment but do not contribute to pass/fail decisions. Thus, there has become a clear distinction between assessment that 'counts' towards passing or failing (which is called summative assessment), and formative assessment, which does not. Although in many instances similar methods can be used for both types of assessment, their psychometric requirements are (potentially, at least) significantly different. For example, high-stakes assessments such as final MB or royal college Membership or Fellowship examinations must be very reliable so that pass/fail decisions are accurate and defensible. After all, not only do people's careers depend on the results, but so does patient care and safety. Formative assessment, aimed at providing educational information and feedback but without contributing to pass/fail decisions, can justifiably be less reliable. Indeed, it can be argued that they should be less reliable because achieving high reliability requires test conditions, such as using well-constructed items, long testing time, psychometric input, and quality assurance procedures, that would be impractical and unnecessary for formative assessment.

The distinction between formative and summative assessment has been particularly useful during the past couple of decades, for a number of reasons. Most importantly perhaps is that such a distinction emphasized the educational role of assessment. This educational role stems from the fact that assessment is not just about passing and failing. It is also about monitoring progress, identifying areas of difficulty or misunderstanding, and providing feedback. Educational support can be provided in response to any difficulties identified and if all is going well, positive feedback is always encouraging and welcome. Constructive feedback based on the findings of formative assessment can be very helpful to the student, and might also be helpful to the teachers delivering particular aspects of the programme and to those responsible for the programme as a whole.

However, although it has been helpful to distinguish between formative and summative assessment as medical education has developed over the past 20 years, we are now moving towards a situation where some assessments have both a summative and formative function. Not only must assessments themselves be fit for a range of purposes, as PMETB requires[10] (principle 1), but the information gained from some assessments might also be used for a range of purposes. PMETB also requires that assessments must provide feedback[10] (principle 5) and are likely to insist that in future detailed feedback on formal examinations must be available to all candidates, whereas a common practice at present is to provide limited (often very limited) feedback only to failing candidates. Feedback can also be very useful to people other than candidates. For example, feedback on the performance of individual examination items can be communicated to the responsible examiners (in examinations such as

Objective Structured Clinical Examinations – OSCEs, for example) and also to the people who designed the item. It can also be useful to provide feedback on how well various aspects of the curriculum were tackled by the candidate group as a whole, so that topics on which candidates did not perform particularly well could be reviewed by the people who taught them.

Thus, we can see that assessments have a multiplicity of educational purposes. In addition to their traditional pass/fail role, they can provide feedback to guide and encourage the students and provide information for teachers and examiners. However, a single assessment clearly cannot do this, nor can it adequately cover the curriculum. This brings us to another practical consideration of assessment in medical education – assessment programmes.

Assessment programmes

Contemporary best practice contrasts sharply in several respects with what has traditionally been the rule in medical education. This is true of curricula, teaching, and assessment at both undergraduate and postgraduate level. We have discussed above the differences between formative and summative assessments and noted that today, despite these differences, we are able to use information from assessments for a variety of educational purposes. Also, as we suggested with the example of reliability, different criteria can apply to assessments used for different purposes. Thus, we can select assessment methods depending on purpose, and make compromises (for example, about methods and testing time) that are themselves dependent on context. We shall describe more about this – the utility model – later in this chapter. From this model we can see that rather than confine assessment to just one or two methods used on a very small number of occasions, for medical curricula we need to design a programme of assessments that utilizes a number of methods, is suited to a number of purposes, and provides feedback to a number of different individuals.

Formal assessments

In the traditional model, assessments were typically (and often exclusively) formal, high stakes, and governed by myriad regulations. They were typically concerned with generating numbers as a means of expressing candidates' achievement, and worked on the supposition that competence could be measured as the sum of a number of stable component parts.

The regulations themselves often stretched back over many years and were usually very difficult to change. Among their contents one could often find specifications of the structure and conduct of the examinations. They would set out details of the methods to be used, the time allocated to each, and ways in which marks from different parts of the examination should (or should not) be combined. They often prescribed what the pass mark would be, and many also set a limit on the number of attempts a candidate would be permitted.

However, for all this detail, traditional examination regulations often paid little attention to any form of quality assurance except, perhaps, the opinions of one or two external examiners and of the examination board itself. There was seldom a requirement for any statistical analysis of the examination or for independent quality assurance, and the pass mark was set without regard to the content or difficulty of each diet of the examination. Indeed, pre-set pass marks of this kind cannot take account of content or difficulty because at the time they were established in the regulations the examination itself had not even been written. Moreover, the presumption that every diet of an examination can be exactly as difficult as every other diet is fanciful, to say the least.

It was principally during the 1990s that formal examinations in UK medical education began to embrace defensible principles of measurement and quality assurance. These changes were most widespread in undergraduate medical education and generally came in the wake of the new *Tomorrow's doctors* curricula; new procedures developed in specialist medical education units such as that headed by Brian Jolly at Bart's and The London; increased collaboration with test developers in North America (particularly Geoff Norman, John Norcini, Susan Case, and David Swanson); and the Undergraduate Medical Curriculum Implementation Support Scheme (UMCISS) established by the then Chief Medical Officer, Kenneth Calman. By contrast, throughout the twentieth century few postgraduate medical examinations were supported by any meaningful statistical analysis – the MRCGP being a notable, though not the only, exception.

Despite some significant improvements, most, if not all, undergraduate examinations were still governed by a pass mark set down in the regulations. Some postgraduate examinations, on the other hand, used a norm-referenced system based on, for example, the top 35% of UK-trained candidates. There was, therefore, an inevitable lack of consistency in standards, methods, and practices across medical schools and royal colleges. There was also a lack of consistency in standards within many examining bodies themselves.

Among the improvements that did occur during this decade were the development and introduction of new examination methods. For example, OSCEs, single best answer Multiple Choice Questions (MCQs) and Extended Matching Items came into much more general use and gradually began to replace traditional methods such as essays, multiple true/false MCQs, and unobserved long case examinations. Moreover, the focus began to move from testing knowledge (or, more commonly, factual recall) towards assessing clinical competence. This shift was an important stepping-stone towards the assessment programmes that are being developed today and the transition is particularly well discussed in van der Vleuten's[15] important article on the assessment of professional competence.

Nevertheless, formal assessment was still the predominant, and in most circumstances the exclusive, form of assessment in medical education, and was very clearly seen as a measurement issue focused on whether or not candidates reached the pass mark.

The picture today is greatly improved compared with that towards the end of the last century. Modern assessment methods are used widely – for example, almost every medical school in the UK now uses OSCEs. There is also a much greater use of statistical analysis to inform pass, fail, and borderline decisions, and also to provide a measure of quality assurance for the examinations.

Formative assessment

Although formative assessment had been used in some medical schools, it remained rare in medical education until the new curricula were introduced in the 1990s. Even where it had been used, it often consisted of little more than mock examinations. Very little feedback on progress, as opposed to attainment, was available to students.

Formative assessment was even more unusual in postgraduate medical education and here, again, the RCGP was a notable exception. In many instances 'teaching by humiliation' was far more widespread than providing an educational programme supported by formative assessment and feedback.

Change regarding formative assessment in undergraduate medical education came about mainly through the new curricula. A number of these featured self-directed or problem-based learning (SDL and PBL) and an essential element of these approaches is frequent feedback, so formative assessment became embedded in the curriculum. Moreover, in many instances both peers and teachers provide this feedback, and as a result medical students seem to be becoming increasingly accomplished at critically reviewing their own and their colleagues' work and providing appropriate feedback.

Apart from the few exceptions already mentioned, the use of formative assessment in postgraduate medical education had to wait for the Foundation Programme to commence in 2005. Through its use of workplace-based assessments, formative assessment and feedback became the norm. Indeed, the Foundation Programme uses only workplace-based assessment – there are no formal exams at all in the first two postgraduate years (although one or two of the royal colleges seem to have it in mind to offer their own part 1 examinations during the Foundation years). Early experience has shown that a significant number of Foundation House Officers (FHOs) held back on their workplace-based assessments until almost the end of each year of the programme so as to be more certain of receiving ratings at or above the standard set for completion of each year. However, in doing this they deprived themselves of the benefits of feedback on their progress and also ran the risk that people would be too busy to carry out the required number of assessments in such a short time. Nevertheless, the general picture to emerge is that most FHOs received feedback on their progress and found it to be helpful.

A second stimulus to introducing formative assessment in postgraduate training was the PMETB requirements. As a consequence, all of the assessment programmes currently approved by PMETB have an element of formative assessment and some, such as the curricula for general practice, psychiatry, and most of the physician specialties, have a substantial component of formative assessment.

Looking to the future

There are probably at least two major developments in assessment in medical education and training that can be expected over the next few years. One will occur as the result of statutory requirements, the other through a philosophical shift about professional competence and how it is developed and assessed.

The statutory requirement is that all postgraduate training programmes approved by PMETB will have to be fully compliant with all of its principles of assessment by 2010. These are:[10]

- *Principle 1*: The assessment system must be fit for a range of purposes.
- *Principle 2*: The content of the assessment will be based on curricula for postgraduate training, which themselves are referenced to all areas of Good Medical Practice.
- *Principle 3*: The methods used within the programme will be selected in the light of the purpose and content of that component of the assessment framework.
- *Principle 4*: The methods used to set standards for classification of trainee's performance/competence must be transparent and in the public domain.
- *Principle 5*: Assessments must provide relevant feedback.
- *Principle 6*: Assessors/examiners will be recruited against criteria for performing the tasks they undertake.
- *Principle 7*: There will be lay input in the development of assessment.

- *Principle 8*: Documentation will be standardised and accessible nationally.
- *Principle 9*: There will be resources sufficient to support assessment.

At the time of writing, all approved assessment programmes comply with principles 1, 2, and 5, and several are already compliant with most of the remaining principles. On the other hand, some still have much to do. It is clear to see, though, that full compliance should result in a substantial improvement in the nature and quality of assessment. Moreover, some postgraduate training organizations that do not currently need to meet PMETB standards and principles, such as the Dental Faculties of the Royal College of Surgeons of England, are nevertheless developing both curricula and assessment programmes that would be fully compliant with them.

The second major area of development is the move away from thinking of assessment (particularly formal assessment) as a measurement issue and instead considering it as a matter of educational design. The distinction is highly significant and has developed alongside the philosophy underpinning the contemporary curricula in medicine and dentistry that are competency-based. In such curricula, the focus is less on the acquisition and recall of a large knowledge base and more on the application of knowledge, the development of professional competencies, and performance – which refers to what the doctor or dentist actually does, day in day out, in the workplace.

From the assessment viewpoint, testing factual recall is comparatively easy. History does show us, though, that in UK medical education examination boards have often made very heavy weather of even this simple matter – usually through the use of inappropriate or unreliable methods, or by assuming predictive validity that is completely unproven. Nevertheless, there is no doubt that the traditional psychometric model has played an important part in improving the quality of medical examinations. Even so, a great deal of potentially useful information remains unused, even in a simple knowledge test. This is partly because the nature of this model is that it is numeric and reductionist, and partly because of the way in which potentially important information is usually discarded. For example, a well-designed MCQ examination can yield information that is useful to the examiners (e.g. item characteristics such as difficulty, discriminant function, the proportion of candidates selecting each option, etc.); to the teachers (common errors and misconceptions); and to the candidates (which topic areas they scored well on and, even more importantly, which they did not). Although in some cases information is fed back to examiners and (much more rarely) teachers, all that most candidates receive is either a pass/fail decision or a single percentage score. Considerable potential educational benefits are therefore wasted through obsessive secrecy and failure to provide good feedback to candidates.

When we wish to assess competence and performance, however, we move into much more complex territory. We not only need some new instruments, but also a different way of interpreting the findings. For example, we need to use much more of the information resulting from assessments. This points to new assessment methods, a new and more effective way to utilize findings, and a new psychometric model to deliver it all.

Why do we need a new model? As Schuwirth and van der Vleuten[16] point out 'the central assumption of the current model is that medical competence can be subdivided into separate measurable stable and generic traits' (p. 296). Therefore, we run into two problems. The first is a growing recognition that competence cannot be subdivided in the way that this model assumes, nor is it stable or generic. Competence is a complex matter, not simply the sum of a number of components. The second problem is that it is difficult to apply the traditional psychometric model to the kind of methods we need to assess competence and performance. The practical consequences of both these factors comes to light when we consider the fact that most doctors who are struck off for incompetence or unprofessional conduct have passed all their examinations.

As performance is demonstrated in the workplace, not in the examination hall, we need to use workplace-based instruments to assess it. Several of these are already in use in the Foundation Programme, as well as in postgraduate and some undergraduate curricula. However, we are still working out ways to overcome some of the problems, particularly those of ratings and timing. For example, we are finding a general reluctance on the part of assessors to give ratings below the benchmark standard in workplace-based assessment, and there is a strong temptation for trainees to leave their assessments until late in their phase of training in the hope of obtaining high ratings. Feedback issues have been partially (but only partially) solved by requiring prompt or immediate personal feedback to the trainee, but this might be of comparatively little value in some cases because of the problems of ratings and timing.

In his excellent paper on the assessment of professional competence, van der Vleuten[15] (*op cit*) sets out a utility model for modern assessment. An extension of the traditional model, which is based on reliability and validity, the new model adds three additional factors: educational impact, acceptability, and cost. A formula is suggested in which each of these five factors is weighted and then they are multiplied together. (Thus, if any one of them has a value of zero, then the utility itself is zero.) However, it is emphasized that this is a conceptual model rather than a practical algorithm. The model and relating issues of the assessment of professional competence are discussed further in two more important papers by van der Vleuten and Shuwirth.[16,17] They describe issues of assessing competencies in greater detail than is possible in this short chapter and reach two important conclusions. First, they support van der Vleuten's earlier call for a utility model of assessment (*op cit*[15]) in which assessment characteristics are differently weighted depending on the purpose and content of the assessment. Secondly, they use this model to illustrate their case that assessment is an instructional design problem. In addressing the problem as one of education rather than measurement, they advocate an integrated and multifaceted assessment programme, as opposed to a collection of methods (see our comments above about prescribed methods and pass marks in high-stakes examinations). The assessment programme should be designed according to the purpose and circumstances and will inevitably involve context-dependent compromises.

Therefore, as we look to the future, we feel that we shall see the development and introduction of specifically designed assessment programmes that provide much more informed feedback to all of the major stakeholders. As circumstances require, these programmes are likely to comprise both workplace-based and formal assessments. In the UK they will have to comply with all the PMETB principles (*op cit*[10]) by 2010, and these specifically require that the methods selected are appropriate (principle 3) and that relevant feedback is provided (principle 5). The overall result should be the development of assessment programmes that are fairer, more transparent, and more suited to their specific purpose.

References

1. GMC. *Tomorrow's doctors*. London: General Medical Council, 1993.
2. Streiner DL, Norman GR. *Health measurement scales: a practical guide to their development and use*. Oxford: Oxford University Press, 1995.
3. Wood R. *Assessment and testing*. Cambridge: Cambridge University Press, 1991.
4. Downing SM, Haladyna TM. *Handbook of test development*. Mahwah, NJ: Lawrence Earlbaum Associates, 2006.
5. Holsgrove G, Davies H. Assessment in the Foundation Programme. In *Assessment in medical education and training* (Eds Jackson N, Jamieson A, Khan A). Oxford: Radcliffe, 2007.
6. Godfrey J, Heylings D. *Guide to assessment*. London: The Medical and Dental Education Network, 1997.
7. Jolly B, Grant J. *The good assessment guide*. London: Joint Centre for Education in Medicine, 1997.
8. Bhugra D, Malik A, Brown N. *Workplace-based assessments in psychiatry*. London: RCPsych Publications, 2007.
9. Jackson N, Jamieson A, Khan A. *Assessment in medical education and training*. Oxford: Radcliffe, 2007.
10. PMETB. *Principles for an assessment system for postgraduate training* (Eds Southgate L, Grant J). London: The Postgraduate Medical Education and Training Board, 2004.

http://www.pmetb.org.uk/fileadmin/user/QA/Assessment/Principles_for_an_assessment_
system_v3.pdf/

11. PMETB. *Standards for Curricula* (Eds Grant J, Fox S, Kumar N, Sim E). London:
The Postgraduate Medical Education and Training Board, 2005.
http://www.pmetb.org.uk/fileadmin/user/QA/Curricula/Standards_for_Curricula_
March_2005.pdf/.

12. GMC *Good medical practice.* London: General Medical Council (developed from
Good medical practice 1995 and 1998), 2001.

13. GMC. *Good medical practice.* London: General Medical Council, 2006.

14. PMETB. *Developing and maintaining an assessment system – a PMETB guide to good
practice* (Eds Holsgrove G, Davies H, Rowley D). London: The Postgraduate
Medical Education and Training Board, 2007.
http://www.pmetb.org.uk/fileadmin/user/QA/Assessment/Assessment_system_guidanc
e_0107.pdf/.

15. van der Vleuten CPM. The assessment of professional competence: developments,
research and practical implications. *Adv Health Sci Educ* 1996; **1**: 41–67.

16. Shuwirth LWT, van der Vleuten, CPM. A plea for new psychometric models
in educational assessment. *Med Educ* 2006; **40**: 296–300.

17. van der Vleuten CPM, Shuwirth LWT. Assessing professional competence:
from methods to programmes. *Med Educ* 2005; **39**: 309–17.

Chapter 10

Selection methods for medicine: core concepts and future issues

Fiona Patterson, Pat Lane, and Victoria Carr

Getting the right people into the right roles is probably the most expensive activity an organization undertakes and mistakes are costly – both financially and in human terms. Although there is almost a century's research literature on selection and recruitment issues across most occupational groups, there has been relatively little published exploring the methods to select doctors. There is a growing body of research examining selection methods for medical school admissions. By contrast, there is limited evidence exploring methods for entry into postgraduate training and senior medical appointments.

This chapter outlines core concepts underpinning the design, implementation, and validation of selection methods. We suggest evaluative standards for selection followed by a summary of research evidence on the relative accuracy of various selection tools. A brief case study illustrates the issues surrounding the utility and cost-effectiveness of selection methods and finally, an agenda for future research is presented.

Selection into training for medicine

In medicine, examinations are most often used to assess end-of-training capability and in theory, all candidates can pass the 'examination'. In selection, if the number of applicants outweighs the number of posts, the selection methods are used to rank the applicant pool effectively. If competition is very high, as is often the case in postgraduate selection, competent candidates may not be awarded a post. The 'cut score' reflects the selection ratio and so differs from standard setting approaches often used in examinations. For large volume recruitment the process may comprise several stages (e.g. long-listing, short-listing, interview). Unlike other job roles the potential cost of making a 'mistake' in medicine is exceptionally high.

In principle, selection is aimed at *predicting* from a pool of applicants who will become a competent doctor (i.e. identify individuals who will successfully complete training) *before* training commences. Selection into medical school (*pre-employment*) and into postgraduate training (*employment*) may have different goals, e.g. medical schools may select primarily on academic ability and focus on passing the course, whereas postgraduate selection focuses more on job fit.[1] Notably, there is specific law governing selection practices, and this differs significantly across the world. In summary, the parameters for designing and validating a robust selection system are somewhat different to other assessment settings and the criteria used to judge the effectiveness of a system are potentially more complex.

Evaluative standards for selection methods

Developing a robust selection system is no easy task – over time selection systems evolve. Before judging how well selection methods work, it is necessary to understand the criteria used to determine best practice. Evaluative standards for judging the quality of selection methods have been proposed,[1] which should be reviewed when designing any selection system. In overview, selection methods should be *reliable, valid, standardized*, administered by trained professional(s), and monitored. Evaluation is essential to ensure that methods are *fair, defensible, cost-effective*, and *feasible*. Figure 10.1 outlines the main phases in a selection process. The process starts with a thorough job analysis to define criteria and choice of selection method(s). Once selection decisions are made, validation studies allow the quality of the system to be monitored and improved over time.

The importance of job analysis to identify selection criteria

Research consistently shows that the foundation to an effective selection system is a thorough analysis of the relevant knowledge, skills, abilities, and attitudes associated with performance in the target role, as this enables accurate identification of selection criteria. Job analysis studies use various methods, such as direct observation, and interviews with job incumbents and other stakeholders.[2] Outputs from the analysis should detail the job responsibilities and the competencies and attributes required of the job holder. Having defined these criteria at an appropriate level (e.g. entry to specialty training), the information is used to construct a person specification (and job description if appropriate) and to choose which selection methods will best elicit relevant behaviours. Job analysis is particularly important when exploring potential differences between medical specialties. For example, recent job analysis studies suggest that communication skills is top priority for paediatrics but

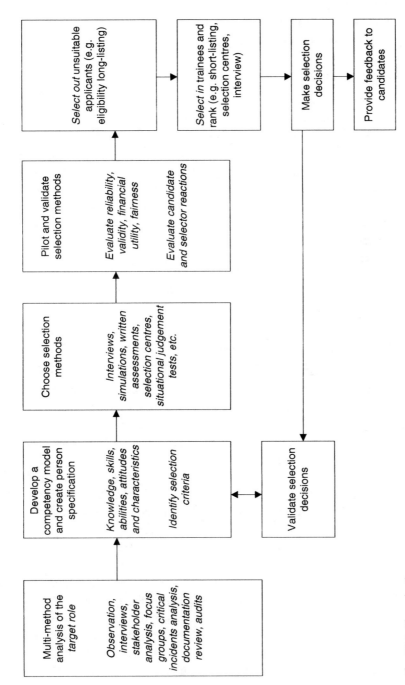

Fig. 10.1 The selection process.

vigilance is the top priority for anaesthesia.[3] Despite job analysis being a core element of best practice selection, research shows that many organizations fail to conduct job analysis effectively.

Making selection decisions

Given the complexity of the doctor role that encompasses high-level cognitive functioning in addition to a range of behavioural skills, it is likely that multiple methods are used for selection purposes. The relative weighting of criteria must be defined, e.g. must candidates score highly on all criteria (*non-compensatory*) or can high scores on some make up for low scores on others (*compensatory*). For particularly important criteria, it may be appropriate to 'select out' candidates who do not achieve a certain minimum standard (such as practical skills for surgeons). If there are few candidates applying and there are many posts available, selection 'cut-offs' will focus on candidates meeting a specified minimal level of competence to be appointed. When there are many more candidates than posts, the choice of selection methods becomes very important in ensuring that the most suitable candidates are accurately identified and ranked.

Validation studies and evaluation

Evaluating candidate reactions to the selection process is essential, especially in gauging perceptions of fairness.[4,5] After selection, we need to ask how well do selection scores predict future work performance? This involves predictive validity studies by collecting predictor information (e.g. interview ratings) for candidates, then following up to gather criterion (outcome) data on their performance (e.g. work-based assessments, exams). Predictive validity is assessed by examining the correlation between scores at selection (Time 1) and data collected at Time 2. Research shows it is unusual in field studies to obtain validity coefficients in excess of $r = 0.5$ and coefficients of considerably less than +1.0 can provide a basis for improved selection practices.[6,7] As most selection systems combine several predictors (selection tools), a key question is how much does adding a further predictor increase the accuracy of the process? This is known as *incremental validity*. Information on incremental validity allows organizations to conduct a cost–benefit analysis of using additional selection tools. In practice, validation studies are difficult to conduct as they present a variety of problems in tracking performance over several years. Accessing appropriate outcome data can be problematic and importantly, recruiters must decide what information should be collected; i.e. what is the selection system actually designed to predict? This is known as the 'criterion problem' in selection.[8] Measures of job and training performance often do not match the criteria used in selection. Further, some selection tools may be more effective at predicting training criteria rather than work performance (and vice-versa).

Accuracy of selection methods

There are thousands of research articles published on the relative accuracy of different selection methods across many different occupational groups. As selection criteria differ enormously across occupational groups, sectors, and levels providing a single and definitive validity coefficient for each method is simply not feasible. For example, the role of cognitive ability required to conduct a job with competence differs significantly depending on the nature of the job role. As a result, researchers have tended to use results from meta-analytic studies, where the results of many validity studies are combined. Table 10.1 summarizes research evidence from meta-analytic studies on the predictive validity of different selection methods across all occupational groups (so interpretation should be guided with caution). This includes an estimate of candidate reactions. Also note that there are international differences in the extent of usage for various methods (which is also governed by differences in employment law).

Application forms

Application forms are often used in long-listing candidates (eligibility information such as educational qualifications) and short-listing candidates as an alternative to curriculum vitae. Information obtained through application

Table 10.1 The relative accuracy of different selection techniques.

Selection method	Evidence for criterion-related validity	Applicant reactions	Extent of use
Structured interviews	High	Moderate to positive	High
Cognitive ability	High	Negative to moderate	Moderate
Situational judgement tests	High	Moderate	Moderate
Personality tests	Moderate	Negative to moderate	Moderate
Work sample tests	High	Positive	Low
Selection centres	High	Positive	Moderate
Handwriting	Low	Negative to moderate	Low
References	Low	Positive	High

forms is collected in a systematic way, making it easier for recruiters to objectively assess and compare candidates' suitability for the post.[9] Application forms may include questions on biographical information, educational background, work experience, and competencies identified through job analysis. Application forms are a crucial part of the selection process and the quality of information obtained varies according to the design of the form. Research shows that structured application forms can provide valid information if they are based on appropriate selection criteria obtained through a job analysis.

Graphology

Some research has explored the use of graphology in selection (i.e. the analysis of handwriting) as a sign of an applicant's personality attributes. There is no single theory or method that dominates the study of graphology. Some researchers have focused on isolated signs in handwriting as specific indicators of personality, whereas others have sought to make subjective interpretations based on a total impression of a person's handwriting. Some recruiters ask that applicants complete the application form by hand as a broad indication of written communication skills. Unfortunately for the graphologists, no clear correlation between handwriting behaviour and basic personality patterns has been found. Research has almost uniformly shown that graphology has no predictive validity in selection.[10]

References

Although employers value references as they contain information on attendance records and health records, ratings often tend to be poor at differentiating fairly between candidates. In principle, references are useful if information in an application form requires verification. However, unless the reference report is in a structured format, decisions about what information to include are left to the referee. References generally contain subjective information so they are open to error and bias. Large empirical studies consistently show that references tend to be unreliable and ineffective at predicting job performance.[11–13] Despite this, references are widely used in selection, and are likely to continue to be used as additional information in the selection process.[14] Research suggests that the reliability of references can be improved if they are in a structured format and validity is improved if the criteria used match the criterion behaviours.[15,16] In the UK, references are used for undergraduate applicants. However, the reliability is questionable given changes in data legislation that remove the confidentiality that existed previously. Ferguson and colleagues[17] showed that references did not predict pre-clinical and clinical performance.

However, medical schools differ in terms of the weight they place on these references.[18]

Interviews

Over many years, research has consistently shown that interviews are ubiquitous in the selection process in many professions.[19] Interviews can be used at different stages of the process, as the sole selection method or in conjunction with others. Interviews vary in terms of their purpose; duration; medium (e.g. telephone); number of interviewers (e.g. panel); and degree of structure (e.g. whether questions and scoring criteria are consistent across candidates and interviewers). Research consistently shows that structured interviews, when based on thorough job analysis with validated scoring criteria, tend to have much higher criterion-related validity than unstructured interviews.[20–23] Meta-analytic studies have found that structured interviews are valid predictors of job performance.[24] Evidence also suggests that structured interviews have incremental validity over cognitive ability tests,[25,26] generally yield smaller ethnic group differences[27,28] and may be more likely to withstand legal challenge.[29]

Academic records

For selection into medical school, academic criteria and school-end examinations are obviously weighted heavily in the decision-making process. One problem with using school-end grades for selection is discriminating among students who obtain similarly high grades and some have argued that such criteria may also reflect social class.[30] In those countries where applications to medical school is at postgraduate level (as in the USA, Canada), academic grades (e.g. GPA) remain the main selection criterion, although they are usually considered in combination with other predictors. Some research has shown that academic criteria correlate with drop-out rates, career progression, postgraduate membership, and fellowship exams.[32] While pre-admission academic grades are undoubtedly related to academic performance at medical school, their relationship with long-term job performance measures is less obvious, partly because of the practical problems in conducting validation studies.[33]

General mental ability and aptitude tests

Research shows that tests of general mental ability (GMA) and cognitive ability tests are robust predictors of job/training performance across a wide range of occupations.[34] However, several studies have raised concerns over fairness with marked racial differences in performance.[35] Aptitude tests are typically defined as standardized tests designed to measure ability to develop skills or acquire knowledge and are used to predict future performance in a given activity. Aptitude tests measure performance across a range of mental abilities, including more specialized abilities (e.g. spatial reasoning) to predict job performance. Aptitude tests are increasingly popular in medical school admissions but are rarely used at postgraduate level, as most candidates have already passed an aptitude test for medical school and some argue there is a danger of obtaining redundant information.[9]

Personality inventories

For many occupational groups the use of personality testing in selection has increased in recent years. Research has demonstrated important relationships between personality and job/academic performance[36] often showing personality tests having incremental validity over knowledge-based assessments.[37] However, the use of personality measures to assess job applicants remains controversial. Critics argue the predictive validity of personality measures for job performance is often low and badly understood. Often there is limited expertise available to choose appropriate tests and some have argued that faking responses could compromise their predictive validity.[38] Best practice is to use personality measures to inform focused questioning at interviews, and that they are not used in isolation to make selection decisions.

Work sample tests and situational judgement tests

Work sample tests have high face validity and meta-analytic studies have shown them to have good criterion-related validity, although they can be expensive to develop as they must be tailored to the job.[1] Work sample tests vary in their physical fidelity to reality. Situational Judgement Tests (SJTs) are a well-established measurement method designed to assess a candidate's judgement regarding a situation encountered in the workplace.[39] Candidates are presented with depictions of hypothetical scenarios and asked to identify an appropriate response from a list of alternatives. SJTs can be designed to measure a variety of constructs (both cognitive and non-cognitive). SJTs have high face and content validity, and have demonstrated significant incremental criterion-related validity above tests of cognitive ability.[40] An SJT has recently been introduced for selection into general practice in the UK and has been shown to have good validity.[41,42]

Selection centres

Selection centres involve a combination of selection techniques (e.g. written exercises, group exercises, various work simulations) using a multitrait, multimethod (MTMM) approach. Selection centres are different to OSCEs (Objective Structured Clinical Examinations) as multiple criteria are assessed in one exercise and a candidate sits *multiple* situations to demonstrate each key skill, and so are observed by several selectors. Thus a fairer (multiple opportunities to perform) and more reliable (multiple observations of key behaviours by multiple observers) judgement can be made. With careful design, the increased reliability should equate to greater validity and more positive candidate reactions.[1] Research shows that a carefully designed and well-run selection centre can be highly effective at predicting job performance across a wide range of occupations[43] showing incremental validity over cognitive ability tests.[44,45] Some researchers have questioned the construct validity of some selection centres so careful design is essential for the process to live up to its reputation and to be cost-effective.[46]

Currently, in all sectors over half of recruiters, and over 95% of large organizations employing more than 10 000 individuals, use selection centres in recruitment. However, it is only recently that this approach has been used in medicine. In the UK, Patterson and colleagues have pioneered the use of selection centres, initially in selection for general practice training followed by several secondary care specialities such as obstetrics and gynaecology, and paediatrics. Results have shown good predictive validity. More recently, this process has been piloted in surgery and for graduate entry to medical school in the UK. Note that most of these selection centres were used in addition to academic tests and interviews.[47–51]

Utility and cost-effectiveness

Best practice selection processes can be costly to design and implement and presenting arguments to spend resource developing new tools can be (on face value) difficult to justify. We present a case study of calculating the cost–benefits of using multiple selection tools. The case is selection into UK general practice, which uses a machine-marked short-listing test followed by a selection centre approach at final stage selection. The case study compares the costs of different approaches used at different locations and examines the cost–benefits of using a short-listing test followed by a selection centre methodology. In summary, the case study clearly illustrates the costs of suboptimal selection significantly outweighs the costs of designing a robust selection process.

Future directions

With increased numbers of students graduating from medical schools across the world, competitive selection at postgraduate level training will be an

Box 10.1 Calculating the cost of selection: a case study of GP selection in the UK

Those responsible for selecting candidates who think they can spot a winner against all the evidence by gut feeling in an interview without delving into personal qualities, behaviours and skills more deeply, potentially expose the organisation to increased employment costs by their failure to utilise a well-constructed and validated selection process.

The adoption of most sophisticated selection approaches (such as a selection centre) does require extra resources during the developmental stages, principally in terms of time, the training of assessors, and the cost of evaluating process and outcomes. The benefits, however, soon outweigh the costs of recruiting the wrong person for the job.

The average recruitment cost, per appointed trainee to GP training, has not been published. Prior to 2000 the majority of GP vocational training schemes advertised and recruited biannually and this incurred very significant costs. The introduction of a single portal to GP training with a successful web-based application service and supporting National Recruitment Office has reduced the costs to NHS Trusts and has received favourable feedback from over 90% of applicants.

In 2005 the Committee of Directors of Postgraduate General Practice Education (COGPED) commissioned an internal cost analysis comparing different methods of selection into training for general practice. The overall cost per appointed candidate was:

♦ South Yorkshire and South Humber Deanery: £390 (three selection exercises + MCQ paper).

♦ Oxford Deanery: £430 (interviews only).

♦ West Midlands Deanery: £448 (two panel interviews, simulation exercise + MCQ paper).

Gross annual training costs per appointed GP trainee (including salary, allowances, supplements, and education costs) were about £87 000 in 2006, which amounts to £261 000 for a 3-year programme. Thus the prevention of one failure recoups the cost of recruiting over 580 doctors on to the training programme (at £448/doctor). With the development of the machine marked assessment for short-listing for 2007, significant savings have been made reducing costs, for example, in the South Yorkshire and South Humber Deanery to £309 per appointed doctor.

The UK recruits about 2600 doctors into GP training each year. If the failure rate to achieve a PMETB certificate is reduced by five doctors per annum

Box 10.1 Calculating the cost of selection: a case study of GP selection in the UK *(continued)*

or the need for extended training is reduced by 30 doctors per annum across the UK – all recruitment costs would be saved.

Nationally in the UK, about 4.5% of doctors have failed to reach the required summative assessment standard within a normal training programme. Almost 1% of these doctors are still unsuccessful after a 6-month extension to training.

In the South Yorkshire and South Humber Deanery, prior to selection by the current selection centres about 1.5% of trainees were failing to achieve a JCPTGP/PMETB certificate (even after extended training). In the past 4 years this attrition has reduced to less than 0.5%. The reduced failure rate is attributed to three factors:

1. Doctors appointed to GP training are more thoroughly assessed in clinical and behavioural terms by using a selection centre approach.

2. The information from the selection process is fed into their training programmes via the first trainer (to be incorporated into education plans).

3. If difficult problems emerge during training, important information is usually found in the selection documentation that gives a good steer towards the planned content of remedial training.

---

increasingly important issue. Therefore, design and validation of selection methods is a critical issue. Selection methods focusing on behavioural competencies are increasingly important. People are often 'hired for what they know and fired for how they behave'. The process of self-selection using accurate careers counselling information is crucially important and further research is critical in this area.

More research is needed to explore the best selection methods for more senior level appointments in medicine. At the consultant level, the competencies required include leadership of teams, resource management, and political awareness, among others.

Future research should explore how a selection system is best designed across the whole training pathway. There may be generic skills required across all specialities but there are likely to be specialty differences. The predictive validity of selection tools may vary depending on the stage in the career path. The real challenge is to integrate this knowledge and to develop selection systems that are reliable from medical school admissions through to specialty training.

References

1. Patterson F, Ferguson E. *Selection into medical education and training*. Understanding Medical Education Series. ASME Publications, 2007.

2. Patterson F, Ferguson E, Lane PW, Farrell K, Martlew J, Wells, A. A competency model for general practice: implications for selection, training and development. *Br J Gen Pract* 2000; **50**: 188–93.

3. Patterson F, Ferguson E, Thomas S. Using job analysis to identify core and specific competencies for three secondary care specialties: Implications for selection and recruitment. 2008, *Med Educ*, in press.

4. Hausknecht, JP, Day, DV, Thomas SC. Applicant reactions to selection procedures: An updated model and meta-analysis. *Pers Psychol* 2004; **57**: 639–83.

5. Anderson N, Born M, Cunningham-Snell N. Recruitment and selection: applicant perspectives and outcomes. In *Handbook of industrial, work and organizational psychology* (Eds Anderson N, Ones DS, Sinangil HK, Viswesvaran C), Vol. 1. London: Sage, 2001; pp. 200–18.

6. Salgado JF, Viswesvaran C, Ones D. Predictors used for personnel selection: an overview of constructs, methods, and techniques. In *Handbook of industrial, work and organizational psychology* (Eds Anderson N, Ones DS, Sinangil HK, Viswesvaran C). London: Sage, 2001; **1**: pp. 165–99.

7. Anastasia A, Urbina S. *Psychological testing*, 7th edn. Upper Saddle River, NJ: Prentice Hall, 1997.

8. Schmitt N, Chan D. *Personnel selection: A theoretical approach*. Sage, 1998.

9. British Medical Association Board of Medical Education. *Selection for specialty training*, Report. London: BMA, November 2006.

10. Cooper D, Roberston I, Tinline G. *Recruitment and selection: a framework for success*. Thomson Learning, 2003.

11. Arnold J, Silvester J, Patterson F, Robertson I, Cooper C, Burnes B. *Work Psychology*, 4th edition, Pearson Books, 2004.

12. Muchinsky PM. The use of reference reports in personnel selection: A review and evaluation. *J Occup Psychol* 1979; **52**: 287–97.

13. Of good character: supplying references and providing access. *IRS Employment Rev* 2002; **754**: 34–6.

14. Ryan AM., McFarland L, Baron H, Page R. An international look at selection practices: Nation and culture as explanations for variability in practice. *Pers Psychol* 1999; **52**: 359–93.

15. Jones A, Harrison E. Prediction of performance in initial officer training using reference reports. *J Occup Psychol*, 1982; **55**: 35–42.

16. McCarthy JM, Goffin RD. Improving the validity of letters of recommendation: An investigation of three standardized reference forms. *Military Psychol* 2001; **13**: 199–222.

17. Ferguson E, James D, O'Hehir F, Sanders A. A pilot study of the roles of personality, references and personal statements in relation to performance over the 5 years of a medical degree. *BMJ* 2003; **326**: 429–31.

18. Parry JM, Mathers JM, Stevens AJ, Parsons A, Lilford R, Spurgeon P, Thomas H. Admissions processes for five year medical courses at English schools: review. *BMJ* 2006; **332**: 1005–9.

19. CIPD annual recruitment survey reports. http://www.cipd.co.uk/subjects/recruitment/general/_recruitment.html

20. Campion MA, Pursell ED, Brown BK. Structured interviewing: raising the psychometric properties of the employment interview. *Pers Psychol* 1988; **41**: 25–42.

21. Goho J, Blackman A. The effectiveness of academic admission interviews: an exploratory meta-analysis. *Med Teach* 2006; **28**: 335–40.

22. McDaniel MA, Whetzel DL, Schmidt FL, Maurer S. The validity of employment interviews: a comprehensive review and meta-analysis. *J Appl Psychol* 1994; **79**: 599–615.

23. Wiesner WH, Cronshaw SF. A meta-analytic investigation of the impact of interview format and the degree of structure on the validity of the employment interview. *J Occup Psychol* 1988; **61**: 275–90.

24. Huffcutt AI, Arthur W Jr. Hunter and Hunter (1984) revisited: interview validity for entry-level jobs. *J Appl Psychol* 1994; **79**: 184–90.

25. Cortina JM, Goldstein NB, Payne SC, Davison HK, Gilliland SW. The incremental validity of interview scores over and above cognitive ability and conscientiousness scores. *Pers Psychol* 2000; **53**: 325–51.

26. Schmidt FL, Hunter JE. The validity and utility of selection methods in personnel psychology: practical and theoretical implications of 85 years of research findings. *Psychol Bull* 1998; **124**: 262–74.

27. Bobko P, Roth PL, Potosky D. Derivation and implications of meta-analytic matrix incorporating cognitive ability, alternative predictors and job performance. *Pers Psychol* 1999; **52**: 561–89.

28. Huffcutt AI, Roth PL. Racial group differences in employment interview evaluations. *J Appl Psychol* 1998; **83**: 179–89.

29. Posthuma RA, Morgeson FP, Campion MA. Beyond employment interview validity: a comprehensive narrative review of recent research and trends over time. *Pers Psychol* 2002; **55**: 1–81.

30. McManus IC, Powis DA, Wakeford R, Ferguson E, James D, Richards P. Intellectual aptitude tests and A levels for selecting UK school leaver entrants for medical school. *BMJ* 2005; **331**: 555–9.

31. Ferguson E, James D, Madeley L. Factors associated with success in medical school: systematic review of the literature. *BMJ* 2002; **324**: 952–7.

32. McManus IC, Richards P. Prospective survey of performance of medical students during preclinical years. *BMJ* 1986; **293**: 124–7.

33. McManus IC. From selection to qualification: how and why medical students change. In *Choosing tomorrow's doctors* (Eds Allen I, Brown P, Hughes P). London: Policy. Studies Institute, 1997; pp. 60–79.

34. Salgado JF, Anderson N, Moscoso S, Bertua C, de Fruyt F, Rolland JP. A meta-analytic study of general mental ability validity for different occupations in the European community. *J Appl Psychol* 2003; **88**: 1068–81.

35. Kehoe JF. General mental ability and selection in private sector organizations: A commentary. *Hum Perform* 2002; **15**: 97–106.

36. Barrick MR, Mount MK, Judge TA. Personality and performance at the beginning of the new millennium: What do we know and where do we go next? *Int J Select Assess* 2001; **9**: 9–30.

37. Ferguson E, Sanders A, O'Hehir F, James D. Predictive validity of personal statements and the role of the five factor model of personality in relation to medical training. *J Occup Org Psychol* 2000; **73**: 321–44.

38. Tett RP, Jackson DN, Rothstein M, Reddon JR. Meta-analysis of bi-directional relations in personality-job performance research. *Hum Perform* 1999; **12**: 1–29.

39. Chan, D. & Schmitt, N. Situational judgment tests. In *Handbook of selection* (Eds Anderson N, Evers A, Voskuijil O). Oxford: Blackwell, 2005; pp. 219–42.

40. Lievens F, Buyse T, Sackett PR. The operational validity of a video-based situational judgment test for medical college admissions: illustrating the importance of matching predictor and criterion construct domains. *J Applied Psychol* 2005; **90**: 442–52.

41. Patterson F, Baron H, Carr V, Plint S, Lane P. Evaluation of three short-listing method-ologies for selection into post-graduate training: the case of General Practice in the UK. *Med Educ* 2008 (in press).

42. Plint S, Gregory S, Evans G. Recruitment to GP specialty training 2007. *BMJ Career Focus* 2007; **335**: gp73–gp75.

43. Damitz M, Manzey D, Kleinmann M, Severin K. Assessment centers for pilot selection: construct and criterion validity and the impact of assessor type. *Appl Psychol* 2003; **52**: 193–212.

44. Krause DE, Kersting M, Heggestad E, Thornton GC. Incremental validity of assessment center ratings over cognitive ability tests: a study at the executive management level. *Int J Select Assess* 2006; **14**: 360–71.

45. Lievens F, Harris MM, Van Keer E, Bisqueret C. Predicting cross-cultural training performance: the validity of personality, cognitive ability, and dimensions measured by an assessment center and a behavior description interview. *J Appl Psychol* 2003; **88**: 476–89.

46. Woodruffe C. *Development and assessment centres: identifying and developing competence.* London: Institute of Personnel and Development, 2000.

47. Patterson F, Ferguson E, Norfolk T, Lane P. A new selection system to recruit general practice registrars: preliminary findings from a validation study. *BMJ* 2005; **330**: 711–14.

48. Randall R, Davies H, Patterson F, Farrell K. Selecting doctors for postgraduate training in paediatrics using a competency based assessment centre. *Arch Dis Child* 2006; **91**: 444–8.

49. Randall R, Stewart P, Farrell K, Patterson F. Using an assessment centre to select doctors for postgraduate training in obstetrics and gynaecology. *Ostetr Gynaecol* 2006; **8**: 257–62.

50. Patterson F, Rowley D. The right choice; A pilot scheme to select surgeons of the future. *Surgeons News* October 2007.

51. Kidd J, Fuller J, Patterson F, Carter Y. Selection Centres: Initial description of a collabo-rative pilot project. *Proceedings for the Association for Medical Education in Europe (AMEE) Conference*, September 2006, Genoa Italy.

Chapter 11

Continuing professional development

Neil Johnson and David Davies

Knowledge and people don't stand still. The twenty-first century doctor is working in an ever-expanding field of medical science – the requirements for continuous updating of knowledge place increasing demands on clinical decision making.[1] In short there is too much to learn with too little time to learn it and this places a major burden on clinicians as they aim to maintain their knowledge in their field of expertise. Alongside this, while doctors typically occupy their career posts for 30 years many of them will want to, or be expected to, develop their careers to take on a variety of additional roles (such as management, teaching, or politics). Consequently, there is huge interest in how doctors learn once they have completed their formal training for their clinical role. The term now widely used for this activity is 'Continuing Professional Development' (CPD).

This chapter has two main sections. First, we explore key factors influencing CPD – both the drivers for CPD and the theoretical or philosophical approaches that we believe underpin successful CPD – and through that we consider the future of medical CPD. In the second part we offer guidance on how doctors can best approach the planning of their CPD, going on to consider in detail how they can make good use of technologically supported approaches to learning (e-learning). Although the focus of this chapter is UK practice, the lessons are generalizable to doctors in most areas of the world.

Drivers for Continuing Professional Development

We have identified four groups of drivers for CPD in doctors.

First, there are **professional** drivers. Doctors are expected to maintain and update the knowledge and skills needed for their current and future work.[2] This has recently been formalized in the appraisal process, which is now a requirement for all doctors.[3] CPD is also driven by the professional desire of groups of doctors to ensure ever-increasing levels of expertise in their field – a desire to move the curve of expertise to the right.

Related to this are a series of **regulatory** drivers. No longer is it acceptable for doctors to use their undergraduate and postgraduate training as the sole demonstration of competence – the demonstration of effective learning as established practitioners is becoming essential.[4] There is also an increasing focus on the measurement of performance of doctors in their actual role (i.e. what is 'habitually done when not observed' rather what the doctor 'is able to do'[5]), to ensure that this reaches or exceeds the necessary standards. In the UK these are both encapsulated in a system of relicensure and recertification.[6,7]

Fortunately, considerable work has been done to clarify the expectations of doctors in both of the above areas. There are now explicit descriptions of the general expectations on doctors (supported by specialty-specific interpretations of this guidance for established doctors)[2] and specific statements relevant to doctors in training.[8] Together these documents provide a comprehensive framework for doctors at any point in their career to plan their learning needs.

There are also **personal** drivers. Doctors may follow an internal drive to explore and extend their knowledge, may feel pressure from their peers, or seek to improve in response to incidents that arise;[9] they may also respond to financial incentives.[10,11]

Finally, there are **organizational** drivers – those that stem from the needs of the organization to ensure that its workforce can undertake its current functions satisfactorily and allow future goals to be achieved.[12]

The complexity inherent both in each of these individual drivers and in the possible combinations of them mean that there is unlikely to be a single, unifying, constant driver motivating doctors; instead it is much more likely that there will be a complex interaction of internal and external drivers of differing strengths that varies not only between doctors but also over time within an individual. A key implication of this is that simple mechanistic approaches to planning and delivering CPD are unlikely to succeed.

Principles underpinning effective Continuing Professional Development

Of the wide range of theories of learning[13] we believe that there are three that have particular relevance to CPD. These are summarized in Box 11.1.

The changing picture of Continuing Professional Development

CPD is changing. We have moved from a position where the content and process of CPD has been largely determined by providers[10] and the level of

Box 11.1 Theoretical underpinnings to Continuing Professional Development

◆ *Adult learning theory*: as adults experienced clinicians need to feel in control of their learning, to relate their learning to their existing experience and to the context in which they work, and are practical and focused in their learning.[14] Thus their learning must be centred on their needs. As consequences, over a career clinicians need to move from the relatively fixed externally prescribed initial training curriculum to a more flexible curriculum determined by their changing needs; the approach to learning will move from 'push-driven' to 'pull-driven' learning.

◆ *Constructivist* and *situated learning theories*: the constructivist[15] and situated[16] theories of learning have in common the notion that learning does not have to be an active process – people develop new ideas or concepts from their current or past knowledge and from their day-to-day experiences without actively seeking to learn from them. In particular they are strongly influenced by the lessons learnt from experience – a process termed 'reflection-in-action' by Schon.[17] This means that learning is a continuous inevitable process and not always planned and/or purposeful; it is sometimes serendipitous, frequently immediate, typically embedded within everyday practice rather than in separate activities, and therefore relatively invisible to others. For CPD this means that: reflection on experience is vital and should be encouraged; it is not possible to pre-determine all learning; a wide range of resources are needed to support learning; and learners need to be able to assess the quality of those resources to determine the reliance they place on them.

◆ *Social learning theory*: clinicians are strongly influenced by their peers – by 'observing others one forms an idea of how new behaviors are performed, and on later occasions this coded information serves as a guide for action'.[18] Thus learning is particularly effective when people learn from each other and/or with the support of one another, usually supported by facilitation to maximize learning.

It should be noted that adult, constructivist and social learning come together in the notion of 'communities of practice' – 'informal networks ... among members of a particular specialty or work group.... (who) have developed a common sense of purpose and a desire to share work-related knowledge and experience'.[19]

uptake by personal factors to a point where learning is increasingly prospectively 'managed' through the identification of needs and prospective plans made for addressing those needs.[20] This is most clearly exemplified by the 'personal development plan' (PDP); its inclusion as a key part of the appraisal process and documentation[3] signifies the importance now attributed to the process of 'personal development planning'.

As CPD continues to evolve, bearing in mind the principles outlined in the previous section, we believe that the following changes to CPD should be encouraged:

1. Reflecting both the wide variety of approaches to learning among established doctors and an increasing acceptance that 'there is no single correct or best way of doing CPD',[21] there should be both a wide range of approaches to *planned* CPD, and greater use of *unplanned* learning.

   (a) *Planned learning* – some content is mandated (e.g. resuscitation training) – here planning is primarily about identifying the most effective learning process and timing. However, for most CPD both content and process will be negotiated, taking into account the individual (their approach to learning, the role they undertake and their future aspirations), their specialty, and the needs of their employing organization. In negotiating the plan we would urge that full use is made of the wide range of ways in which doctors can learn;[20] many approaches (such as mentoring or shadowing) can be very valuable but are currently used infrequently.

   (b) *Unplanned learning* – we believe that 'windfall learning' and 'just-in-time' learning have an important place in CPD – the key is to recognize and make effective use of them and to integrate them appropriately with planned learning. Windfall learning (e.g. conversations or journal reading) is desirable for a number of reasons: for individuals it can highlight previously unrecognized needs or offer new ways of approaching a problem; on a broader scale it may stimulate groups to consider entirely new ways of thinking and thereby provide a basis for step changes in care. Just-in-time learning is based on the doctor 'pulling' the learning that they need; it requires the doctor to be questioning and to have the skills to search for possible sources of answers and the systems to access those resources.

2. With the drive for relicensure and recertification comes the need to demonstrate that *effective* learning is taking place. While in part this can be addressed through effective quality assurance of learning events, we see personal evaluation by individuals of the effectiveness of their learning becoming increasingly important – particularly at the level of whether or

not their learning is enabling them to practise effectively. This requires new approaches to evaluation (described in more detail below).

3. Further maturation of the PDP processes and documentation are needed. Planning learning, merging unplanned learning, and assessing effectiveness need to be robust but flexible. The associated documentation will therefore need to be sophisticated if it is to reflect the complexity of those processes – it must support the recording of needs and resulting plans, enable integration of those plans with learning that is picked up along the way, enable effectiveness to be evaluated, and provide a transparent record of how that learning is relevant for the doctor, their organization and the licensing and certificating bodies. It is most likely to take the form of a 'portfolio' (described in more detail below).[22]

4. Improving patient outcomes will continue to be the key driver for CPD. However, as patient care is increasingly provided by teams learning will increasingly be team-based.[23] This is discussed in more detail in Chapter 19.

5. The range of possible sources of learning is expanding rapidly. This is particularly true for technology-based approaches. There are two significant consequences to this. First, doctors need to become adept at making good use of these resources. Secondly, as greater use is made of a wide range of sources methods for assuring their quality become crucial. We foresee two approaches to this. For planned learning doctors will increasingly use sources that are credible and subject to robust quality assurance processes (e.g. Royal colleges or universities). For unplanned learning we envisage that doctors will seek sources accredited by credible bodies, or that they will need to develop skills themselves to assess the quality of their sources.

It is this last change that we believe will be the biggest, and certainly the most rapid, change in CPD in the foreseeable future. Whereas only a decade ago access to world-class knowledge and best available evidence was in the realm of the few, the democratizing effect of the Internet and the ease of access to e-learning is bringing a consistency of experience to all parts of the globe and to all professionals in healthcare. There is therefore an opportunity for healthcare professionals to look beyond conventional methods such as attending formal teaching sessions with their inherent time and space restrictions, and instead use new communication technologies and embrace distance or e-learning.

For the purposes of this chapter, e-learning will be used as a term to encompass technology supported learning in all its forms, including distance or online learning including the Internet.

As the Internet is now a commonplace, almost an everyday tool for most of us then it is no surprise that information sources are increasingly available online. Indeed in the example of libraries, most journals and increasingly textbooks are consulted in their online version outside of a physical library. The references for this chapter (and, the authors suspect, for most of the chapters in this book) were researched and consulted online, even if the final copy was read after being printed on a cheap office printer. It is the ever-increasing rich sources of information that are making e-learning, either as formal courses or as a method of enabling informal learning almost as commonplace as the Internet itself; furthermore we consider the definition of e-learning broad enough to encompass the fulfilment of an instant thought or immediate learning need by consultation with Medline or the BMJ online.

Planning Continuing Professional Development

The issues identified in the first part of this chapter have a number of implications. In this section we consider these implications when planning or providing CPD. We consider in detail the planning and evaluation of an e-learning approach.

When planning CPD – or supporting others to plan their CPD (for example as an educational supervisor or appraiser) – attention needs to be given both to the subject areas and to the best methods to achieve effective learning. Identification of one's learning needs can come from internal and external sources (see 'drivers' in earlier section). Externally, the need for updating one's professional knowledge and skills, as well as drivers towards professional revalidation creates a learning framework of competencies upon which the learner hangs his/her own knowledge, skills, and attitudes. In the UK and elsewhere, there are the formal competency frameworks mentioned earlier. It is relatively easy therefore for an individual learner to identify using such a framework their knowledge, skills, and attitudes yet to be acquired. The subject areas chosen should reflect a balance across all the drivers for CPD – attention shouldn't be paid solely to some drivers (typically the personal and professional ones) at the exclusion of others; a key role of supervisors and appraisers is to encourage and ensure that colleagues develop a broad understanding of their needs.

In deciding what methods to use it is important to select methods that fulfil the principles that underpin effective CPD (outlined above). Doctors should be encouraged to use a wide range of approaches – not just the conventional lecture or conference. Together these should allow the doctor to gain new knowledge, understand how that might apply to his/her particular setting, implement change and encourage reflection on what more general lessons can be learnt. In a formal education setting this might be called taking a 'blended learning' approach. In deciding on methods, account should be taken of individual preferences for methods – but in doing so, it is crucial both to recognize that preferences do change over time (reflecting factors such as the level of pre-existing knowledge and experience and the nature of the subject) and to avoid selecting methods solely because they require little effort or are not personally challenging.

A structured approach to planning personal learning is particularly important if doctors are to manage the massive information overload resulting from the digital revolution. It is possible to imagine that one day within the lifetime of us all the sum total of human knowledge will be available for download via the Internet; as companies such as Google attempt to make all this information easily accessible to everyone, tomorrow's doctor needs to be able to survive this tsunami of information (see Figure 11.1). We believe that the setting of clear goals for information needs, based upon learning needs, allows doctors to select intelligently from the information available that which they really need.

The range of learning needs, the variety of approaches taken by doctors to their learning, and the vast range of resources now available to support learning require that doctors and their appraisers (or educational supervisors) will need to use the PDP process flexibly. In particular they will need to make effective prospective plans for CPD while allowing for and integrating unplanned learning. Alongside this they will need to maintain a record of learning that demonstrates not only what learning has taken place but how this has enabled the doctor to develop personally and professionally, how it will help them in their particular role in their organization(s),

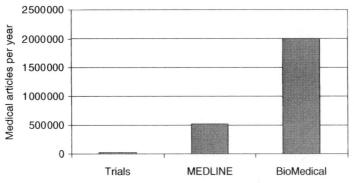

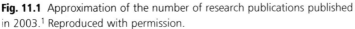
Fig. 11.1 Approximation of the number of research publications published in 2003.[1] Reproduced with permission.

and how it contributes to their relicensure and recertification. To do this effectively we recommend that doctors maintain their record of learning continuously.

Portfolios, either traditionally kept on paper in a learning diary or log, but more commonly now kept online as an e-portfolio, provide learners with a means for creating a plan for learning that specifically demonstrates that the requirements of revalidation are being met. Because libraries and other information providers are increasingly using metadata (data that describe the content and potential use of other data) to identify potential learning resources or opportunities that adopt the same competency frameworks as classification systems the potential for immediate identification of suitable resources to address identified needs is being realized. Thus a learning need to understand current approaches to the management of the diabetic patient with cardiovascular disease can automatically link to the current best available evidence in a patient pathway system such as the Map of Medicine (Map of Medicine)[24] widely available in the NHS in England (Figure 11.2).

The same e-portfolio that is used to plan CPD is also used to record activity and attainment. Thus the e-portfolio becomes the hub of the learner's activity and can be a means for others to verify that learning has taken place by sharing the learning record with a learning mentor or peer.[25]

Finding good e-learning

So where does the learner engaged with CPD find good e-learning opportunities? Typically the first step is the use of a search engine – 'Googling' for information. The difficulty with this approach, though, is the separation of the good from the bad from those sources identified by the search. However, the developments set in train by the GMC and MMC in the UK[2,8] have resulted in formal bodies traditionally associated with specialty training such as the Medical Royal Colleges increasingly engaging in the production and endorsement of e-learning content; just as the colleges are helping to prescribe the competencies required for their specialties increasingly they are helping to meet these requirements with accredited e-learning. Similarly, other respected education providers are offering suitable places to begin to search. The provenance of bodies such as the Medical Royal Colleges and other professional bodies, universities, and reputable publishers who are now producing highly professional, peer reviewed and accredited e-learning content offers some assurance of quality to doctors looking for an appropriate place to start. Excellent examples of such initiatives

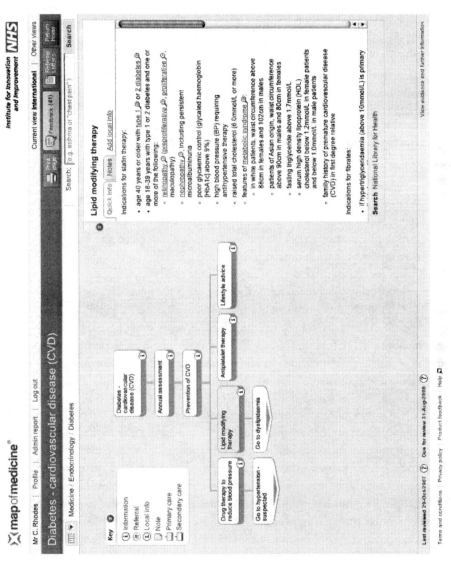

Fig. 11.2 Evidence-based patient pathways for managing the diabetic patient with cardiovascular disease (copyright Map of Medicine Ltd., 2008). Reproduced with permission.

include the Radiology Integrated Training Initiative (R-ITI)[26] collaboration between the Royal College of Radiologists, the Department of Health and the NHS and the BMJ Learning portal aimed at general practitioners in the UK.[27] A further example from an international perspective is the International Virtual Medical School (IVIMEDS).[28] This group is attempting the address the international dimension of medicine and healthcare by collaboratively developing e-learning materials to address the continuum of medical education, from undergraduate medical school to CPD. In the USA the MedEdPortal[29] developed by the Association of American Medical Colleges is creating a rich repository of peer-reviewed e-learning materials.

Evaluating the effectiveness of e-learning

How will we know when e-learning has been effective? Are there ways in which we can measure the impact that e-learning and CPD has had on the individual and the environment in which they work? Evaluation of e-learning effectiveness can follow Kirkpatrick's model[30] for evaluating any training programme (see Box 11.2). Essentially, the effectiveness of e-learning can be measured initially by the impact of the experience, and ultimately by the changes in behaviour brought about and the improvement of patient outcomes.

In practice evaluation of the immediate impact of the e-learning experience may be conducted in the manner in which the learning tool takes place – that is on-line. Conducting evaluation administration online can often save time when collating, processing, and analysing responses. Immediate feedback from the learner to the e-learning provider may be in the form of an online evaluation questionnaire accompanying the e-learning material. This part of the evaluation cycle may lead to improvements in the structure, content, and delivery of e-learning in the same way that conventional evaluation of classroom teaching may lead to improvements.

Evaluating the effect of e-learning on the learner's knowledge, skills and attitude is best measured through the formative or summative assessments that will inform re-licensure and re-certification. Alternatively, reflection by the learner on what has been learnt may be sufficient as an initial goal. Feedback from peers or a learning mentor can also give the learner insight into the impact on behaviour and attitudes, perhaps as part of a 360° evaluation. The personal learning portfolio or e-portfolio is a good place to record such reflections.

Finally impact on the organization, at its broadest the healthcare system, is best measured by an analysis of the effect on patient outcomes.

Box 11.2 The four-stage Kirkpatrick model for evaluation

1. *Reaction*: how participants have reacted to the programme. This element of evaluation is best described as feedback to the learning provider on the utility of the learning. It includes the learners intellectual and emotional response to the material as well as some of the practical elements such as how it was presented, etc. This aspect of evaluation helps improve the e-learning materials for future use.

2. *Learning*: what participants have learnt from the programme. What knowledge, skills or attitudes has the learner acquired as a result of using these materials? How did they meet the identified learning needs and attainment of the intended competencies?

3. *Behaviour*: whether what was learnt is being applied on the job. Learning abstract knowledge may have its rewards in the broadest sense but unless observable and measurable differences result from learning then in the context of health service provision learning has been at best unsuccessful or at worst misplaced.

4. *Results*: impact on the environment. How the learning has affected the learner in the context of the environment he/she works, including the institution (hospital, health service) and especially the impact on patient outcomes. Without the context of improved patient outcomes CPD has little relevance to the health service. It is important to acknowledge that the range of factors affecting patient outcomes does mean that it can be very difficult to attribute changes in outcome directly to individual learning activities.

Conclusions and remaining challenges

We have observed a significant shift from provider-driven learning to managed learning, but with limited account being taken of the force of unplanned learning; we believe that both planned and unplanned learning are needed. We also believe that a blend of methods to support learning should be used, with much greater use of e-learning but without the loss of the social interaction that is crucial for behavioural change. We believe that methods for evaluating the effectiveness of learning at the individual level, particularly ones suitable for e-learning, are needed (although we accept that the impact of learning on patient outcomes may be difficult to demonstrate). We also believe learning should frequently be team-based, particularly when changes that will affect many team members are being considered. Together these will require sophisticated approaches to the planning, recording, and quality assurance of CPD.

However, even if these changes take place, there remain some continuing challenges to CPD. We believe three are particularly important:

♦ How can individual clinicians, and whole teams, be best prepared for very rare contingencies (for example, managing a clinical problem that you may see only once or twice in a career)?

♦ How can effective learning from one another – especially learning from those who may have the answer to your problem but with whom you are not in direct contact – be best enabled?

♦ How can technology be used to improve learning about interpersonal interactions – particularly those between clinicians and patients or between clinicians?

As a result we would encourage clinicians and educators not only to try to make the current system better in the way we have outlined, but also to work together to consider how these continuing challenges can be addressed.

References

1. Glasziou P. Evidence-based practice. Available at: http://www.cebm.net/index.aspx?0=1416 (accessed 28 September 2007).
2. General Medical Council. *Good Medical Practice.* London: General Medical Council, 2006.
3. Department of Health. *Appraisal.* London: DoH, 2003.
4. Irvine DH. Everyone is entitled to a good doctor. *Med J Aust* 2007; **186**(5): 256–61.
5. Epstein RM. Assessment in medical education. *N Engl J Med* 2007; **356**(4): 387–96.
6. Chief Medical Officer. *Good doctors, safer patients: proposals to strengthen the system to assure and improve the performance of doctors and to protect the safety of patients.* London: Department of Health, 2006.
7. Sutherland K, Leatherman S. Does certification improve medical standards? 2006; **333**: 439–41.
8. PMETB. Curricula. Available at: http://www.pmetb.org.uk/index.php?id=curricula (accessed 19 September 2007).
9. Allery LA, Owen PA, Robling MR. Why general practitioners and consultants change their clinical practice: a critical incident study. *BMJ* 1997; **314**: 870–4.
10. Kelly MH, Murray TS. Motivation of general practitioners attending postgraduate education. *Br J Gen Pract* 1996; **46**(407): 353–6.
11. Heath KJ, Jones JG. Experiences and attitudes of consultant and nontraining grade anaesthetists to continuing medical education (CME). *Anaesthesia* 1998; **53**(5): 461–7.

12. Pitts J, Curtis A, While R. Practice professional development plans: general practitioners' perspectives on proposed changes in general practice education. *Br J Gen Pract* 1999; **49**(449): 959–62.

13. Kearsley G. Explorations in Learning & Instruction: The Theory Into Practice Database. Available at: http://tip.psychology.org/ (accessed 13 July 2007).

14. Knowles M. *The adult learner: a neglected species*. Houston, TX: Gulf Publishing, 1984.

15. Bruner, J. *Toward a theory of instruction*. Cambridge, MA: Harvard University Press, 1966.

16. Lave J, Wenger E. *Situated learning: legitimate peripheral participation*. Cambridge: Cambridge University Press, 1990.

17. Schon D. *The reflective practitioner: how professionals think in action*. London: Temple Smith, 1983.

18. Bandura A. *Social learning theory*. New York: General Learning Press, 1977.

19. Sharp J. *Communities of practice: a review of the literature*. Available at: http://www.efriend.com/cop-lit.htm (accessed 13 July 2007).

20. Grant J, Chambers E. *The good CPD guide: a practical guide to managed CPD*. London: Joint Centre for Education in Medicine, 1999.

21. du Boulay C. From CME to CPD: getting better at getting better? *BMJ* 2000; **320**: 393–4.

22. Mathers NJ, Challis MC, Howe AC. Portfolios in continuing medical education – effective and efficient? *Medical Education* 1999; **33**: 521–30.

23. Department of Health. *Working together, learning together: a framework for lifelong learning for the NHS*. London: DoH, 2001.

24. Map of Medicine. Available at: http://www.mapofmedicine.com/ (accessed 15 September 2007).

25. Royal College of General Practitioners. The ePortfolio for nMRCGP: a guide for trainers. London: RCGP, 2007.

26. Radiology – Integrated Training Initiative. Available at: http://www.rcr.ac.uk/index.asp?PageID=969 (accessed 21 September 2007).

27. BMJ Learning. Available at: http://learning.bmj.com/ (accessed 28 September 2007).

28. IVIMEDS. Available at: http://www.ivimeds.org/ (accessed 14 September 2007).

29. Association of American Medical Colleges. MedEd Portal. Available at: http://www.aamc.org/mededportal (accessed 20 September 2007).

30. Kirkpatrick DL. *Evaluating training programs: the four levels*. San Francisco, CA: Berrett-Koehler, 1994.

Chapter 12

Medical leadership

Isobel Down and John Clark

Healthcare in the twenty-first century requires skilled and competent doctors to deliver safe, high quality clinical care while working as part of a multidisciplinary team. However, as the political and organizational system in which doctors' practise becomes ever more complex, so the need to respond with a wider set of medical competencies increases. Improving the health of the population, and the delivery and effectiveness of health and social care services, depends heavily on the support and active engagement of all doctors, not only in their practitioner activities but also in their managerial and leadership roles.

Over the past decade, public sector services including the health system have seen an unprecedented focus on service improvement in terms of quality, productivity, and costs. The National Health Service (NHS) has seen significant additional investment during the initial years of a decade of reforms as outlined in *The NHS plan*.[1] Like most other developed countries, the UK has an increasingly elderly population within a more technologically opportunistic society where new treatments and drugs offer improvements in quality and duration of life. The associated demands and expectations of our society are leading to spiralling costs of healthcare, which has resulted in a quest for greater efficiency and effectiveness. The involvement of the medical profession is central in developing a leadership response to the challenges that face the health service.

The changing nature of medicine as a profession

There is widespread acknowledgement of the changing nature of medicine as a profession. Writing from an Australian perspective, Dowton's comments equally apply to the UK.[2] He recalls the traditional role of the medical profession being defined through long-standing legislative canons coupled with the status accorded to individual doctors by society and societal contracts, as well as deeply entrenched cultural systems arising principally from the influence of professional craft groups. Dowton identifies a number of external influences that have now altered doctors' autonomy and the hierarchies within which they practise. These include a greater demand for accountability for the safety of patients, quality and efficacy of healthcare, and public access to medical information. He concludes that despite leadership roles being critical, inadequate attention has been paid to developing individual leaders and new models of leadership within the medical profession.

Perhaps the most important contribution to the discussion over the changing nature of the medical profession has come from the profession itself. In particular, through a report by the Royal College of Physicians (RCP) entitled *Doctors in society: medical professionalism in a changing world.*[3] The report defines medical professionalism as 'a set of values, behaviours and relationships that underpin the trust the public has in doctors' (p. 56). It also mentions the need to strengthen leadership and management skills and to develop clinical leaders for the future. Specifically, it argues for the incorporation of leadership and management competence within a doctor's training, and urges the General Medical Council (GMC) to include these skills as key competencies of professional practice.

Medical training has consistently focused on the knowledge and skills necessary to develop clinically skilled practitioners, but it is increasingly important that doctors are not only competent clinicians, but additionally demonstrate leadership and management competence within the non-clinical aspects of their role.

In 1993 the GMC published a key document called *Tomorrow's doctors*, which included recommendations to support a framework for UK medical schools to use for curriculum design and schemes of assessment.[4] Revised in 2003, the document identifies the required knowledge, skills, attitudes, and behaviours expected of medical graduates. The document reinforces the principles set out in *Good medical practice*[5] and places them at the centre of undergraduate education. In 2005, the GMC consulted on strategic options for medical education and received further suggestions on the enhancement of the undergraduate curriculum, including several relating to the idea that the concepts of leadership and management should be a crucial part of redefining professionalism. A further revision of *Tomorrow's doctors* is anticipated in 2008 and it is expected that this will strengthen the requirement for doctors to be competent in both leadership and management.

As part of its published strategy for 2006–10, the Postgraduate Medical Education and Training Board (PMETB) is committed to consult on the curriculum content and learning outcomes to be achieved in all specialties.[6] There are currently 58 specialty curricula that have been developed to deliver both core and specialty specific learning. The current content relating to management and leadership is variable and predominantly refers to knowledge, skills, and behaviours contained within the arena of clinical management or professionalism. In the future, it is likely a common set of generic standards will be applied across all 58 specialties. These will include a core set of management and leadership competencies that must be attained in order to secure a Certificate of Completion of Training.

Leadership in the NHS: the theory

Within the increasingly complex health system in the UK, leadership is often cited as imperative yet there remains confusion about its definition and application. The topic of leadership has occupied the thinking of many over time, from the early Greek philosophers to the relatively recent explosion of leadership gurus and management theorists. For most of the twentieth century, leadership theory centred on traits, qualities, and behaviours of the individual leader. With the advent of the concept of transformational leadership in the last decade, organizations placed increasing emphasis on the ability of its leaders to be change agents, with highly developed interpersonal skills. The agenda of reform within the health service required transformational leaders at the helm, to lead by example and to drive change. However, more recently, the focus on individual leadership has come to be regarded as too short term to deliver sustainability to organizations. The NHS has witnessed Chief Executives come and go, often leaving behind them more significant challenges for the organization to cope with.

From the work of organizational theorists such as Henry Mintzberg,[7] healthcare organizations can be described as professional bureaucracies that are characterized by dispersed or distributed leadership. These are organizations where professional groups derive authority from professional expertise and credibility, and have a large measure of control over their work. The characterization of the health service as a professional bureaucracy has implications for leadership.

The notions of team or distributed leadership, where responsibility is dissociated from the organizational hierarchy, move us away from the development of individual leadership qualities towards the recognition of collective tasks of leadership and the development of adaptive and effective leadership processes. Leadership therefore becomes everyone's business, not confined to those with explicit roles within the organizational structure. The definition of leadership remains a complex construct; influenced by social, organizational, and personal processes. However, the concept of team or distributed leadership feels appropriate to the healthcare sector and supports the view that all doctors have a leadership role and responsibility as part of a professional bureaucracy.

Doctors and managers

The GMC document 'Guidance on Management for Doctors' states that 'all practising doctors are responsible for the use of resources; many will also lead teams or be involved in the supervision of colleagues; and most will work in managed systems, whether in the NHS or in the independent, military, prison, or other sectors.[8] Doctors have responsibilities to their patients, employers, and those who contract their services. This means that doctors are both managers and are managed.

Attempts to engage doctors in management have historically been through the establishment of organizational structures, such as the creation of clinical directorates. These became the preferred mode of organization of acute hospitals in the UK following the 'Griffiths NHS management inquiry report',[9] which stated that hospital doctors 'must accept the management responsibility which goes with clinical freedom' (p. 18). Clinical Directors have typically been senior doctors, selected for their ability and enthusiasm but also on the grounds of seniority or peer acceptability, who have taken responsibility for a unit of management while retaining their clinical duties.

Reinersten *et al.* emphasize the complexities and difficulties in the relationships between doctors and managers.[10] They point out that doctors tend to have an individualized focus on the clinical management of patients, which may at times conflict with managers' focus on system improvement. The authors stress the importance of involving doctors in management, and imply that change will not happen without their engagement with the wider organizational context.

While clinical directorate structures attempted to integrate clinicians into management, Davies *et al.* report that clinical directors were 'the least impressed with management and the most dissatisfied with the role and influence of clinicians' (p. 627).[11] This is perhaps understandable, given the expectations placed on clinical directors who as practising clinicians had little prior access to leadership and management training. While the health service has responded to this through the development of clinical director training opportunities, these measures have been largely remedial.

The NHS has historically been characterized by a culture whereby senior leaders mainly come from business management and non-medical clinical professional backgrounds. Few doctors seek Chief Executive positions although in June 2007, the Chief Executive of the NHS (England) told a conference of doctors 'Within two years, we want a doctor applying for every Chief Executive post advertised'.[12] This aspiration clearly provides an opportunity for the medical profession, should it choose to take it, to build on the work already underway to develop management and leadership skills for doctors at every level.

There is a distinction between the management and leadership competencies required of all doctors to be effective practitioners, and those required for wider organizational and system leadership roles. Indeed, not all doctors will have the necessary leadership skills to be effective leaders at the latter level. Seniority should not be the criteria by which such roles are filled.

Some international perspectives

The UK is not alone in seeking to increase the engagement of the medical profession in the leadership of its health services. Many other countries are committed to redefining the role of the doctor and to establishing training programmes to support the development of leadership skills.

Arrangements for the involvement of doctors in leadership roles vary. For example, in Japan and Turkey only doctors can be appointed as Hospital Chief Executives. In contrast, within many Nordic countries the drive for reform has strengthened the role of managers, resulting in a weakening of the leadership role of doctors. Denmark features as an exception to this and is influencing a number of European countries, including the UK, in reinforcing the managerial and leadership role of a doctor. In Denmark, all clinical departments are required to have a physician leader, and there is a medical director post on every hospital board. Based on the Canadian Model (CanMEDS), the Board of the National Union of Consultants in the Danish Medical Association have developed a set of eight roles for the future specialist:[13]

- Medical expert
- Professional
- Leader/manager
- Academic
- Collaborator
- Communicator
- Promoter of health
- Advisor

These roles underpin all aspects of postgraduate training and development programmes and doctors are expected to demonstrate competence in all eight roles as part of the appointment criteria for specialist appointments.

Leadership competencies for doctors: no longer an optional extra

The importance of engaging doctors in managing, leading, and transforming services is now fully recognized by the medical profession, the government, and the wider NHS. New definitions of professionalism and lessons from other countries aim to ensure that doctors are more effectively involved in the leadership of health services. This is influencing changes in the competencies required of doctors at all levels of training and careers.

Competency approaches to leadership development and assessment originated in the late 1970s within the United States and were widely adopted within the UK as a basis for management education from the mid-1980s. Boyatzis defined job competency as 'an underlying characteristic of a person which results in effective and/or superior performance in a job' (p. 21).[14]

In future, the acquisition of management and leadership competency, and the ability to contribute to the development of quality healthcare services, will be compulsory elements of a doctors' training. Morgan contends that 'good management and leadership should be regarded as essential a part of professionalism as are clinical skills'.[15]

Over the lifetime of a medical career, there are several phases and different emphases in relation to management and leadership (see Table 12.1).

A new medical leadership competency framework

A project on medical engagement and leadership is being undertaken by the NHS Institute for Innovation and Improvement and the Academy of Medical Royal Colleges, in conjunction with all medical regulatory, professional, educational, and service bodies. The aims of the project are to:

- ◆ Create cultures within NHS organizations that positively encourage medical engagement and leadership.
- ◆ Strengthen the role of doctors in leadership and management.
- ◆ Develop a framework of management and leadership competencies for doctors to be used to support career-long development (i.e. from undergraduate education, during postgraduate education and throughout employment as a specialist or career grade doctor).

A framework for assessing leadership and management competence, which will be adopted by all medical educational and regulatory bodies, was developed as part of the project. The framework aims to describe the areas

Table 12.1 Phases and different emphases in relationship to management and leadership.

Medical students	Every student needs to be aware of the management and leadership skills that will help them develop their ability to work in teams and deliver high-quality care.
Foundation level to specialist registrar	Every doctor needs to have the knowledge and skills to be effective members of multidisciplinary teams, and to be involved in improving the quality of care provided as well as understanding the impact of their clinical decisions on the wider systems of care.
Early years of appointment to specialist registrar and career grade doctors	Every doctor needs to supplement the development of clinical skills with management and leadership competencies. Leadership abilities will help all doctors to become more effective clinicians and to work with colleagues to develop the service.
Roles in managing and leading the work of peers	A growing number of doctors may wish to extend their skills and practice to include leadership responsibility for a particular service, organization or function.
Roles at a corporate level	Some doctors will take on top-level corporate medical leadership roles in, for example, NHS trusts, medical professional or educational bodies.
Chief Executive or National Leader	A few doctors will develop and apply high-level strategic thinking demanding specialized knowledge and leadership skills.

and levels of competence to be attained by all doctors at three defined career stages:

+ *Stage 1*: the end of undergraduate training.

+ *Stage 2*: the end of postgraduate training or at defined stages of a career grade doctor's career.

+ *Stage 3*: no later than 5 years post-registration and at further defined stages of a career grade doctor's career.

The framework was developed using a highly inclusive approach, which involved semistructured interviews with a wide variety of medical education-alists, medical and non-medical leaders, students, and trainee doctors. Current coverage of leadership within existing curricula was reviewed, and was found to be at best patchy at all career stages. Within the undergraduate curriculum, there were some examples of student-selected modules intended to introduce the concepts of leadership and management, outside the core curriculum. In addition, most medical schools did provide some relevant learning oppor-tunities such as communication skills or teamwork, in general defined under the broad banner of professionalism. At postgraduate stage, most deaneries offered short, locally provided, courses in leadership and management. For more senior doctors, there were a number of leadership training opportunities identified, but issues of cost and quality assurance were identified during the interviews conducted.

In addition to the comprehensive inquiry carried out with stakeholders in the UK, a critique of existing national and international competency frameworks was undertaken. Further, consideration of the existing NHS Leadership Qualities Framework (LQF), which is designed to support executive leadership development influenced the development of the Medical Leadership Competency Framework.[16]

The Medical Leadership Competency Framework has five overall domains relating to the effective delivery of care in service. Each of the five domains is subdivided into four elements, and each of these into four further competency outcomes. Proposed sets of skills and knowledge underpin the attainment of competence for each domain, and illustrative examples for the three career stages are included. The competency statements themselves have been written in a way that incorporates the important aspects of attitudes, expertise, and behaviours.

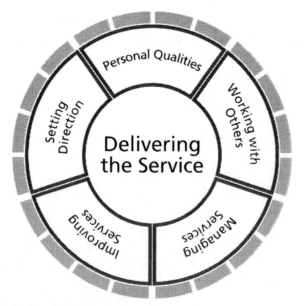

Fig. 12.1 Medical Leadership Competency Framework.

Building on the many valuable sources of advice and information, the framework will be refined to ensure the language used within it is appropriate and meaningful to the medical profession, and supports the embedding of leadership and management skills within the doctor's education and career. It is crucial that the framework is able to support the development of learning opportunities that are timely and relevant to all medical students and doctors. In accepting that the acquisition of leadership and management skills are core for all doctors, the framework affords the possibility to deliver appropriate learning outcomes within core clinical training, rather than as a peripheral or extracurricular activity.

The success of this component of the overall project should not be measured in the short term or indeed even in the medium term. Implementation of a competency based approach to leadership and management for doctors will inevitably take time and will evolve alongside other competing demands within medical education. The application of the framework within medical schools, deaneries, and health service organizations will require further development of appropriate assessment methodologies, and an ongoing commitment by the medical education community and regulatory bodies to pursue a competency based approach to examination and accreditation of leadership skills for all doctors.

The broader focus of the project, aimed at creating a culture that encourages medical engagement in leadership and management, will depend in part on the acceptance of this paradigm by the non-clinical leadership of the health service. Further development of the medical leadership framework to explore joint management and leadership development opportunities for clinicians and managers will facilitate the process of cultural change, and may also be of benefit to other clinical professions. Indeed, the successful introduction and application of competency based leadership and management education and training in the UK may provide a useful model for other countries to adopt elsewhere.

The future

The requirement for leadership and management competencies within the portfolio of a doctor's skills is widely acknowledged by the medical profession, including those involved in the design and delivery of medical education, and by the bodies with responsibility for its regulation. Doctors have key roles to play in the delivery and development of improved health services for patients and populations, alongside their other clinical professional and managerial colleagues.

The acquisition of leadership and management competencies will no longer be accepted as an optional extra for doctors in the twenty-first century. The introduction of relevant and mandatory competencies within medical education and training aims to encourage greater medical engagement with the leadership and management agenda. All doctors will have greater opportunity to be involved in decisions affecting their service and personal roles, and some doctors will be further encouraged to pursue significant leadership roles in the future.

References

1. Secretary of State for Health. *The NHS plan: a plan for investment, a plan for reform.* London: Her Majesty's Stationery Office, 2000.
2. Dowton BS. Leadership in medicine: where are the leaders? *Med J Aust* 2004; **181**: 652–4.
3. Royal College of Physicians. *Doctors in society: medical professionalism in a changing world.* Report of a Working Party of the Royal College of Physicians of London. London: RCP, 2005.
4. General Medical Council. *Tomorrow's doctors: recommendations on undergraduate medical education.* London: GMC, 2003.
5. General Medical Council. *Good medical practice.* London: GMC, 2006.
6. Postgraduate Medical Education and Training Board. *Strategy document: 2006–2010.* London: PMETB, 2005.
7. Mintzberg H. *The structuring of organizations.* Englewood Cliffs, NJ: Prentice-Hall, 1979.
8. General Medical Council. *Guidance on management for doctors.* London: GMC, 2006.
9. Department of Health and Social Security. *Griffiths NHS management inquiry report.* London: Her Majesty's Stationery Office, 1983.
10. Reinertsen J, Gosfield A, Rupp W, Whittington J. *Engaging physicians in a shared quality agenda.* Cambridge, MA: Institute for Healthcare Improvement, 2007.
11. Davies HTO, Hodges C, Rundall T. Views of doctors and managers on the doctor-manager relationship in the NHS. *Br Med J* 2003; **326**, 626–8.
12. Day M. The rise of the doctor-manager. *Br Med J* 2007; **335**: 30–1.
13. Frank JR (Ed.). *The CanMEDS 2005 physician competency framework. Better standards. Better physicians.* Better care. Ottawa: The Royal College of Physicians and Surgeons of Canada, 2005.
14. Boyatzis RE. *The competent manager: a model for effective performance.* New York: Wiley, 1982.
15. NHS Institute for Innovation and Improvement. *Management, leadership and doctors: enhancing engagement in medical leadership project* [pamphlet]. London: NHS Institute for Innovation and Improvement, 2007.
16. NHS Institute for Innovation and Improvement. *Leadership Qualities Framework.* Available at: http://www.nhsleadershipqualities.nhs.uk/ (accessed October 2007).

Chapter 13

Learning from other countries

Geoff Meads

Purpose

The theme of this chapter is transferable learning. The perspective of the chapter is global and contemporary. Its principal aim is to identify alternative international approaches to medical education that can be applied appropriately to developments in the UK, and possibly elsewhere. A framework of 'Modernization' is used to help ensure that there is an authentic comparability between the UK and the other countries so that they may be regarded as relevant resources for this purpose. Accordingly, in each case the democratic nation states referenced are undertaking reforms of their health systems during the post-Millennium period, which are characterized by such common characteristics as new forms of clinical and corporate governance, participation and regulation, and stewardship strategies for public health. In each 'modernizing' health system the model of medical education is itself undergoing significant change. Indeed, despite the strong professional resistance that is internationally a consistent factor in such change, the development of novel curricula is usually an important and integral element of a state's overall policies for the positive transformation of health and healthcare relationships.

Specifically for medical education the 'modernizing' principles of decentralization and partnership are those which have the most powerful impact. Together they pave the way for the much wider involvement of different community interests and non-professional groups in curricula design and delivery. These principles have also been the most prominent and explicit in successive policy statements in the UK since the incoming central government of June 1997 declared its intention of re-creating a new and dependable National Health Service (NHS).[1-3] In the pages that follow we shall therefore focus particularly on those countries where there are both novel forms of local resource management and collaboration, and educational innovations designed deliberately, or sometimes by default, to support the new organizational developments. Because the emphasis on decentralization and partnership often finds its expression in primary care agencies, as practice-based commissioning and primary care trusts in England readily illustrate, many of the international initiatives cited below will be derived from this service sector.

The data for this chapter are mostly derived from a 2007 literature review and international fieldwork over the 2001–06 period. This took place in 24 countries where new forms of primary care were being developed in response to national policies that emphasized the benefits of both decentralization and new cross-boundary partnerships. This research was commissioned by the UK Health Foundation and Department of Health, which were keen to identify and draw on global best practice in those areas of the NHS where central policymakers recognized significant shortfalls. One of these was in the area of community-based healthcare education. The whole research programme has been widely reported elsewhere, with the peer-reviewed publications,[4,5] including those specifically dedicated to relevant 'modernizing' educational developments in other countries.[6,7]

Context

The essential values expressed in this chapter are those of parity and reciprocity. They represent the normative context for transferable learning between countries in relation to medical education. They also constitute important contemporary values for those learning to become doctors today. As such they belong to the modern international idiom of relational healthcare, which views the quality of relationships as the conduit for converting formal health status into an actual sense of well-being.

This is a view frequently expressed by those leading the development of medical education in economically disadvantaged countries, where financial stringencies serve to restrict the growth of specialist scientific disciplines. Cost containment is, for example, a critical factor at the University of San Jose in Costa Rica where students at the Medical School are taught Social Development as a statutory responsibility, and the director of postgraduate studies is also titled Head of Social Action. The relational viewpoint is also, however, growing in its influence in the UK and some of the more economically developed and market-oriented countries. Here too there are growing pressures for increased financial controls over the use of expensive new therapies and clinical techniques, and these pressures coincide with an understanding that such therapies and techniques can only be managed effectively by doctors who acquire skills of communication with not just individual patients but with whole communities as well. In Costa Rica virtually all of its 1800 community-based doctors have attended one of the San Jose Medical School's five local campuses to gain a 14-module local healthcare management qualification. This underpins not only the contracts for medical provision in nationwide Social Action Development agreements between the university and the central Department of Social Security, but also their joint development of telemedicine as a community-oriented training resource. This is available daily to trainee doctors and their supervisors at the local *ebais* clinics throughout the country. For an NHS of foundation trusts and Public–Private Partnerships (PPPs) in England, the future parallel with this development in Central America may well lie in the relationship between university medical and business schools and the joint development of social marketing and community development modules for their combined students.

This comparison of Costa Rica and the UK points to the pivotal principle of international exchange in relation to any aspect of health systems development. Always adapt; never adopt. Seek to emulate; do not try to imitate. Context is all important, and this is especially true for medical education where sensitivity to cultural constraints – and opportunities – is overwhelmingly important. The case example of Costa Rica may stimulate new ideas, or it may act as a warning sign. It may even inspire; but it cannot simply be copied. The model of medical education of one state cannot successfully be imposed in the different environment of another. A vivid illustration of this statement is that within 5 years of the Berlin Wall being dismantled the Soviet *Semashko* model was almost unrecognizable throughout many of the former Russian satellite states.

This imperial reference is especially relevant to the UK where colonial traditions cast a long shadow over the mindsets of those leading medical education, even in the 'modernizing' post-Millennium era. The historical legacy is that of an independent sovereignty, which has often bordered on a sense of overweening superiority. For the NHS as an institution, and for British medical schools in particular, there is still the risk in the future of this past bequeathing an insularity that inhibits genuine two-way learning with other countries. Such an attitude, for instance, would be unthinkable at their Costa Rican counterparts where the Millennium Development Goals of the United Nations and World Health Organization[8] are formative influences in the shaping of learning objectives. In the UK Global Health remains a foreign subject[9] and, indicatively, even since 2000 standard texts for general medical practice trainees and trainers from one of the country's most established healthcare publishers contain virtually no international references beyond those to WONCA.[10,11] A popular official handbook for medical course organizers, issued long after the General Medical Council signalled its intention of ensuring that tomorrow's doctors would be more multifaceted and primary care oriented,[12] continues to refer to international settings solely in terms of a final chapter's set of warnings on the risks faced by medical students if they should venture into Africa, Eastern Europe or, as the worst scenario, any of the countries of the Middle East.[13] Much of the text reads as if it could have been written, if not in Victorian times, at least half a century ago.

For the UK medical education has been a one way street. Other countries learn from us. The medical schools of London, Manchester, Southampton, and Edinburgh have been seen in the UK as the basic reference points for the rest of the world: setting the standards and sustaining a professional infrastructure of Royal Colleges in the many different specialities of medicine that has spawned successor bodies across the world, from Thailand to Latvia and from Portugal to the West Indies. A willingness to be open to ideas and innovations from other countries has only come relatively recently. Ironically, this change of attitude has in part taken place among the British as a reaction to a new imperialism represented by the USA and the export of its health maintenance and managed healthcare models. The educational requirements needed for effective performance within these are no longer derived from vocational or personal orientations with self or internal regulatory mechanisms. Rather they follow what has been identified as a growing trend in Western countries towards learning as certificated 'repeat production' with external regulation that is bureaucratic in character and focused on details and procedural compliance.[14]

With the mantra of 'evidence-based medicine' the new American service models have their academic origins in Californian, Minnesota, and New England medical universities, where there has been the backing of powerful pharmaceutical and life science corporate interests. In the UK many medical professionals and educationalists, and central policy makers, have felt an urgent need to counterbalance these. A new interest in alternative approaches to community participation, combinations of health and social care services, health promotion, and interprofessional practice has arisen as a result as part of this reaction. With this new interest has come a willingness to learn from those countries where these components of contemporary health systems appear to be more advanced and, of course, effective in terms of maintaining medical status.

Transferable learning

Systems of medical education and healthcare do not automatically align. Indeed a creative tension between the two can generate a powerful and positive dynamic. In Chile, for example, there are some of the most multiprofessional healthcare teams in the world and the Catholic University in Santiago has been instrumental in their development. Its crucial role over 2003–06 was to redesign medical curricula to support six initial zonal health centres in which nutritionists, dentists, physical and occupational therapists, drugs dispensers and psychologists train and work alongside general medical practitioners, all responding to referrals triaged by an integrated community welfare and nursing team. The university role only crystallized, however, after the country had withstood two general strikes in which medical unions played a leading role; and significantly, the chief academic architects of the new curricula include immigrant medical educators from such countries as Germany, Ecuador, Bolivia, and even the UK. In a similar fashion the San Jose Medical School of Costa Rica cited (p. 182) drew on the legitimacy and stimulus provided by its enduring external links with McGill University in Canada and the Karolinska Institute in Sweden to help push through the quality assurance arrangements and primary care placements required for the implementation of its Social Action educational and ethical research programmes.

Without such levels of support and skilled facilitation the political balance between medical education and practice can easily be lost. In modern Britain there has been the danger of a cultural dissonance between the two comparable with that of New Zealand in the 1990s. Here the attempts to promote market competition in both the healthcare and higher educational sectors in tandem backfired as universities forged ahead while Crown Enterprise hospitals and mixed public–private status primary health organizations, sensitive to the needs of the indigenous Maori and other minority populations, lagged far behind. The result was a reversion over time to a more localized and less market oriented model of medical education, although with a stronger continuing emphasis on workplace learning.[15]

A similar gap between the curriculum and clinic has undermined successive attempts in Canada to roll out several otherwise internationally impressive developments in social medicine. The professional control of the former at provincial level, where the interests of independent practices and specialist consultants in hospitals tend to prevail, has successfully checked both local and national attempts to disseminate, for example, Quebec's approach to community health centres and Ontario's family health networks.[16] Indonesia, Zambia, and Thailand are among the other countries that have endured parallel experiences,[17] while the paramount importance of integrating major structural developments in medical education and healthcare practice has been demonstrated by the highly successful Ugandan Sector Wide Approach to both AIDS/HIV and malaria epidemics. In Uganda policymakers have consciously sought to adhere to the tenets of the World Bank's Comprehensive Development Framework, by establishing universal primary education as the platform for universal health promotion.[18,19]

The danger of medical education and medical practice being in not only a dissonant but also even a destructive relationship because of a lack of alignment with national health systems points to the need to define clearly the latter and their development. Even for parallel national systems being re-engineered in accordance with the 'modernizing' principles of partnership and decentralization there are substantial variations in organizational form. From a primary medical care organizational perspective the recent Warwick University research was able to recognize five types worldwide,[20] and with each of which a specific style of medical education can be associated as an appropriately applied pedagogy. These are set out below with examples of universities where medical educators are internationally – but not exclusively – recognized as leaders in the particular mode of learning.

For the UK the extended general practice would seem at first glance to be the organizational model that is most evident in the NHS environment. Certainly such medical schools as those of Leicester, Sheffield, and Exeter Universities have been closely associated with both the development of inter-professional practice based teams and the adoption of problem-based learning (PBL) approaches.[21–23] The two are mutually reinforcing. The PBL approach is to focus on the person of the patient, not just the symptoms; and the perception of the patient of his or her illness, rather than more narrowly on a scientific definition of the clinical condition. This opens the way for a range of professionals to contribute from their different sources of expertise and experience to the negotiation of diagnostic meaning and alternative intervention options. PBL is very much in the British tradition of family doctoring with loud echoes of one of its founding fathers, Michael Balint, who was writing at the time when the first Department of General Practice was established in a UK university medical school in Edinburgh.[24]

Closer examination of the organizational models in Table 13.1, however, quickly leads to the appreciation that the extended general practice is not the only modern international health system rooted in decentralization and partnership relevant to the UK. Indeed, it soon becomes apparent that they all are. Indeed, on reflection, it may well appear that the educational approaches attached to some of the newer primary care organizations are likely to exert the most powerful influences over future curriculum developments in medicine. As a result there is a clear logic in suggesting that they may well then also lead to more efficacious processes in healthcare delivery itself for collaboration and local resource management.

It is not difficult, for example, to recognize that the managed care enterprise finds its expression today in the NHS primary care and foundation trusts and the promulgation of practice-based commissioning. Given the strong political

Table 13.1 International systems of healthcare delivery and education.

Primary care organization	Educational model	Curriculum leaders	Host nations
Extended general practice	Problem-based learning	Maastricht, Kuopia, Linjöping Universities	The Netherlands, Finland, Sweden
Managed care enterprise	Evidence-based medicine and management	Minneapolis, Metropolitan (Mex), Auckland Universities	USA, Mexico, New Zealand
Polyclinic	Transdisciplinary/ values-based	Londrina, Santiago (Catholic), Newcastle (NSW) Universities	Brazil, Chile, Australia
Community development agency	Civil society/ citizenship approach	Chiclayo, El Alto, San José Universities	Peru, Bolivia, Costa Rica
District health system	Community based education and service	Moi, Gezira, Western Cape Universities	Kenya, Sudan, South Africa

and economic ties of the two countries a two-way relationship between the UK and the USA is scarcely a surprise, with the latter already claiming to possess by the turn of the century over 28 000 scientifically endorsed clinical guidelines as a teaching resource for the evidence-based medicine, and management approach.[25] Similarly, the hybrid organizational developments that characterize healthcare franchises in such countries as the Philippines and Colombia, where institutional outreach services are often the norm, have their Western counterparts now in the growing number of mixed public–private status social enterprises.

For both the growing movement towards values-based education in medicine (VBM), at such universities as far apart as Warwick in England and Newcastle in Australia, helps underpin and legitimize the often commercially oriented changes taking place. At the heart of VBM is a liberal educational impulse that seeks to ensure that new doctors are more sensitive than their predecessors to very different ethnic, social, and generational expectations of what comprises health, who constitutes an effective healthcare practitioner and where treatments take place. It is an impulse designed to help those involved in both the teaching and learning of medicine acquire the skills and mental attitudes required to practice successfully in a globalized and multicultural society. Its logic of tolerance also paves the way for novel organizational models in which, for example, hospitals are no longer largely closed institutions but hub and spoke models and patients are consumers and customers as well.

Greece offers a role model for such a style of development with its multiple forms of healthcare in its 17 geographic health regions, in all of which the Presidents also hold academic appointments in university medical and health-care faculties.[26]

Both VBM and evidence-based medicine are pedagogic developments that internationally have a particular appeal to medical schools in the private sector. They can both be understood as market oriented and focused on the individual user. As such they are attractive to sponsors, from the pharmaceutical industry and elsewhere, and are still seen as socially responsive and responsible. Globally such educational developments are paving the way for a major growth in the number of private medical schools, in relatively few of which is general medical practice or family medicine included in the curriculum. The figure for example is less than 50% in four of the countries cited above: Chile, Colombia, Greece, and the Philippines; and similarly low proportions apply in such other countries as Slovakia, Mexico, and Thailand where the private sector expansion of medical education seems synonymous with additional profit-oriented medical specialties.

For the UK some of the most interesting developments in medical education are taking place in the 'modernizing' countries of Sub-Saharan Africa and Latin America. Their relevance to the UK arises from their peculiar strengths in relation to participation, not least in terms of course design. In both parts of the world the relationship between medical education and medical practice is more interactive than it is in either Europe or North America. The development of service and curricula go hand in hand. Doctors do not simply train and then do medicine. Education and practice are in a concurrent not consecutive relationship. They are not seen as sequential. They continuously shape each other. The outcome can be a real dynamism in medical teaching and learning.

The community development agency has been the principal organizational model recently espoused by most 'modernizing' policy makers in Latin American healthcare. Its most obvious characteristic is the inclusion of substantial and sometimes majority lay representation on the management boards of medical service units. Among these representatives, almost invariably, are university academics from a range of healthcare and non-medical disciplines. In return university decision making structures are heavily weighted in favour of local community representatives. These changes need to be understood in the cultural context of a continent in which the regeneration of professions and the relationship between professions is part of a widespread move to create new civil societies, often in response to catastrophic civil conflict and breakdown.

The community development model can be found as part of the *Progresa* programme in Mexico aimed at extending primary care to five million more people partly through 1-year rural training and work placements for final year medical students; as part of the nationwide *Misiones* in Venezuela where voluntary local health cooperatives have been instrumental in the development of a new 5-year integrated family and social medicine qualification; and, of course, in Brazil with its 5000 new local community health and welfare centres where the transdisciplinary approach to medical education is most apparent in the mix of health and social care students training together. Among the various initiatives taking place in Latin America Peru, however, remains the exemplar of the modern civil society approach to medical education and practice.

By 2003 there were 760 *Comunidades Locales de Administracion de Salud* (CLAS) in Peru responsible, under the terms of the Ministry of Health's 2002 decentralization laws, for the management of over 1200 local clinics and hospitals.[27] A CLAS managing committee usually consists of a medical director and six lay members, of whom three are elected by the local community and three selected by local social organizations, including educational establishments. Each member has a designated lead role for a community health education priority. Nationally the CLAS come together in the regional and national assemblies of *ForoSalud*, a forum for civil society development that promotes holistic health and well-being principles and cross-sectoral collaborations. Its intellectual leadership comes from the social sciences, and much of its funding from liberal grant making foundations in the USA. The outcome for medical education is a national 'Future Generations' programme based on 'Social Managerialism', with medicine inextricably linked to issues of social control.

Existing Peruvian doctors did not originally want this. The changes only came after the debate about medical practice and its educational prerequisites was brought together in what were termed 'Service circles' that embrace, in particular, local women's movements and seniors' groups alongside health and education professionals. A supportive policy and financial framework was provided from 1991 to 1997 by the government's National Fund for Social Development and Cooperation, which sought explicitly to 'overcome medical opposition and resistance'. This has had its counterparts in Nicaragua, Bolivia, Mexico, Chile, and Costa Rica. In each of these today university medical schools have ownership of and accountability for up to 10% of the countries' healthcare facilities, with local community support. These facilities are the sources of ongoing curriculum change and testify to the scale of change taking place in Latin America through the implementation of a global 'Towards

Unity for Health' (TUFH) paradigm that postulates a five-way equivalence and interdependence between local communities, medical professions, national politicians, higher education, and private businesses.[28]

The TUFH philosophy has been endorsed by the World Health Organization. In Sub-Saharan Africa this has worked alongside the World Bank and the UK Department for International Development to support the district health system model and sector-wide approach to strategic aid and development. Based usually on population units of about 500 000 both demand a new multistakeholder approach to medical education, with non-governmental organizations especially influential because of the economic reliance on external charities and benefactors. In Uganda, for example, the creation of a combined curriculum for nursing, pharmacy, dentistry, and medicine through the local outreach training centres of Makerere University has been dependent on generosity of the Rockefeller Foundation, CAFOD, Action Aid and other donors. Parallel developments for trainee doctors can be identified throughout South Africa, Kenya, Tanzania, Malawi, and the Sudan. In each there are differences of emphasis in curriculum development. In South Africa the subject of rehabilitation is a recurrent feature of, for example, the 'Shared Community Based Practice' programme of the Western Cape University where trainee doctors and physiotherapists undertake placements together, while at the Durban Medical School a PBL approach is utilized in trainees' community attachments across Kwa-Zulu, Natal in which budding occupational therapists are especially prominent. In the Sudan meanwhile, at Gezira University's Faculty of Applied Medical Sciences in Khartoum, it is health psychology that supplies the topic on which medical students come together to learn as undergraduates with counterparts from all the other healthcare disciplines.

The African model of medical education with the widest international reputation is that of the 'Community Based Education and Service' pioneered in northern Kenya by Moi University. Based on a series of partnership arrangements between the medical school and the people of Eldoret, after an initial induction visit, students spend from year 2, a minimum of 3 weeks a year located in a community health facility as part of an interprofessional team working with local people to identify needs and to develop programmes to address specific healthcare priorities. The focus is on disease prevention and neighbourhood capacity building. Medical and other healthcare students do not simply have the chance to test and extend their learnt clinical skills outside hospital settings, they also learn as doctors how to become integral to the process of defining health, planning services, and locally respond to identified needs, which can range from new vaccination campaigns to freshwater jars and daycare schemes. As a result in Kenya the concept of medicine in Kenya is genuinely multistakeholder, incorporating not just intra- and interprofessional learning but community education as well.

Conclusions

The examples from Sub-Saharan Africa illustrate again the importance of locating medical education in its cultural context, even at a time when there is greater scope for transferable learning between countries because of the comparability of contemporary healthcare reforms based upon organizational principles of partnership and decentralization. Sensitivity to particular context remains still of crucial significance in medical education, where developments 'precipitated' by top-down structural initiatives are often counter productive. As the recent experience of many countries, including both the UK and Canada indicates, an awareness of the 'enabling' historic, social, geographic, and, above all, political determinants of a health system continues to be the platform on which progressive interprofessional and community-oriented changes in curricula can be built.[29,30] However, it is now evident that this awareness should incorporate international perspectives, sometimes from previously unlikely locations; and that there is clearly a potentially rich resource for UK medical schools to draw upon in other countries.

References

1. Secretary of State for Health. *The new NHS – modern, dependable.* Cm 3807. London: The Stationery Office, 1997.
2. Secretary of State for Health. *The NHS plan – for investment and reform.* London: Department of Health, 2000.
3. Hargadon J, Staniforth M. *A health service of all the talents: developing the NHS workforce.* London: Department of Health, 2000.
4. Meads G, Iwami M, Wild A. Transferable learning from international primary care developments. *Int J Health Plann Manage* 2005; **20**, 253–267.
5. Meads G. *Primary care in the twenty first century: an international perspective.* Oxford: Radcliffe Publishing, 2006.
6. Wild A, Meads G. Practice teaching in a global world. *J Practice Teaching* 2004; **5**(3): 5–19.
7. Ashcroft J, Meads G. *The case for interprofessional collaboration in health and social care.* Oxford: Blackwell Publishing, 2005.
8. World Health Organisation. *Health in the millennium development goals.* 2007. http://www.who.int/mdg/goals/en/print.html/.
9. McKee M. A UK global health strategy: the next steps. *Br Med J* 2007; **35**: 110.
10. Middleton P, Field S. *The GP trainer's handbook.* Oxford: Radcliffe Medical Press, 2001.

11. Gear S. *The complete MRCGP study guide*. Oxford: Radcliffe Publishing, 2006.

12. General Medical Council. *Tomorrow's doctors: recommendations on undergraduate medical education*. London: GMC, 1993.

13. McEvoy P. Educating the future GP. Oxford: Radcliffe Medical Press, 1998.

14. Entwistle NJ, Peterson ER. Conceptions of learning and knowledge in higher education: relationships with study behaviour and influences of learning environments. *Int J Educ Res* 2004; **41**: 407–28.

15. Mutch C. Educational policy for dynamic change in New Zealand. *Int J Educ Res* 2004; **41**: 553–63.

16. Beland F. Preventive and primary care access systems. In *Health care systems in transition* (Eds Powell FD, Wessen AF). London: Sage, 1999; pp. 173–98.

17. Miller Franco L, Bennett S, Kanfer R. Health sector reform and public sector health worker motivation: a conceptual framework. *Soc Sci Med* 2002; **54**, 1255–66.

18. Okuonzi SA, Birungi H. Are lessons applicable from the education sector applicable to health care reforms? The case of Uganda. *Int J Health Plann Manage* 2000; **15**, 201–19.

19. Njie H. Poverty and ill health: the Ugandan national response. *Development* 2001; **44**: 93–8.

20. Meads G. Family medicine: future issues and perspectives. In *Family medicine at the dawn of the 21st century* (Eds Garcia-Peña C, Muñoz O, Duran L, Vazquez F). Mexico DF: Instituto Mexicana del Seguro Social, 2005; pp. 17–34.

21. Anderson LA, Persky NW, Whall AL *et al*. Interdisciplinary team training in geriatrics: reaching out to small and medium sized communities. *Gerontologist* 1994; **34**, 833–8.

22. Poulton BC, West MA. Effective multidisciplinary teamwork in primary health care. *J Adv Nurs* 1993; **18**: 918–25.

23. Pereira Gray DJ, Goble RE, Openshaw S *et al*. Multiprofessional education at the Postgraduate Medical School, Exeter University. *Ann Community-Oriented Educ* 1993; **6**: 181–90.

24. Balint M. *The doctor, his patient and the illness*. London: Pitman Medical, 1964.

25. Niessen LW, Grijseels EW, Rulten FF. The evidence-based approach in health policy and health care delivery. *Soc Sci Med* 2000; **51**: 859–69.

26. Tountas Y, Karnaki P, Pavi E. Reforming the reform: the Greek national health system in transition. *Health Policy* 2002; **62**: 15–29.

27. Iwami M, Petchey R. A CLAS act? Community-based organisations, health service decentralisation and primary care development in Peru. *J Public Health Med* 2002; **24**(4): 246–51.

28. Boelan C, Haq V, Hunt M *et al*. Improving health systems: the contribution of family medicine. Geneva: WONCA, 2002.

29. Abelson J. Understanding the role of contextual influences on local health care decision making: case study results from Ontario, Canada. *Soc Sci Med* 2001; **53**: 777–783.

30. Meads G. *Walk the talk: sustainable change in post-2000 interprofessional learning and development*. London: UK Centre for the Advancement of Interprofessional Education, 2007.

Chapter 14

Maturing learners

Ed Peile

We don't grow old: when we stop growing, we become old.

Deepak Chopra (1993)[1]

Introduction

Medical educationalists currently focus the bulk of their attention on learners in the age range 18–65, with the most intensive activity being registered in the young adult decade from 18 to 28 years. Continuing professional development predicates that the education of doctors will continue until retirement, and the combined pressures of an increasing emphasis on revalidation and updating, and a trend towards later retirement mean that we will see more demand for medical education of doctors in their sixties and seventies.

This chapter will examine some of the considerations for medical education as learners mature. Maturation happens over time and, initially at least, moves forward chronologically so that we mature with age. There are many differences between ageing, which advances until death, and maturing, which is a process that may peak and arrest. We need to examine the intertwined influences of physical and psychological development, of incremental life experience, social change, and of changes in ethos and moral perspectives on learning as the clock ticks on. Maybe this should read as the clocks tick, because there is something asynchronous about the *zeitgebers* of maturation.

The concept of maturity

Like age, maturity is a value-laden concept. Just stop and think for a moment about some of the epiphenonema of maturity in the parallel worlds of law, agriculture, human biology, and education. Maturity has been defined as the time when growth has stopped and the body is developed – and the inevitable consequence is a concept of biological peaking with the 'prime of life' coinciding with optimal athleticism and sexual prowess around 20 and decline thereafter. Maturity has other implications, however; in the financial world it is also the time when an obligation must be repaid (bonds and insurance policies mature) and in law, the time when one is deemed to be competent – competent enough to make decisions or to purchase poisons. Mature wines are worth more, as there is a ripening process, and the better the wine, the longer it will benefit from maturation, but beware that which has gone brown at the edges. The concept emerges that maturing is a finite process: there comes a time when one has matured.

This concept needs to be questioned in an educational context. There is reason to consider that maturation may be a continuous process of psychological development, and one that is only arrested by a decline in cognitive faculties.

By and large, maturity has, I suggest, a more positive connotation than age. To be described as a mature doctor is perhaps more complimentary than to be called an old doctor, indeed the latter descriptor might trigger reference to the laws against age discrimination in the UK. We should therefore unpick what is valued about maturing in medicine and what are the implications for learning.

Maturing learners in educational theory

At the beginning of the last century, Pavlovian theories of behaviourism dominated educational theorising with Watson, Thorndike, Skinner, and others writing about conditioning responses in learners. There was little emphasis on maturation in their writings. John Dewey, the noted pragmatist, was really responsible for the shift in emphasis on to the importance of experience for learning. Laying the foundations for subsequent theorizing about learning cycles,[2] Dewey's system, postulated experience as always the starting point of an educational process; never the result.

For Dewey, all genuine education comes about through experience. Other key concepts in his work were democracy, continuity, and interaction.[3]

With the emphasis on experience and on interaction, comes a supposition that there must be an element of maturation in the learning process. Jean Piaget, a Swiss Developmental psychologist, emphasised the development of logical reasoning in early childhood experience and viewed progression towards 'adult mastery' as happening in stages.[4]

Lev Vygotsky defined the zone of proximal development as 'the distance between the actual developmental level as determined by independent problem solving and the level of potential development as determined through problem solving under adult guidance, or in collaboration with more capable peers.'[5] Notice that Vygotsky drew his definition widely enough to accommodate adolescent and adult learners as well as children. Rom Harre, the philosopher, argued meanwhile that childhood cannot be regarded as a pathway to maturity.[6] He defines adulthood in terms of prevailing social conventions and 'moral orders' rather than construing a maturing process that approaches a state of completion. For Harre and the social constructionists following in the wake of Vygotsky, social interaction is the essential component of meaningful learning through experience, and maturing occurs only through processing of interpersonal interaction.

Adult learning and androgogy

Writing in 1926, Edouard Lindeman[7] described his key assumptions about adult learners:

1. Adults are motivated to learn as they experience needs and interests that learning will satisfy.
2. Adults' orientation to learning is life-centred.
3. Experience is the richest source for adults' learning.
4. Adults have a deep need to be self-directing.
5. Individual differences among people increase with age.

The novelty of Lindeman's approach lay in the connection of the previously disconnected activities of learning for career advancement and learning for self-actualization. His influence can be detected over 40 years later in the five basic hypotheses of Carl Rogers.

1. We cannot teach another person directly, we can only facilitate his learning.
2. A person learns significantly only those things that he perceives as being involved in the maintenance of, or enhancement of, the structure of self.
3. Experience that, if assimilated, would involve a change in the organization of self, tends to be resisted through denial or distortion of symbolization.
4. The structure and organization of self appear to become more rigid under threat and to relax its boundaries when completely free from threat. Experience that is perceived as inconsistent with the self can only be assimilated if the current organization of self is relaxed and expanded to include it.
5. The educational situation that most effectively promotes significant learning is one in which (a) threat to the self of the learner is reduced to a minimum, and (b) differentiated perception of the field is facilitated.

A crucial difference, however, is that Rogers, writing 'Freedom to Learn' in 1969,[8] did not confine his theorizing to adults. In between the time of Lindeman and Carl Rogers' seminal work had come Malcolm Knowles and his theory of androgogy. Knowles had taken issue with a pedagogical model, designed for teaching children, whereby teachers take full responsibility for all decision making about the learning content, method, and timing of the curriculum. He felt that the 'submissive' learners of childhood did not represent adult learning, and he derived an 'androgogical' model focused on the education of adults. Knowles' precepts of androgogy are:

- adults need to know why they need to learn something;
- adults maintain the concept of responsibility for their own decisions, their own lives;
- adults enter the educational activity with a greater volume and more varied experiences than do children;
- adults have a readiness to learn those things that they need to know in order to cope effectively with real-life situations;
- adults are life-centred in their orientation to learning;
- adults are more responsive to internal motivators than external motivators.

Other processes of learning requiring 'adult' maturity were soon built on the foundations of androgogy. The notion arose that adult education programmes should seek to help adult learners transform their very way of thinking about themselves and their world – what Mezirow calls 'perspective transformation'.[9] Brookfield[10] proposes that this can be achieved through the development of competence in 'critical reflectivity', and put this forward as a maturing competence.

Wlodowski[11] suggests that adult motivation to learn is the sum of four factors:

1. *Success*: adults want to be successful learners.
2. *Volition*: adults want to feel a sense of choice in their learning.
3. *Value*: adults want to learn something they value.
4. *Enjoyment*: adults want to experience the learning as pleasurable.

Wlodowski's work built on expectancy theory,[12] a classic theory of adult motivation in the workplace that suggests that an individual's motivation is the sum of three factors:

1. *Valence*: the value a person places on the outcome.
2. *Instrumentality*: the probability that the valued outcomes will be received given that certain outcomes have occurred.
3. *Expectancy*: the belief a person has that certain effort will lead to outcomes that get rewarded.

One of the earlier attempts to explicate multiple intelligences was Horn and Cattell's theory of *fluid* and *crystallized* intelligence.[13] Crystallized intelligence is a function of experience and education, and increases in adult years. The presumption was that any loss in fluid abilities was compensated for by crystallized intelligence in stable environments. In fact, adults do show some loss of fluid abilities, particularly on speeded tasks. But, they also become better at using the knowledge they have, and this may be deemed a maturing aspect of learning.

Bright reviewed the many criticisms of androgogy in 1989,[14]

> It is suggested that the study of adult education attempts the impossible by over-identifying with the academic, theoretical model of the intrinsic disciplines. It is not being suggested that there are no differences between adults and children. On the contrary, there are probably many, but, whatever the nature and extent of such differences, it is very doubtful whether they can be accurately described and encapsulated within gross and simplistic dichotomies such as those suggested by Knowles.

Perhaps the most trenchant criticism of androgogy came from Geoff Norman[15] 'Nowhere did Knowles ever lift an experimental finger to test any of his assumptions.'

Not only did androgogy, as a collection of propositions, spark intense debate, but it also induced a focus on adult learning in the social sciences and led to considerable research activity among clinical and developmental psychologists, sociologists, educationalists, and philosophers.

Houle[16] categorized learners as follows:

1. The *goal-oriented learners*, who use education for accomplishing fairly clear-cut objectives.

2. The *activity-oriented*, who take part because they find in the circumstances of the learning a meaning that has no necessary connection – and often no connection at all – with the content or the announced purpose of the activity.

3. The *learning-oriented*, who seek knowledge for its own sake.

Maturing in ability to reflect

Williams[17] defines reflection after Boyd and Fales,[18] 'Reflection ... is the process of internally examining and exploring an issue of concern, triggered by an experience, which creates and clarifies meaning in terms of self, and which results in a changed conceptual perspective' (p. 30).[17]

An intelligent 'pause for thought' was recognized by Harvey Siegel as an essential component of learning and 'Critical thinking'.[19] Williams adopted the concept of the 'reflective glance' from Schutz[20] commenting that this

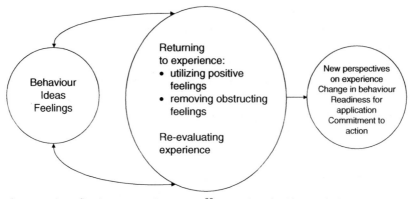

Fig 14.1 The reflection process in context.[22] Reproduced with permission.

glance will penetrate more or less deeply into the lived experience, which is at the centre of professional learning.[17] This concept had earlier been adopted by the Further Education Unit: 'The individual's experience needs to be followed by some organised reflection. This reflection enables the individual to learn from the experience, but also helps identify any need for some specific learning before further experience is acquired' (p. 21).[21]

Boud *et al.*[22] mapped out this reflection process, emphasizing the individual and unique perception of each learner.[23]

There has to be an iterative process between knowledge and experience for learning to occur. Adult learners, who develop competence in 'critical reflectivity',[10] can transform their very way of thinking about themselves and their world.[9]

Donald Schön, working with Chris Argyris in Harvard consultancy, did much to identify the relevance of reflection to medical learners, distinguishing the importance of reflection-in-action from the reflection-on-action that comes after the event.[24–26]

Carl Rogers, as a humanistic psychologist, did not limit his observations on autonomous self-directed learning to adults, and indeed much of his writing shows the influences of his early work with children. His work on development of personality remains one of the most important contributions to the understanding of maturing learners.[8] He described principles rather than stages of learning, and he focused on the 'fluid and changing gestalt' in the development of self-concept. Famously, he saw 'unconditional positive regard' as the key to self-actualization,[27] which is a fundamental attribute of lifelong learning, and has been endorsed by Heron[28] in his work on helping medical learners to mature in reflection.

Reframing is an important construct in the process of using knowledge acquired in courses, workshops, and conferences, and one that probably needs practice in the art of mediating between theory and practice, in order to reveal new meanings in theory and new strategies for practice.[29] This is an example of a skill in reflective learning that is a candidate for proxy marker status in estimating a learner's maturity in the art of reflection.

Implications for the medical teacher of conceptualizing the maturing learner

Uncertainty in the mind of the learner may be denied by medical learners[30] but when recognized, it presents opportunities for the facilitative teacher[31] and as many authors have pointed out,[32–34] there is no firm demarcation between where case learning finishes and professional supervision starts. Often, in educational meetings, the facilitator has the role of a professional supervisor. Howkins and Shohet[33] described three categories of supervision: educational, supportive, or managerial.

Pratt[35] examined the issue of learner dependency and proposed a four-quadrant model to reflect combinations of needs for high or low direction or support. By implication, the maturing learner will require less direction and lower levels of support. But it is important to remember that however mature the learner, there will never come a time when they can exist without any support. Judicious combinations of support and challenge will always be needed to promote the learner's development, and many educators find it useful to remember the axiom: 'One *supports being* … One *confronts doing.*'

As regards the value of challenge to learners, it has been argued that controlled exposure to challenge can enhance participants' psychological resilience. An adventure learning supports this claim, demonstrating significantly greater gains in psychological resilience for 41 young adults participating in 22-day Outward Bound programmes than in a control group.[36]

It was Gerald Grow[37] who helpfully derived a taxonomy of stages in learner autonomy, which related the student stage to an appropriate related tutor behaviour.

For the dependent learner in Grow's model, the most appropriate tutor is the authority expert. Think of the new doctor working in an unfamiliar clinical environment – he is only too grateful to have an expert at hand to guide him safely through the first day, be she nurse or senior doctor! Dependent status of the learner may be a relatively fixed personality attribute, or it could be a stage of development on the road to self-direction. Either way, whether we are dealing with a 'maturing learner' process or merely encountering

Table 14.1 Grow's stages in learning autonomy.[37] Reproduced with permission.

Stage	Student	Teacher	Examples
Stage 1	Dependent	Authority, coach	Coaching with immediate feedback, drill. Informational lecture. Overcoming deficiencies and resistance
Stage 2	Interested	Motivator, guide	Inspiring lecture plus guided discussion. Goal-setting and learning strategies
Stage 3	Involved	Facilitator	Discussion facilitated by teacher who participates as equal. Seminar. Group projects
Stage 4	Self-directed	Consultant, delegator	Internship, dissertation, individual work or self-directed study group

different types of learner, it behoves the clinical educator to adapt to the learner stage, and not to induce mismatches, as Grow illustrates.

Progressive independence is a highly effective model in medical education,[38] and one that has been long recognized.[39]

Boltanski and Thevenot's sociology of critical capacity[40] revises Durkheim's theory of moral fact[41] and constructs a taxonomy of motivation around the concept of orders of worth, which in considering adult learning is perhaps more useful than Kohlberg's often cited work on development of moral reasoning in childhood.[42]

Boltanski and Thevenot's work has relevance for adult learning in medicine. If tutors can understand the relative contributions of a learner's drivers

Table 14.2 Match and mismatch between learner stages and teacher styles.[37] Reproduced with permission.

	T1: Authority expert	T2: Salesperson, motivator	T3: Facilitator	T4: Delegator
S4: Self-directed learner	Severe mismatch students resent authoritarian teacher	Mismatch	Near match	Match
S3: Involved learner	Mismatch	Near match	Match	Near match
S2: Interested learner	Near match	Match	Near match	Mismatch
S1: Dependent learner	Match	Near match	Mismatch	Severe mismatch students resent freedom they are not ready for

Table 14.3 Boltanski and Thevenot's orders of worth.

Domestic	Values of family, community, and tradition
Civic	Values of public benefit, common will, the good of all and equality
Inspired	Values of personal growth, creativity, and spontaneity
Market	Values of material wealth, competitiveness, and short-term gain
Industry	Values of productivity, efficiency, functionality
Opinion	Values of recognition by others, fame, celebrity status

towards the 'human qualifications' of creativity as opposed to authority, celebrity, or expertise, they can work more in the respective emotional, or anecdotal, semiotic, or criterion-referenced/statistical information formats.

Carl Rogers[27] focus on unconditional positive regard is a powerful reminder to medical educationalists, versed in the 'positive first' routines of Pendleton, and the need to separate the person from the behaviours in feedback on professionalism, of the importance for the continued maturation of the learner of a fundamental humanistic respect by the teacher for the learner as an individual. A fully functioning person, according to Rogers[27] has a growing openness to experience – a prerequisite for experiential learning.

Peile *et al.*[43] categorized the behaviours by trainers that have been shown to be helpful to learners in general practice up to 10 years later.

Other aspects of maturing as medical learners

Several eminent medical educationalists, Schmidt *et al.*[44] and Regehr and Norman[45] among them, have examined the literature on educational development in respect of medical learners. Others have examined the evidence on what forms of continuing medical education impact on postgraduate medical learners and have related this to theories of adult learning.[46]

Meserve *et al.*[47] questioned whether 'clever nihilism' could be a developmental stage of cynicism that develops as evidence-based medicine learners progress from 'naïve empiricism' to 'mature pragmatism'. They admit, however, that it could also be an inherent, often latent, learning style.

Nath and colleagues[48] have looked in dental education at the possibility that professionalism may to some extent be related to the degree of maturity of the learner in healthcare fields. They comment that: 'The perception and significance of professionalism are likely to reflect one's maturity level, one's progression through the profession, or the distinction between actually "practicing a profession" and learning the "practice of a profession."' (p. 826).[48]

Their study indicated that perceptions of professionalism vary most with level of education and age and, to a lesser extent, with healthcare discipline and gender. They do, however, comment that their results may 'reflect a maturation process or an acceptance of the predominant values and mores of the professional group to which one belongs'.[48]

Ashley[49] is an enthusiast for apprenticeship learning in medicine, to maximizing the benefits of role modelling in medical learning by means of apprenticeship placements, and he refers to evidence that humans learn best by watching and copying.[49] Apprenticeship learning is predicated to a large extent on learner maturation processes – in time the diligent apprentice can achieve mastery.

Hayes *et al.*[50] looked for evidence that maturity reduces anxiety among medical students. The authors, citing adult learning theory, assumed that graduate entry students have potentially: higher motivation (career change and self-funding issues); more mature learning skills; increased self-direction; and more 'life experience'.

There is anecdotal support for a high level of motivation in graduate-entry students, and for a perception among clinical teachers that these students are more internally driven to learn which, in turn, motivates the clinicians to teach.[51,52] The whole question about medical students' motivation to learn has been discussed by Misch.[53] Older students have stronger motivation towards career choices in medicine.[54]

The evidence on learning styles suggests that they are determined at secondary school and although medical curricula can encourage different styles there is relatively little change.[55] Deep learning styles, whereby comprehension and contextualization is an essential component of learning, is the preferred style of educationalists wishing to prepare students for lifelong learning, although the value of 'strategic' learning styles, which accommodate some rote learning of material that is only of temporary value to medical students, is also recognized.[56] However, current evidence is that even with curriculum change, it is difficult to influence medical students' learning styles.[57]

One other attribute of maturity in learners may be their assertiveness as consumers of medical education. To combat the potential for disillusionment, schools must become learning organizations wherein double loop learning leads to learning about learning.[58] The introduction of GEM in Australia and London has been researched as a case study to examine the 'dynamic, complex and open' processes of change management.[59]

Maturing 'learning organizations' in medicine

Maturity as a learning organisation is measured by quality assurance indices: higher levels of maturity are taken to imply that an organisation has progressed further along the learning pathway.[60] There are recognized models of maturity that appear to assume not only that maturity is a measurable quality but also that higher levels of maturity lead to better process outcomes. An example of such a model is the e-learning Maturity Model (eMM), a quality improvement framework for e-learning in higher education consisting of 35 processes, subdivided into five process areas, each used to define a key aspect of the overall ability of an institution to deliver e-learning effectively.[61] The eMM, developed in New Zealand is being trialled by University of Manchester in the Higher Education Academy Benchmarking Pilot.

Graduate entrants to medicine

For many years graduates from other degree courses have studied medicine as undergraduates. In 2000 the UK followed Australia and USA in offering places on shortened fast-track courses for graduates entering medicine.[51,52]

The predictive value of A levels for performance at medical school by school-leavers could reflect their assessment of knowledge, motivation, or study habits.[56] Lower grades in A levels are also a predictor of early drop-out from medical school[62,63] so we can presume that factors that cause students to struggle at the later stages of secondary education persist into tertiary education. Is there a maturation process whereby such factors been filtered out by the time that students have demonstrated their ability to obtain a moderately well classified first degree? We do not yet know, and it will be some time before there are enough UK doctors who have graduated by the fast-track route to ascertain if A levels remain a predictor of success on graduate-entry medicine courses. The evidence that they are a predictor of success at post-qualification membership examinations[56] suggests that they are unlikely to have lost their predictive power at the graduate stage, and also hints at motivation as being an important component factor.

Personality measures have also been shown to predict success in UK school-leaver courses[56] as have learning styles.[56,64] The point of interest here is the apparent resistance to change of learning styles; there is little to support a process of maturation with such evident trait stability.

Early indications about maturing processes from graduate-entry programmes

It seems likely that in schools with a mixed entrance policy, graduates without science degrees do not struggle more than science-trained colleagues in early assessments.[65] If this is confirmed, it may suggest that for graduate entrants the experience of having 'learnt how to learn' at university is more important than the subject learning that took place. Early work from Australia demonstrates that tracking doctors qualifying from a medical school offering both graduate-entry medicine and school-leaver courses has shown that graduates are at least as well prepared for work as a junior doctor as their counterparts from conventional courses.[66]

Domains where graduates did feel better prepared included: interpersonal skills, confidence, collaboration, holistic care, and self-directed learning.[66] This may be partly attributable to type of education, but it is also possible that either greater age or maturity could account for some of these factors. There is, moreover, evidence that this is not simply an age phenomenon: another Australian study on perceived preparedness for junior doctor years found older graduates to be less confident on patient management than their younger peers.[67]

Despite the expectation that older (more mature) students will be advantaged by adult approaches to learning,[68] the experience at St Georges is that some can be disadvantaged by fixed learning approaches, greater financial concerns, and a scientific background that may be suboptimal for their learning progression.[50] Graduate-entry students have been found to make greater use of library facilities than fellow undergraduates on a 5-year course.[69]

Perhaps one of the most important attributes to be related to maturity is staying-power. A study in Leeds (not on graduate-entry courses) suggested that mature students had a lower than average attrition rate.[70]

Unfortunately, much remains to be answered both about the effectiveness of graduate-entry schools in relation to school-leaver education, and about influence of maturity.[71,72] Citing Oakeshott[73] 'what university has to offer is not information but practice in thinking', Horton asks, 'Can we put our hand on our heart and say that this is one of the chief concerns of those running medical schools today?'.[74]

A study on curriculum showed that course design differences accounted for more of the anxiety exhibited by medical students than any differences in maturity between student groups.[50] However, in another study from Australia, very early clinical exposure appeared to make no difference to graduates' perceptions of their basic practical skills and patient management.[67]

Mature medical learners

Perhaps most significant for medical education in considering the ongoing maturation of learners in continuing professional development is the work of Dreyfus and Dreyfus[75] and Benner[76] in categorizing the stages of maturation from novice to expert and in Benner's study, demonstrating who learns from whom in the clinical workplace. The expert, functioning at an unconsciously competent level, is not the easiest person to learn from.

Newman and Peile[77] considered some of the attributes of mature learners in medicine, and identified some of the appropriate strategies to address the challenges presented by learners who are entering roles at an advanced level of maturity.

The concept of 'biographical learning' may be helpful here. It is defined as 'a self-willed, 'autopoietic' accomplishment on the part of active subjects, in which they reflexively 'organize' their experience in such a way that they also generate personal coherence, identity, a meaning to their life history and a communicable, socially viable lifeworld perspective for guiding their actions' (p. 17).[78]

Mark Taylor points out the difficulty for senior doctors as mature learners to engage with learning that goes past the end-point of confirming a previously held view and engages with the often painful process of changing perceptions. He emphasizes that mature learners who take responsibility for the reflective, questioning entry step into learning cycles are better able to adapt to ensuing change.[79]

Conclusions

In this chapter we have looked at some of the evidence about maturing learners. Building on the work of the social constructionists, there appears to be considerable evidence to support the notion that the ability to increase the value of experience by meaningful reflection is a skill that can increase with maturity. Appropriate support to learners appears critical to this development, as is appropriate challenge, which contributes to learner resilience increasing. Medical learners who have both built up more experience on which to reflect, *and* matured at least to the point where they can admit uncertainty are likely to continue progressive growth in their learning, to the benefit of their patients.

References

1. Chopra D. *Ageless body, timeless mind: the quantum alternative to growing old*. New York: Crown Publishing, 1993.
2. Kolb D, Fry R. Towards an applied theory of experiential learning. In *Theories of group processes* (Ed. Cooper C). London: Wiley, 1975; pp. 33–57.
3. Dewey J. *Experience and education*. New York: Collier Books, 1938.
4. Piaget J. *The construction of reality in the child*. New York: Basic Books, 1954.
5. Vygotsky LS. *Mind and society: The development of higher psychological processes*. Cambridge, MA: Harvard University Press, 1978.
6. Harre R. The conditions for a social psychology of childhood. In *The integration of a child into a social world* ((Ed. Richards MPM). Cambridge: Cambridge University Press, 1974.

7. Lindeman E. *The meaning of adult education.* New York: New Republic, 1926.

8. Rogers C. *Freedom to learn.* Columbus, OH: Merrill, 1969.

9. Mezirow J. A critical theory of adult learning and education. *Adult Educ* 1981; **32**: 3–27.

10. Brookfield S. *Understanding and facilitating adult learning.* San Fransisco, CA: Josey Bass, 1986.

11. Wlodowski R. *Enhancing adult motivation to learn.* San Francisco, CA: Jossey-Bass, 1985.

12. Vroom V. *Work and motivation,* Revised Edition, San Francisco, CA: Jossey-Bass Classics, 2007.

13. Horn J, Cattell R. Refinement and test of the theory of fluid and crystallised intelligence. *J Educ Psychol* 1966; **53**: 253–70.

14. Bright B (Ed.). *Theory and practice in the study of adult education: the epistemiological debate. Radical forum on adult education.* London: Routledge, 1989.

15. Norman G. The adult learner: a mythical species. *Acad Med* 1999; **74**: 886–889.

16. Houle C. *Continuing learning in the professions.* San Francisco, CA: Jossey-Bass, 1980.

17. Williams P. Using theories of professional knowledge and reflective practice to influence educational change. *Med Teach* 1988; **20**: 28–34.

18. Boyd EM, Fales AW. Reflective learning: key to learning from experience. *J Humanistic Psychol* 1983; **23**: 99–117.

19. Siegel H. *Educating reason: rationality, critical thinking, and education.* New York: Routledge, 1988.

20. Schutz A. *The phenomenology of the social world.* Evanston, IL: Northwestern University Press, 1967.

21. FEU. *Experience, reflection, learning.* London: British Further Education Council Curriculum and Development Unit, 1981.

22. Boud D, Keogh R, Walker D. Promoting reflection in learning: a model. In Reflection: Turning Experience into learning (Eds Boud D, Keogh R, Walker D). London: Kogan Page, 1985.

23. Freire P. *Pedagogy of the oppressed.* London: Penguin, 1996.

24. Schön D. *The reflective practitioner: how professionals think in action.* New York, Basic Books, 1983.

25. Schön D. *Educating the reflective practitioner: towards a new design for teaching and learning in the professions.* San Francisco, CA: Jossey-Bass, 1987.

26. Schön D. *The reflective turn: case studies in and on educational practice.* New York: Teachers College Press, 1991.

27. Rogers C. *On becoming a person: a therapists view of psychotherapy.* London: Constable, 1961.

28. Heron J. The role of reflection in co-operative enquiry. In *Reflection: turning experience into learning* (Eds Boud D, Keogh R, Walker D). London, Kogan Page, 1985; pp. 128–138.

29. Russell T. Reframing: the role of experience in developing teachers professional knowledge. In *The reflective turn: case studies in and on educational practice* (Ed. Schön D). New York: Teachers College Press, 1991; pp. 114–187.

30. Katz J. Why doctors don't disclose uncertainty. In *Professional judgement: a reader in clinical decision making* (Eds Dowie J, Elstein A). Cambridge: Cambridge University Press, 1988; pp. 544–565.

31. Germana J, Lancaster R. Brain dynamics, psychopathological uncertainty and behavioural learning. *Integr Physiol Behav Sci* 1995; **30**: 138–50.

32. Gardiner D. *The anatomy of supervision: developing learning and professional competence*. Milton Keynes: Open University Press, 1989.

33. Hawkins P, Shohet R. *Supervision in the helping professions*. Milton Keynes: Open University Press, 1989.

34. Hughes L, Pengelly P. *Staff supervision in a turbulent environment. Managing process and task in front-line services*. London: Jessica Kingsley Publishers, 1997.

35. Pratt D. *The research lens: a general model of teaching*. Melbourne, FL: Kreiger Publishing Company, 1998.

36. Neill J, Dias K. Adventure education and resilience – the double-edged sword. *J Adventure Educ Outdoor Leadership* 2001; **1**: 35–42.

37. Grow G. Teaching learners to be self-directed. *Adult Educ Q* 1991; **41**: 125–49. Expanded version available online at: http://www.longleaf.net/ggrow/.

38. Kennedy TJ, Lingard L, Baker GR, *et al*. Progressive independence in clinical training: a tradition worth defending? *Acad Med* 2005; **80**: S106–11.

39. Irby DM. Clinical teacher effectiveness in medicine. *J Med Educ* 1978; **53**: 808–15.

40. Boltanski L, Thevenot L. The sociology of critical capacity. *Eur J Soc Theory* 1999; 2(3) 359–77.

41. Durkheim E. *The division of labor in society*. New York: The Free Press Reprint [1893]1997.

42. Kohlberg L. Moral education in the schools: a developmental view. *School Rev* 1966; **74**: 1–30.

43. Peile E, Easton G, Johnson PN, *et al*. The year in a training practice: what has lasting value? *Med Teach* 2001; **23**: 205–11.

44. Schmidt H, Norman G, Boshuizen HP, *et al*. A cognitive perspective on medical expertise. Theory and implications. *J Acad Med* 1990; **65**: 611–21.

45. Regehr G, Norman G. Issues in cognitive psychology: implications for professional education. *J Acad Med* 1996; **71**: 988–1001.

46. Davis M, Thompson M, Oxman AD *et al*. Changing physician performance: a systematic review of the effect of continuing medical education strategies. *JAMA* 1995; **274**: 700–5.

47. Meserve C, Kalet A, Zabar S, Hanley D, Schwartz MD. Clever nihilism: cynicism in evidence based medicine learners. *Med Educ Online* 2005; **10**: 4. www.med-ed-online.org/.

48. Nath C, Schmidt R, Gunel E. Perceptions of professionalism vary most with educational rank and age. *J Dent Educ* 2006; **70**: 825–34.

49. Ashley EA. Medical education – beyond tomorrow? The new doctor – Asclepiad or Logiatros? *Med Educ* 2000; **34**(6): 455–9.

50. Hayes K, Feather A, Hall A, *et al*. Anxiety in medical students. *Med Educ* 2004; **38**: 1154–63.

51. Carter Y, Peile E Graduate Entry Medicine; high aspirations at birth. *Clin Med* 2007; **7**: 143–7.

52. Carter Y, Peile E. Graduate entry medicine: curriculum considerations. *Clin Med* 2007; **7**: 253–6.

53. Misch DA. Andragogy and medical education: are medical students internally motivated to learn. *Adv Health Sci Educ* 2002; **7**: 153–60.

54. Wilkinson T, Wells J, Bushnell J. Are differences between graduates and undergraduates in a medical course due to age or prior degree? *Med Educ* 2004; **38**: 1141–4.

55. McManus I, Keeling A, Paice E. Stress, burnout and doctors attitudes to work are determined by personality and learning style: a twelve year longitudinal study of UK medical graduates. *BMC Med* 2004; **2**(29): 1–12.

56. McManus IC, Smithers E, Partridge P. A-levels and intelligence as predictors of medical careers in UK doctors: 20-year prospective study. *BMJ* 2003; **327**: 139–42.

57. Reid WA, Duvall E, Evans P. Can we influence medical students approaches to learning? *Med Teach* 2005; **27**: 401–7.

58. Davies HTO, Nutley SM. Developing learning organisations in the new NHS. *BMJ* 2000; **320**: 998–1001.

59. Prideaux D, McCorie P. Models for the development of graduate entry medical courses: two case studies. *Med Educ* 2004; **38**: 1169–75.

60. Neefe C. Comparing levels of organisational maturity of colleges and universities. University of Wisconsin MSc Thesis, 2002.

61. UTDC. University Teaching Development Centre, Victoria, New Zealand. http://www.utdc.vuw.ac.nz/research/emm/index.shtml (accessed 6 December 2007).

62. Peers I, Johnston M. Influence of learning context on the relationship between A-level attainment and final degree performance: a meta-analytic review. *Br J Educ Psychol* 1994; **64**: 1–17.

63. Bekhradnia B, Thompson J. *Who does best at university?* London: Higher Education Funding Council, 2002.

64. McManus I, Richards P, Winder B. Clinical experience of UK medical students. *Lancet* 1998; **351**: 802–3.

65. Rushforth B. Life in the fast lane: graduate entry to medicine. *Student BMJ* 2004; **12**: 368–70.

66. Dean SJ, Barratt AL, Hendry GD, Lyon PM. Preparedness for hospital practice among graduates of a problem-based, graduate-entry medical programme. *Med J Aust* 2003; **178**: 163–7.

67. Hill J, Rolfe I, Pearson S. Do junior doctors feel they are prepared for hospital practice? A study of graduates from traditional and non-traditional medical schools. *Med Educ* 1998; **32**: 19–24.

68. Kaufman DM. Applying educational theory in practice. *BMJ* 2003; **326**: 213–16.

69. Martin S. Impact of a graduate entry programme on a medical school library service. *Health Inform Libr J* 2003; **20**: 42–9.

70. Simpson KH, Budd K. Medical student attrition: a 10-year survey in one medical school. *Med Educ* 1996; **30**: 172–8.

71. Searle J. Graduate entry medicine: what it is and what it isnt. *Med Educ* 2004; **38**: 1130.

72. Prideaux D, Teubner J, Sefton A, Field M, Gordon J, Price D. The consortium of graduate medical schools in Australia: formal and informal collaboration in medical education. *Med Educ* 2000; **34**: 449–54.

73. Oakeshott M. The study of politics in a university In: *Rationalism in politics and other essays*. Indianapolis: Liberty Fund, 1991; pp. 184–218.

74. Horton R. Why graduate medical schools make sense. *Lancet* 1998; **351**: 826–8.

75. Dreyfus HL, Dreyfus SE. *Mind over machine: the power of human intuition and expertise in the era of the computer*. Oxford: Basil Blackwell, 1986.

76. Benner P. *From novice to expert: excellence and power in clinical nursing practice*. Menlo Park CA: Addison-Wesley, 1994.

77. Newman P, Peile E. Valuing learners experience and supporting further growth: educational models to help experienced adult learners in medicine. *BMJ* 2002; **325**: 200–2.

78. Alheit P, Dausien B. The double face of lifelong learning: two analytical perspectives on a silent revolution. *Stud Educ Adults* 2002; **34**: 3–22.

79. Taylor CM. Education and personal development: a reflection. *Arch Dis Child* 1999; **81**: 531–7.

Chapter 15

The European Working Time Directive and Postgraduate Medical Training: challenge or opportunity?

Michael J Bannon

Introduction

Junior doctors in training (as well as many of their seniors) have for generations worked long hours. In fact, until recently, there was a cultural acceptance among doctors of the need, especially in the acute specialties, to
work 80–100 hours per week with no guaranteed periods of rest or time off
following periods of on-call. It was argued that that this working pattern
offered not only many hours of exposure to multiple clinical scenarios
but also provided ample opportunities to undertake practical procedures.
In addition, there were perceived additional benefits for patients in terms of
continuity of care. Following on this, prolonged contact with patients allowed
for *continuity of training* in the sense that doctors could follow the clinical
progress of individual patients from admission, to treatment, and eventual
outcome. However, working long hours over prolonged periods of time
results in tiredness and fatigue and concern about doctors' working hours
has been expressed for many years. Concern may be summarized under
three headings:

1. The first area of concern relates to patent safety. It has been conclusively
    demonstrated that lack of sleep along with chronic fatigue on the part
    of doctors produces significant impairment of clinical judgement and
    in reaction time to emergencies.[1] The impact of sleep deprivation has
    been shown to be equivalent to that of consuming several units of alco-
    hol.[2] The effect may be subtle in that tired doctors may overtly appear to
    be functioning in a competent manner but more precise psychomotor
    testing will reveal significant deficiencies of certain aspects of their clinical
    performance.

2. There is some evidence from around the world to suggest that doctors who have been deprived of sleep following long periods of duty are at a significant risk of subsequent involvement in road traffic accidents.[3]

3. More recent observational studies have challenged the previously held beliefs regarding the educational benefits of working for long periods of time without appropriate levels of rest. It has now been shown that fatigued doctors do not learn as efficiently as when they are rested. In addition, they demonstrate poor retention of any new knowledge gained when they are tired.[4]

As a result of the above there is now a growing body of opinion worldwide that it is no longer appropriate for junior doctors to continue with their previous patterns of working. The arguments revolve around issues of patient safety, junior doctor well-being, and also their clinical training.

New Deal and European Working Time Directive

Two initiatives have attempted to address the issue of junior doctors' working hours: the New Deal for Doctors in the 1990s and more recently, the European Working Time Directive (EWTD). The Minister for Health in 1990 convened a working group in order to define a way forward with respect to improving the working lives of junior doctors. The resulting negotiations and debate undertaken between representatives of the medical profession, the Department of Health and the NHS resulted in the *New deal for junior doctors*.[5] This represented a package of measures aimed at improving working conditions for doctors in training. An initial target of 72 hours per week was set for those working to on-call rotas. Furthermore, limits were determined for maximum continuous hours of duty. However, initial progress towards achievement of the targets set by the New Deal was relatively disappointing. For example, 84% of junior doctors were alleged to be in breach of the standards set by the New Deal in August 2003. Perhaps this lack of compliance was a reflection upon the fact that implementation of the New Deal was not enforced by legislation.

The other significant influence in this respect resulted from the EWTD. The latter was devised to ensure the welfare of workers and also to protect the public. The Working Time Directive of the European Union was defined within Council Directive 93/104/EC on the 23 November 1993[6] and was subsequently amended by the Directive 2000/34/EC of the European Parliament and by its Council held on 22 June 2000. EWTD refers to a set of regulations that limit the numbers of hours worked with the aim of ensuring the health and safety of workers. Key features include limiting the maximum length of the working week to 48 hours within 7 days, and a minimum rest period of 11 hours in each 24 hours. EWTD regulations were extended to include junior doctors in training from 1 August 2004. In keeping with other European Directives, EWTD requires EEA member states to include its provisions within national legislation. A gradated implementation of EWTD among junior doctors was planned in the UK:

Timetable for full implementation of European Working Time Directive (Table 15.1)

However, full compliance with EWTD includes more than an estimation of average hours worked by junior doctors over a period of time. Further challenges for doctors' employers were set the SiMAP judgment in Spain (2000)[7] and the Jaeger judgment in Germany (2003).[8] The SiMAP judgment declared that the time spent by trainees in a clinical setting should be considered as actual working hours. The Jaeger judgment confirmed that this was the case even if the was allowed to sleep while on call. Both judgments continue to have legal status across the EEA.

August 2004 represented a date in time when an interim target of 58 hours per week for trainees was set in the UK. The majority of NHS Trusts met this target and to a large extent maintained compliance since 1 August 2004. This was achieved by means of a number of initiatives. These included:

+ Employment of more doctors in non training grades.

+ Revision of rotas, including cross-cover of several services by one individual or team.

+ Re-organization of clinical services.

+ Use of other health professionals to undertake tasks previously performed by doctors.

+ However, perhaps the most significant development from the junior doctor's point of view was the relatively sudden and almost universal

Table 15.1 Timetable for implementation of European Working Time Directive (EWTD).

Date	Deadline
June 2000	A timeframe was agreed to incorporate junior doctors into EWTD
August 2004	An interim 58-hour maximum working week was set Rest and break requirements become enforceable by law
August 2007	A further interim of a 56-hour maximum working week was set
August 2009	By this date a 48-hour maximum working week will be legally required

implementation of shift working in nearly all of the acute clinical special-ties. This has represented a radical change for many trainees in specialties where full on-call rotas (i.e. working a full day followed by a night resident on call during which time the trainee would have varying amounts of rest or sleep and would be expected to work some or all of the next day) have represented a more familiar pattern of working. It was not unusual until relatively recently for entire clinical teams to be on call together, i.e. consultant, registrar as well as more junior grades. This traditional firm structure rapidly disappeared with the arrival of shift patterns of working.

It is clear that implementation to date of EWTD has had a profound impact on junior doctors' working lives as well as on their life-style. A particular feature of clinical training of doctors in the NHS is that is embedded in service delivery. Any change in the way in which clinical services are organized will therefore also have implications for doctors' training. This was discussed at the House of Lords[9] when it was declared:

> We were surprised to learn that training hours had been reduced from 30,000 hours to about 8,000 hours since the early 1990s … further reduction in 2009 would cut this training time to 6,000 hours. We say more time is needed to work out a common-sense compromise that improves doctors' working conditions without putting standards of patient care at risk or harming medical training.

It is fair to say, however, that a distinction should be made between the over-all hours worked by junior doctors and the actual training that they receive. However, the key concern was that a reduction in doctors' working hours would by necessity also result in a reduction in time for their training.

International perspective

The number of hours worked by junior doctors and their patterns vary across the world. However, the issues and concerns are similar to those raised in Europe with a commitment in many countries to reduce the average number of hours worked per week by doctors.

- ◆ Europe:
  - • Allegedly Scandinavia has already achieved a 40-hour week for junior doctors. Norway has limited the length of the working day to 8 hours for the past 80 years while a 37-hour week is what is in place in Denmark. Danish medical training includes what is termed 'off site training' to a total of 300 hours over a 7-year training programme. While this approach undoubtedly facilitates a shorter working week, clinical contact with patients is reduced.

- The Netherlands has apparently successfully implemented WTD but does not include educational activities within the hours counted as work. In addition, a modular approach to training is promoted in that country.
- A varied and confusing picture is apparent across the rest of the European Economic Area with various member states claiming that compliance is achieved (a fact that has been refuted by informal surveys undertaken among trainees in those countries).

- Australian junior doctors do not work more than 40 hours per week.
- In New Zealand, junior doctors were limited to a maximum of 72 hours per week and 16 hours of consecutive work per shift since 1985; in fact New Zealand was one of the first countries in the world to implement a reduction in junior doctors' hours.
- In the USA, the Accreditation Council for Graduate Medical Education (ACGME) implemented an 80-hour week for junior doctors averaged over a 4-week period. Juniors must have at least one complete day off in every seven. While continuous periods of 30 hours on call are allowed, junior doctors are not allowed to admit new patients after 24 hours of duty.

Working Time Directive 2009

The changes to services provision and to doctors working hours (i.e. a further reduction to 48 hours per week) required by 1 August 2009 are imminent. The questions to be asked are:

1. Can we achieve the compliance required by WTD by 1 August 2009?
2. If yes to the above, can we do so and at the same time maintain high standards of care and patient safety?
3. Finally, can we not only maintain but actually protect appropriate standards of postgraduate medical training in what is in effect a shorter working week with shift working?

There is some evidence that challenges 1 and 2 above are achievable but at a cost. For several years, the Department of Health for England has implemented a series of pilot studies that have explored almost every possible aspect of EWTD implementation. The relevant website (http://www.healthcarework-force.nhs.uk/workingtimedirective.html) is a rich resource of findings from various pilot studies along with conclusions from regional and national conferences. Pilot studies have explored ways by which compliance might be achieved from a number of dimensions. The outcomes from the 17 pilots studies that looked at compliance for 2004 were published in 2005.[10]

The results were encouraging. Nearly all pilot studies enabled compliance with a 58-hour week for junior doctors. Furthermore, nearly half demonstrated additional benefits in patient care in terms of reduced waiting times for investigation and treatment as a result of more streamlined processes out of hours. A reduction in clinical errors by junior doctors was also claimed. Innovative solutions have been found for both the type of hospital providing care (teaching, specialist, large district general, rural/remote) and for different clinical specialties. Predictably there has been a tendency to provide cross-cover for several related specialties such as general surgery and trauma and orthopaedics. Cross-cover from other specialties is more difficult for paediatrics and obstetrics. Both are acute and highly specialized with limited possibilities of cover from other specialties. Pilot studies have also explored the feasibility of new clinical roles (healthcare workers undertaking tasks previously considered to those that should be completed by medical staff) along with newer and more flexible ways of working. Key overall themes from the 2004 EWTD pilots include the need for effective team working and flexibility of roles between doctors and other healthcare workers.

A further series of pilots have been commissioned in order to develop solutions for EWTD 2009 compliance. Three key areas have been identified:

1. 'Cooperative solutions', which refers to the development of cooperative and integrated solutions between organizations and agencies across a regional area.

2. 'Team working, handover and escalation', which ensures that effective handover between clinical teams takes place after each shift and that clinical teams have the skills to prioritize their input to urgent clinical situations when required.

3. 'Taking Care 24:7' represents a further a set of pilot studies that will explore new ways of working over the full 24-hour day. This will include the use of various healthcare staff to reduce the dependence on junior medical staff during the full working day.

Hospital at Night (H@N)

Another initiative that is complementary to EWTD and which has gained increased acceptance is the Hospital at Night Project or H@N.[11] The H@N project has gradually evolved over the last 10 years. It has been observed for many years that the traditional model for a medical on-call team was not based upon an objective assessment of volume and patterns of work or even upon patient need. The team structure was built around models of hierarchy with the most senior members of the team on call from home and the most junior being resident on call. Even in specialist hospitals it was not unusual to find multiple teams on call, many of them non-resident. In many cases, patients who became acutely unwell at night time were first assessed by the most junior member of the team who was often not fully empowered to make definitive therapeutic or diagnostic decisions. More senior members of staff would be called who would assess the clinical situation later. Delays in the diagnostic process and duplication of effort (especially the phenomenon of multiple clerking) were common. The H@N approach represents a radical paradigm shift. In essence, a dedicated multiprofessional, multidisciplinary team provides essential out of hours clinical cover. The team is small but experienced enough to rapidly assess and deal with acute clinical problems as they arise. It should be noted that for most specialties, there is a reduction in clinical activity requiring strictly medical input after midnight. This is especially the case for acute surgery. The Hospital at Night (H@N) concept proposes the establishment in hospitals of one or more multiprofessional teams who between them have the full range of skills and competencies to meet patients' immediate needs.

Key components of the H@N approach are:

1. Doctors work as part of a multidisciplinary team that has the competencies to deal effectively with emergency care out of hours. Importantly, this includes the ability to recognize when help from other professionals (such as the surgeon on call) may be urgently needed. The team co-ordinator is usually a senior nurse and the composition and skills of the team are determined by the patient case mix.

2. 'Low level' tasks (phlebotomy, form filling, venepuncture, phoning for bed availability) for doctors in training are reduced and are undertaken by other members of the team.

3. An effective bleep policy is implemented to ensure that doctors (and other members of the team) are not disturbed unnecessarily. Often this requires all bleeping request to be processed and approved by one senior member of the H@N. (One hospital has introduced an innovative approach to this problem known as *I-Bleep* by issuing all junior doctors with personal data assistants that not only act as bleeps but also contain information on patients as well as hospital protocols and formularies).

4. Effective patient management and flows of information results in a reduction in duplication of tasks.

5. Effective use of new technologies, such as digital imaging, e-prescribing, and electronic records where available also helps with above objectives.

Findings from the first survey of Hospital at Night implementation in the NHS since 2004 are encouraging.[12] By late 2007 nearly half of English NHS trusts in England had implemented H@N in some form and most reported benefits. In most cases, WTD 2009 compliance was achieved or at least managers felt that achievement of a 48-hour week for junior doctors would be feasible by 2009. There were additional apparent advantages. Several hospitals declared a reduction in reported clinical incidents and considered that this was directly attributable to the H@N project. Furthermore, H@N allowed for new opportunities to enhance and extend nursing roles. It is now accepted that H@N is not only a key component in the overall strategy WTD 2009 compliance but also an opportunity to enhance patient care.

Can Working Time Directive 2009 be achieved?

Experience to date would indicate that WTD 2009 compliance may only be achieved by a combination of integrated strategies. A team from Essex Workforce Confederation[12] devised a useful checklist has defined the 10 critical elements needed by hospitals and other healthcare providers.

1. Leadership commitment:
   - there are management and clinical leads with clearly defined roles and lines of accountability;
   - a project plan is agreed and implemented across the organization.

2. Management of change:
   - the changes needed for successful WTD 2009 implementation are change required to deliver WTD 2009 are identified and managed.

3. Rota design:
   - information on each specialty is collated with areas of non-compliance documented;
   - effective engagement of clinical staff (especially junior doctors) is undertaken.

4. New ways of working:
   - this includes definition of new roles, replacement roles, and extension of existing roles so that tasks previously undertaken by junior doctors are effectively assigned to other healthcare workers.

5. Training and development:
   - strategies are identified for the protection of medical training.

6. Technological solutions:
   - there is a need to exploit in a co-ordinated fashion the benefits of new technologies that include electronic patient records, prescribing, mobile computing along with network solutions.
7. Service redesign:
   - this includes service reviews that include patient pathways, process mapping, and analysis, H@N, and re-configuration of service delivery, such as separation of emergency and elective services.
8. Workforce plan:
   - a baseline overview of the current staff is defined that includes their competencies, age, grades, and retirement dates. The workforce needed for successful WTD 2009 implementation is calculated and a plan undertaken reconfigure to the new model.
9. Finance:
   - the financial implications of achieving compliance across the organization are identified and secured.
10. Communications:
    - this is essential but often overlooked. Active communication between all interested parties is self-evident but often absent.

Trainee welfare and the European Working Time Directive

Shift working has been in place for many professional groups for generations. For most junior doctors, this way of working represents a new and unfamiliar experience and a radical change from the relatively recent past. Concern has been expressed that junior doctors had not been adequately prepared in 2004 for the challenge of working night shifts and the resulting life-style changes. The Royal College of Physicians (London) has published guidance in this respect for junior doctors.[13] The key message was for doctors to understand the principles of what has been termed 'sleep hygiene' and to prepare well before a night shift. Night working generates what is accepted to be a sleep debt that increases after each shift. The resulting fatigue impairs concentration, reaction time, and ability to learn. Extra sleep before a night shift is recommended, preferably in the form of a 2-hour afternoon nap. Short naps during the night shift are also of benefit.

The other important issue is that of effective rota design. After 2004, many rotas included seven consecutive 13-hour shifts. This pattern of working has been shown to be dangerous with increased risk of error and accident. There is now a substantial amount of evidence that indicates good practice for rota design and implementation. It is feasible to create rotas that will be compliant in terms of hours worked with both EWTD 2009 and the New Deal. However, a key objective for 2009 will be to design rotas that are not only legal but that are sustainable. Ahmed-Little has outlined the principles for good rota design[14] that include:

+ Consultation with all interested parties (junior doctors, consultants, senior nursing staff, managers) before implementing changes.
+ Identification of local workload with subsequent matching to medical staffing levels.
+ Realistic start and finish times in the normal working day.
+ Recognition of the need for prospective cover for annual leave.

European Working Time Directive and postgraduate medical training

However, what about the implications of EWTD in the broadest sense (shift-working, shorter working week, required periods of rest and loss of traditional firm structure) on medical training? Experience from UK hospital Trusts and from the Department of Health EWTD pilot studies clearly indicate that compliance with the Directive is achievable in principle; that patient care and safety can be assured and that additional positive outcomes in patient care can be accomplished. However, it is true to say relatively scant attention has been specifically directed towards an evaluation of the impact of EWTD on postgraduate medical training. There was insufficient hard information available in August 2004 on this issue apart from almost unanimous resistance from the profession to the Directive. In particular, significant concern was expressed about the adverse effects on training. For this reason, the Department of Health (England) commissioned a research project undertaken by Sheffield University to specifically determine the real as well as the perceived impact of EWTD on postgraduate medical training and to develop models whereby training might be protected after August 2009. The team from Sheffield undertook their research in two phases:

+ A scoping phase that looked at existing evidence on the impact of a shorter working week on medical training by means of reviews of both the medical and organizational psychology literature and qualitative research among key stakeholders (trainees, trainers, and Trust EWTD leads).

♦ A primary research phase that would explore innovative methods whereby training would be enabled post August 2009 (the results of this part of the study are awaited).

The results from the scoping phase are now available.[15] The findings from both literature review and qualitative studies are as follows.

The overall perception from the medical literature is one of significant negative feeling towards the EWTD. In fact in 2004, trainees in several specialties considered that their life-style was worse since the introduction of a 58-hour week and night shifts were especially unpopular. They also lamented the demise of the traditional medical firm structure and some remarked that they no longer felt that they were members of functioning clinical teams. There were also issues regarding loss of training opportunities that were previously available by means of following the patient journey from admission to its end. Of even more concern was the observed reduction of attendance by trainees at structured training events such as grand rounds, journal clubs, tutorials, and clinical pathology meetings. This finding was hardly surprising as most of these training events occur during the day and as such would not be accessible to trainees working night shifts or on time off following a set of night shifts.

The craft specialties (surgery, gynaecology, and some of the more interventional medical and radiological subspecialties) reported a significant reduction in the number of operations and practical procedures that are documented in trainee log books. This finding was of particular concern in the surgical specialties. It was claimed that the total number of hours worked by trainee surgeons had diminished from 30 000 in 1997 to less than 7000 in 2007 with obvious effect on training opportunities. However, factors other than EWTD have resulted in an apparent reduction in out of hour operative experience for junior surgeons. A positive attempt has been made over the last 10 years to actually reduce operations after midnight on reasons of safety. In addition, the institution of Independent Treatment Centres (ISTCs) has resulted in the transfer of several operative procedures such as hernia repair and cataract surgery to outside of the NHS, thus reducing operative opportunities for surgical trainees. It should also be noted that similar concerns have been expressed by the Royal College of Anaesthetists regarding their trainees.

Other negative findings from both the medical literature and focus groups revolve around organizational issues. Many consultant supervisors felt that training is not fully valued by senior hospital managers. NHS service delivery targets (such as 18-week out-patient waits) were also considered to act as a deterrent to training. Some consultant supervisors felt pressurized to meet service commitments at the expense of training juniors. There were other constraints that were not directly linked to EWTD but nevertheless had an adverse effect on the capacity to train. These included perceived reduced funding for education and training, increased workload for consultants and inadequate educational infrastructure.

More positive themes with resulting possible ways forward were evident from the review of the organizational psychology literature. The importance of organizational support for training is well documented. In other words, organizations that support training gain additional benefits in terms of employee commitment and productivity. Those involved in medical education can also learn much from the concept of 'transfer of learning', i.e. ensuring that trainees actually transfer the skills acquired from structured training courses (advanced life support, basic surgical skills, and use of simulation) into the clinical workplace setting.

Putting all this together the project team proposed the following potential solutions for training post-August 2009:

1. Increased support and commitment at senior organizational level for medical education and training.

2. Enhanced educational infrastructure (protected time, support for trainers) to develop training within a clinical setting.

3. Exploiting to the full the educational potential of every moment of clinical time (to include ward rounds, handover, critical incidents).

4. Exploration of the use of simulators and clinical skills laboratories as an adjunct to clinical training.

5. Determine the full extent of transfer of learning for current established courses (such as Basic Surgical Skills and Advanced Life Support) into clinical practice.

It is not as yet clear whether any or all of the above will succeed in the protection of postgraduate medical training after August 2009. In particular, there is significant concern that surgical training will be significantly impaired. Opinion here is divided, however. Some surgeons claim that quality training in this specialty will not be feasible post 2009[16] and call for legislation to be changed or that surgical training should be considered as a special case. Other surgical trainers[17] hold a different perspective and believe that training can be implemented in a 48-hour week without compromise to training. However, urgent action on the part of both healthcare managers and doctors' educators is needed. EWTD 2009 is without doubt a significant challenge. However, the opportunity to improve doctors' working lives as well as patient safety must be embraced.

References

1. Landrigan CP, Rothschild JM, Cronin JW *et al.* Effect of reducing interns' work hours on serious medical errors among interns in intensive care units. *N Engl J Med* 2004; **351**: 1838–48.

2. Dawson D, Reid K. Fatigue and alcohol performance impairment. *Nature* 1997; **388**: 235.

3. Steier S, Vinker S, Bentov N, Lev A, Kitai E. Driver drowsiness – are physicians at a special risk? *Harefuah* 2003; **142**(5): 338–41, 398, 399.

4. Stickgold R. Sleep-dependent memory consolidation. *Nature* 2005; **437**: 1272–8.

5. Delamothe T. Juniors' new deal on hours. *BMJ* 1991; **302**: 1482.

6. European Union, Official Journal L307 (13 December 1993), 18–24.

7. SiMAP judgement: Sindicato de Médicos de Asistencia Pública v. Conselleria de Sanidad y Consumo de la Generalidad Valenciana, 2000.

8. Jaeger judgment: Landeshaupstadt Kiel v Norbert Jaeger, 2003.

9. http://www.publications.parliament.uk/pa/ld200304/ldselect/ldeucom/67/67.pdf/.

10. Department of Health. NHS Modernisation Agency. *Working time directive pilots programme final report.* London: Department of Health, 2005.

11. Bolger G, Walker W. Night moves. *Nurs Stand* 2007;**21**(31): 26–7.

12. Health Care Workforce. Hospital at Night Baseline report (2006). Available at: http://www.healthcareworkforce.nhs.uk/baseline_report_benefits_of_hospital_at_-night.html.

13. Horrocks N, Pounder R. Working the night shift: preparation, survival and recovery – a guide for junior doctors. *Clin Med* 2006; **6**: 61–7.

14. Ahmed-Little A. *Rota masterclass.* 2007; available from www.healthcareworkforce.nhs.uk/option,com_docman/task,doc_download/gid,1019.html/.

15. Davies H, Clarke J, Farrell K, Voelklein C, Paterson F. Impact of the European Working Time Directive on Postgraduate Medical Education (Unpublished report, 2007).

16. Benes V. The European Working Time Directive and the effects on training of surgical specialists (doctors in training): a position paper of the surgical disciplines of the countries of the EU. *Acta Neurochir* 2006; **148**(11): 1227–33.

17. Lim E, Tsui S. Impact of the European Working Time Directive on exposure to operative cardiac surgical training. *Eur J Cardiothorac Surg* **30**(4): 574–7. Health Care Workforce. *The WTD puzzle*

Chapter 16

Doctors in training: their views and experiences

Isobel Bowler

Introduction

This chapter reviews the published evidence from studies exploring the learner perspective on post-basic medical education in the UK. The learner group is all doctors who have completed their undergraduate medical training and who are undergoing foundation and specialty clinical training. This chapter does not look at the views and experiences of medical students or of trained clinicians undertaking continuing professional development. The available evidence is restricted because of recent radical changes in the organization of, and therefore trainee experience of, medical training in the UK.

Recent changes in the experience of doctors in training in the UK

Medical education in the UK has recently undergone a major transformation as a result of the implementation of the Modernising Medical Careers (MMC) Programme.[1] MMC arose from concern that Senior House Officers (SHOs) were largely providing service without having access to structured training.[2] This group was vital to the running of the UK health service, and carried a high clinical workload, but many were not receiving the formal training to help them acquire the knowledge and skills needed to advance their careers. The MMC programme was designed to address this and other key issues in medical training. It has two components. The first is a new 2-year Foundation Training programme for new medical graduates introduced in 2005. The roll out continued with the introduction of revised specialty training programme from August 2007.

Therefore, doctors graduating from medical school in 2004 or before have had a fundamentally different experience of training than subsequent cohorts of medical graduates. The first cohort of doctors undertaking the new foundation training programme completed it in August 2007, so recently that there is very limited published information on their experience.

Even before August 2005 the experience of doctors in training was being transformed as a result of changes to working practices. The main driver was the need to reduce hours worked by doctors to bring the NHS into compliance with the European Working Time Directive. Terms and conditions for all NHS employees have also been improved by the implementation of Improving Working Lives.[3] There have also been changes made to basic and overtime payments, which have affected the remuneration of doctors in training.

The first application round for the new specialty training programme at the start of 2007 was not successfully implemented. This particularly affected recruitment to the secondary care specialties. The difficulties of the Medical Training Application Service (MTAS) led to a legal challenge by a group of affected doctors[4] and resulted in an to an independent review led by Professor Neil Douglas.[5] In the words of the review team's report 'The introduction of the Medical Training Application Service (MTAS) triggered a major crisis in the medical profession'. At this stage views of the specialty training programme are understandably coloured by this recent past. The independent inquiry into MMC reported in January 2008.[6]

Search procedure

A search of the electronic Medline database since 1996 using key words ATTITUDE-OF-HEALTH-PERSONNEL and EDUCATION-MEDICAL-GRADUATE yielded 449 results. Limiting this to studies in Great Britain narrowed this to 71 records. Limiting it to records added since 2002 limited the results to 53. All these records were scanned. In addition hand searches of the last 2 years' contents of the journals *Medical Education* and *Education for Primary Care* was carried out. The recent publications of one of the Oxford Medical Careers group were also scanned.[7] The Department of Health, MMC, and the Postgraduate Medical Education and Training Board websites were searched for relevant documents.

Results

The search above yielded a low number of published reports that covered the views and experience of training. Twelve published papers were identified that had some relevance. Evaluations from pilot MMC projects and the results of a recent national survey of trainees were identified.

Experience and views of pre-registration house officer year

Pre-registration House Officers (PRHOs) are those doctor who have just graduated from medical school and are in the first year of clinical medical training.

As described above PRHOs in the UK are on the first of 2 years of foundation under the MMC reformed curriculum and are sometimes now referred to as foundation year 1 doctors, often shortened to F1 or FY1 doctors.

The Oxford Medical Career Group publishes regular reports on longitudinal surveys of cohorts of doctors,[7] the first postal survey being sent to each cohort as they graduate from medical school. Of recent graduates the 2002 cohort has been surveyed 1 and 3 years after graduation and the 2005 cohort has been surveyed 1 year after graduation. Because of time lag to publication after survey there are at the time of writing no published results of the survey of the 2005 cohort as they completed their first year of foundation training in 2006.

A key theme of the Career Group's work is 'to ascertain the views of doctors about their work, training, career and working environment'. In order to track the impact of the changes already described above, the Group have surveyed PRHOs at the end of their first year of clinical training in 2000, 2001, and 2003 (the sample drawn from UK medical school graduates of 1999, 2000, and 2002). Two papers in particular[8,9] report data on doctors' views of their first year of medical work. The study used closed questions and asked doctors to rate on a 10-point scale their experiences. Questions included 'How much have you enjoyed the PRHO year overall' and 'How satisfied are you with the amount of time the PRHO year has left you for family, social and recreational activities'. They were also asked a series of themed statements where they could agree, disagree or 'neither agree nor disagree'. Issues explored in the themed statements included; satisfaction with the length of working hours, the perceived fairness of remuneration both for basic hours and additional hours worked, satisfaction with their working conditions, their annual leave arrangements, arrangements for induction and hand-over. They were also asked about their satisfaction with the quality of training, educational opportunities, support from senior doctors, supervision of their work, feedback, and breadth of experience of clinical procedures.

The authors report 'some very positive messages about trends in doctors' experiences of the PRHO year'. Compared with the earlier cohorts the 2003 house officers had enjoyed the year more, were more satisfied with the leisure time available to them and were more satisfied with most aspects of work experience surveyed. However, the majority did not agree that their training was of a high standard, or that they were gaining a wide range of experience or receiving constructive feedback on their performance. There was greater dissatisfaction over surgical than medical posts (a theme common across all three cohorts).

Data from the same study published separately[10] reports that although over 90% of UK house offices regarded career advice as important at their career stage only a third agreed they had been able to obtain useful advice. There is a work programme as part of MMC to support newly qualified doctors in career choices. Future studies will show whether this new approach plus the opportunity to work across more specialties will help inform foundation doctors in making career choices.

The 2003 house officer cohort was the first to report on the experience of general practice PRHO placements in sufficient numbers to be analysed.[9] House officers assessed the experience of GP house jobs much more favourably than those in hospital medicine and surgery on a wide range of criteria. This is important because the new Foundation programme includes a general practice placement for 55% of foundation trainees in their second (FY2) year.

Experience of senior house officers in their second foundation year

The first SHO year is now spent in the second year of structured foundation programme training. These doctors are also referred to as Foundation Year 2 doctors (FY2 or F2). There are no published evaluations on the experiences of the first national cohort of FY2 doctors as they have completed the programme too recently for data to be available.

Before the national roll out of the MMC programme there were a number of pilot sites across UK. Some evaluations from these pilots have been published and give an indication of how the new approach is likely to have been received by doctors. A study of the pilot in the Oxford deanery[11] found predominantly positive feedback from the FY2 trainees. Trainees reported overwhelmingly positive views with respect to their first rotation and the programme as a whole. They enjoyed the shorter length of each placement, quality of training and support from supervisors, selection of placements, and breadth of training and experiences. Concerns were expressed about variations in salary between posts, night cover of different specialties, and sometimes feeling out of their depth. Overall, trainees felt the scheme represented a good transition from House Officer to SHO and most trainees felt the training and support they received were excellent.

A study in the Mersey Deanery[12] explored the views of F2 doctors and their educational supervisors to gain an understanding of their perceptions of the available learning experiences, support and supervision. Key findings were that the F2 programme was successful in delivering high levels of support and a good range of experiences provided for trainees. Some respondents believed that the adoption of a 4-month placement rather than the traditional

6-month placement provided the opportunity to sample a broader range of specialties than traditional SHOs were able to, which may be beneficial when making career choices.

Views of doctors in specialty training

The search strategy described above found a number of papers looking at doctors in specialty training. A number of studies identified focused on particular techniques[13] or learning about particular topic areas.[14] While important for those specialties there was little of more general applicability found in this search.

There were some studies with more generalizable results. One looked at views and experience of work life balance among trainees in obstetrics and gynaecology.[15] Half of the trainees (64 of 128, 50%) felt that they had achieved satisfactory work-life balance. Two-thirds of the trainees (83 of 128, 65%) found their work moderately or very stressful. Despite this the majority (85 of 128, 66%) claimed that they would choose obstetrics and gynaecology again if given a second chance. A large number of trainees (110 of 128, 86%) were looking forward to their future in this field. Another study looked urology Specialist Registrars' (SpRs) experience of the record of in-training assessments (RITA) process and its value in preparing them for their chosen consultant careers.[16] The study reported that there has, however, been haphazard delivery of that education due to a lack of objectivity in definition and assessment of the educational goals in individual training years. The authors argue that the RITA process should be more prescriptive in its administration and the setting of annual targeted training objectives should help to optimize the training opportunities for individual SpRs.

In 2006 the Postgraduate Medical Education and Training Board carried out its first of what will be an annual survey of all doctors in training in to include: SHOs in approved posts, Specialist Registrars (SpRs), Locum Appointment Training posts (LATS), Fixed Term Training Appointments (FTTAs)and GP Registrars (GPRs). The results[17] for 2006 indicate that GPRs are the most satisfied with their training (85% satisfaction score). Surgical group SHOs were the least satisfied (70%). Satisfaction with the quality of supervision shows a similar pattern with pathology SHOs and SpRs, psychiatry SpRs, and GPRs showing the highest scores, and SHOs in medicine, obstetrics and gynaecology and surgery showing the lowest scores. Of the surgical SHOs (the least satisfied group) 10% indicated that they were supervised by someone they felt was not competent to do so at least once a month. Out of the surgical SHOs 27% reported feeling force to cope at least once a month with problems beyond their competence or experience. PMETB Survey data were also used to measure the impact of national initiatives on training. As examples, radiology trainees in academies reported higher overall satisfaction with their posts than those not in academies, and trainees working at sites in the Hospital at Night initiative were more likely to report multidisciplinary handovers than trainees who were not.

A separate study of GPRs backs up the high level of satisfaction with training expressed in this survey. A survey of GPRs in London in 2000[18] followed by national surveys in 2003 and 2004[19] found high levels of reported satisfaction with training. GPRs were asked to rate their satisfaction with training on a five-point scale (ranging from 1, very unsatisfied to 5, very satisfied). The average score was 4.12 (SD = 0.761). Asked in an open question to write what they were particularly satisfied with, 41.2% (362 of 878) cited their trainer, 23.6% (207 of 878) their experience generally, 22.7% (199 of 878) the practice/practice team, 21.2% (186 of 878) the VTS half day release, 16.5% (145 of 878) support generally. About three-quarters (75.2%, 771 of 1025) felt that their training had prepared them well or very well for working as a GP. Only 1.2% (12 of 1025) felt that their training had not prepared them well for working as a GP. GPRs were asked to assess their skill level in various aspects of the requirements of the job. The areas where they stated they were least well prepared were practice management and finance (only 17% adequately prepared), and IT (59% felt adequately prepared.

Discussion

It is striking how few studies of trainees' experience and views of their training are available. Where we have generalizable data it is usually headline information that highlights trends over time and issues for trainees. Although this is useful, what is needed in addition is more detailed work that looks at specific aspects of training and seeks to identify 'what works', how it works, and how it might be generalized.

It seems clear that the experience of doctors in their first job (PRHOs) has been greatly improved by the reforms to working hours. However, there remained dissatisfaction with the quality of their training, the breadth of their experience and the careers guidance available to them. These finding pre-date the introduction of the 2-year foundation programme. The findings from the MMC pilots suggest that satisfaction levels should improve in the 2005 cohort, which has undertaken the new programme.

A recurring theme among SHOs is feeling out of their depth or having a workload beyond their experience or competencies. This is nothing new for doctors in training. Without the feedback from their supervisors we cannot know whether they are being given inappropriate tasks or whether they are being stretched in order to learn. This has always been a feature of becoming a skilled doctor. However, lack of perceived support and back up will result in junior doctors feeling anxious and insecure. It may also have a negative impact on patient safety.

The lack of perceived work life balance among trainees in some specialties is a concern. This should be monitored as the effects of reforms to working hours and conditions are felt through the trainee workforce.

Some specialties score worse than others in terms of satisfaction across a number of studies. In particular surgical trainees, especially in more junior grades (SHO), report less positively than GPRs. General Practice scores more highly than other specialties for doctors in foundation training (evidence at this stage from the PRHOs, which can be tested by future reports from F2 doctors).

Comparing surgical SHOs with GPRs is not comparing like with like. The former is a far less experienced doctor, and working in a very different type of job. The 'apprentice' model of general practice training with a close supervisory and support relationship between the GPR and the GP trainer is a highly valued aspect of GP training. It is clearly not possible to replicate this model in the modern hospital setting. However, there may be things to be learnt from how general practice trains new recruits, which can be replicated in other settings and specialties. Surgical training posts also compare poorly with medical training posts in terms of trainee satisfaction across a range of measures. Further work could be undertaken to understand the factors that are leading to these differences in satisfaction. A more detailed understanding could be used to inform changes to surgical training programmes to improve trainee experience.

Conclusions

There is a dearth of good quality detailed studies of the trainees' experience to support those implementing and designing training programmes in the UK. There should be more focus in research on the experiences of doctors in training. In particular good quality detailed studies that produce evidence-based recommendations are to be encouraged. This is particularly important as the reforms to medical education become embedded.

References

1. Department of Health. *Modernising medical careers: the next steps*. 2004. Available at http://www.mmc.nhs.uk/pages/resources/keydocuments (accessed 1 October 2007).

2. Department of Health. *Unfinished business: proposals for reform of the senior house officer grade – a paper for consultation.* 2002. Available at http://www.dh.gov.uk/en/Publicationsandstatistics/Publications/PublicationsPolicyAn dGuidance/DH_4007842 (accessed 1 October 2007).

3. Department of Health. *Improving working lives standard NHS employers committed to improving the working lives of people who work in the NHS.* 2000. Available at http://www.dh.gov.uk/en/Publicationsandstatistics/Publications/PublicationsPolicyAn dGuidance/DH_4010416 (accessed 3 October 2007).

4. Guardian Newspaper. Junior doctors lose court fight over jobs. 23 May 2007. Available at http://www.guardian.co.uk/society/2007/may/23/health.politics (accessed 2 July 2008).

5. Douglas Review Team. *Review of the medical training applications service and selection process.* 2007 (Douglas Review). Available at http://www.mmc.nhs.uk/download_files/final%20reportx.pdf (accessed 1 October 2007).

6. Tooke J. *Aspiring to excellence. Findings and final recommendations of the Independent inquiry into Modernising Medical careers.* 2008. Available at http://www.mmcinquiry.org.uk/ Final 8 Jan 08 MMC all.pdf (accessed 2 July 2008).

7. Oxford Medical Careers Group list of publications available at http://www.uhce.ox.ac.uk/ukmcrg/publications.php (accessed 1 October 2007).

8. Goldacre M, Davidson J, Lambert T. Doctors' views of their first year of medical work and postgraduate training in the UK questionnaire surveys. *Med Educ* 2003; **37**, 802–8.

9. Lambert T, Goldacre M. Doctors' views about their first postgraduate year in UK medical practice: House officers in 2003. *Med Educ* 2006; **40**: 1115–22.

10. Lambert T, Goldacre M. Views of doctors in training on the importance and availability of career advice in UK medicine *Med Educ* 2007; **41**: 460–6.

11. Limbert C, Jones H, Bannon M. Evaluation of MMC foundation year 2 pilot scheme: the trainees' experience. *Br J Hosp Med* 2005; **66**: 534–6.

12. O'Brien M, Brown J, Ryland L, Shaw N, Chapman T, Gillies R, Graham D. Exploring the views of second-year Foundation Programme doctors and their educational supervisors during a deanery-wide pilot Foundation Programme. *Postgrad Med J* 2006; **82**: 813–16.

13. McNarry A, Dovell T, Dancey R, Pead M. Perception of training needs and opportunities in advanced airway skills: a survey of British and Irish trainees. *Eur J Anaesthesiol* 2007; **24**: 498–504.

14. Burke S, Stone A, Bedward J, Thomas H, Farndon P. A 'neglected part of the curriculum' or 'of limited use'? Views on genetics training by nongenetics medical trainees and implications for delivery. *Genet Med* 2006; **8**: 109–1.

15. Thangaratinam S, Yanamandra SR, Deb S, Coomarasamy A. Specialist training in obstetrics and gynaecology: a survey on work-life balance and stress among trainees in UK. *J Obstet Gynaecol* 2006; **26**: 302–4.

16. Pearce I, Royle J. O'Flynn K, Payne S. The record of in-training assessments (RITAs). in urology: an evaluation of trainee perceptions. *Ann R Coll Surg Engl* 2003; **85**: 351–4.

17. Postgraduate Medical Education and Training Board. *National Trainee Survey 2006 – key findings*. 2006. Available at http://www.pmetb.org.uk/uploads/media/NationalTraineeSurveySummary Report.pdf (accessed 2 October 2007).

18. Bowler I, Jackson N. Experiences and career intentions of general practice registrars in Thames deaneries: postal survey. *Br Med J* 2002; **324**: 464–5.

19. Bowler I. *Report on the national GP Registrar Exit Survey Jan–Dec 2004*. Report prepared for COGPED (Committee of GP Education Directors) (unpublished 2005).

Chapter 17

Doctors in difficulty

David Wall

Introduction

This chapter has been written to help in the understanding of how to identify
and manage doctors who run into difficulties, both in the training and career
grades. My personal experience in this role has been in the West Midlands
Deanery, which is a large Deanery with a population of 5.6 million (about
one-tenth of the UK population). In this region I will see about 100 doctors
and dentists in difficulty each year now. Numbers have increased year by year,
and have doubled in the last 4 years. These are referrals made by others who
have concerns about the doctors or dentist, not those who self-refer. Doctors
referred come from both the training grades and career grades. Over the last 4
years the main increases in numbers have been in doctors in the Foundation
Years, and those in general practice, both General Practice (GP) registrars and
GPs in the career grades. The numbers of specialist registrars from hospital
practice have remained fairly steady. Most doctors referred are male (87% in
the 2007–08 year), which is the latest year in my personal series of cases.

This chapter reflects my own experience over many years, and in addition
much of what is written here follows the nationally recommended 11 principles derived from various sources including those from the National Clinical
Assessment Service (NCAS). NCAS in their publication *Handling concerns
about the performance of healthcare professionals: principles of good practice*[1]
described 11 key principles for handling performance concerns. Whatever else
we may do or think it is essential to remember that patient safety is paramount. For this reason patient safety concerns are at the top of the list of the
11 NCAS principles. There are as follows:

1. Patient safety must be the primary consideration.

2. Healthcare organizations are responsible for developing policies and
   procedures to recognize performance concerns early and act swiftly to
   address the concerns.

3. Policies for handling performance concerns should be circulated to all
   healthcare practitioners.

4. Avoid unnecessary or inappropriate exclusions of practitioners.

5. Separate investigation from decision making.

6. Staff and managers should understand the factors that may contribute to performance concerns.

7. Performance procedures should contribute to the organizational programme for clinical governance.

8. Good human resources practice will help prevent performance problems.

9. Healthcare practitioners who work in isolated settings may need additional support.

10. Individual healthcare practitioners are responsible for maintaining a good standard of practice.

11. Commitment to equality and diversity.

Most of all these 11 principles are self-explanatory, but these principles will be expanded within this chapter.

Doctors may run into many problems. Some are remediable by expert help from colleagues in the various organizations such as the Postgraduate Deaneries, NCAS, the British Medical Association, the Medical Charities, and the General Medical Council (GMC). Others are not remediable from such organizations. In order to conceptualize these, we categorize the various problems into four main areas. These are as follows:

♦ Personal conduct

♦ Professional conduct

♦ Competence and performance issues

♦ Health and sickness issues

Personal conduct issues (not related to being a doctor)

The organization be it the GP surgery or the hospital must have within it doctors who operate to the highest of standards of personal conduct. This is also a GMC requirement in *Good Medical Practice*.

Examples of such problems we have encountered include the doctor as perpetrator in terms of theft, fraud, assault, vandalism, rudeness, bullying, racial and sexual harassment, child pornography, and serious traffic offences. The Trust (as the employer of its doctors in the training and career grades) should take the lead under its approved disciplinary procedures. For GPs (most of whom are self-employed) the Primary Care Organization (PCO) may take the lead. Sometimes the police and the courts will be involved. In some situations the GMC will be informed of an offence in this area – unrelated to the practice of medicine. If a doctor in training is involved, then we ask that the employer must inform both the deanery and the trainee in writing at an early stage that he/she may approach the deanery for advice, particularly if there are any concerns that any allegations are as a result of professional issues, and/or education and training difficulties.

The deanery will not be involved in such a disciplinary panel, but will need assuring of the following:

- the Trust will follow an agreed disciplinary procedure
- the trainee has been advised that they may be legally represented (by the BMA, a solicitor, for example)
- national guidelines are followed if a trainee is to be suspended
- pastoral support is provided if needed

Doctors as perpetrators in such trouble do need additional support. However, after reasonable support does not work, dismissal will need to be seriously considered.

Professional conduct issues (related to being a doctor)

Examples of such problems we have encountered include inappropriate breast examinations, claiming qualifications the doctor does not have, plagiarism and research misconduct, failure to take consent properly, prescribing issues, improper relationships with patients, improper certification issues (such as the signing of cremation forms, sickness certification, passport forms), and breaches of confidentiality. Again the Trust should take the lead under its approved disciplinary procedures. For GPs the PCO may take the lead. In some situations the GMC will be informed. Again for trainees, the Deanery will provide an input into such a disciplinary process via the clinical tutor, the GP trainer, the Chair of the Specialty Training Committee (STC) or Regional Adviser (for specialist and now specialty registrars) or other member of the Deanery. Any decision to involve the GMC is a very serious one for the doctor involved and this will be a joint decision between the Trust (or other employer) and the Deanery. The GMC recommends that approved procedures be followed first at the local level, rather than report everything to the GMC at the earliest stage.

Competence and performance issues

Examples of such problems we have seen include a single serious clinical mistake, excessively slow surgical operating, low standard of results clinically (possibly found as a result of audit), persistent bad timekeeping, poor communication and/or consultation skills and repeated failure to attend educational events. More recently, we have seen some very basic problems, including inability to: speak English well enough to be understood or take a history; inability to examine a patient; and almost injuring the instructor with a defibrillator on an Advanced Life Support Course. Hopefully most of these may be dealt with through the educational framework. The Trust or other employer will need to take a lead in some of these problems, if there may have been a complaint from patients or relatives, and the possibility of a legal action. An isolated serious mistake may happen to any of us. If we are honest, many of us have been in this situation at some time in our careers. It usually does not reflect the overall competence of the doctor concerned.

Further considerations of some key domains for doctors in difficulty

Personality, behaviour, and performance

The workplace can accommodate many different personalities and behaviours as long as it does not interfere with patient safety, or the quality of performance of doctors or others, or cause problems with bullying and harassment.

There are several personality characteristics that may cause problems with behaviours and performance.[2] For example, the 'macho' type of behaviour (in both men and women) may lead to problems as such individuals may not recognize their limitations, or when they are heading for problems, and may tend towards authoritarianism and inappropriate behaviour.

Although we might not be able to change an individual's personality, it is often possible to detect and quantify unacceptable behaviours with 360 degree assessment,[3] and to help modify these behaviours with coaching, constructive feedback, and even sanctions.

Education and training

Education of medical students and of doctors in training has undergone major changes since the 1960s and 1970s. There is now much more emphasis on communication skills, both with patients and with colleagues, on team working in a multidisciplinary team, and about attitudes and behaviours appropriate for a doctor. Little of this was taught 30 years ago and beyond. In addition, some doctors still find it difficult to relate to patients and to nurses and other members of the healthcare team, and exhibit authoritarian and condescending attitudes to both patients and colleagues. All doctors now undergo appraisal of some sort, and this needs to be a supportive formative process to encourage education and development.

It has been recognized for some time that the transition from medical student to Foundation Year 1 doctor is a stressful and difficult one.[4,5] Some of these doctors, up to 1–2%, need to undergo remedial training and repeat all or part of the year.[2] In addition, Foundation Year 1 doctors are responsible for a disproportionate number of prescribing errors.[6]

NCAA (then called the National Clinical Assessment Authority[2]) highlighted several early signs of doctors in difficulty in terms of their education. These included:

- *the disappearing act*: not answering bleeps, and disappearing, frequent sick leave
- *low work rate*: slow in doing procedures, clerking patients, dictating letters
- *ward rage*: shouting at the nurses or other colleagues
- *rigidity*: poor tolerance of uncertainty, difficulty making priority decisions
- *bypass syndrome*: nurses and other colleagues avoid asking the doctor to do anything
- *career problems*: examination difficulty, disillusionment with medicine
- *insight failure*: rejection of constructive feedback, defensiveness, counter challenge

Much of all this is identified by 360 degree assessment. The TAB (Team Assessment of Behaviours)[3] is a valid and reliable assessment that measures professional relationships with patients, verbal communication skills, team working, and accessibility. We have encountered all of the above and more, often documented using evidence from 360 degree assessment.

Teamwork

As has been mentioned above, most of us now work in teams, but how many of us work in supportive and effective teams? Working in a clinical area in a multidisciplinary team demands a lot more of us all. For example, the team I have worked in for 30 years delivering care for babies and small children has two health visitors, a practice nurse, a healthcare assistant, a secretary, a lay volunteer, and me as the doctor. This has worked really well for many years, and is a pleasure to work as part of this team. Good teams are rewarding to work in, members are less stressed than when in a poor team, and the sense of support for each member is really important.

We have seen problems in teams where one member has ignored the wishes of others, has behaved in an authoritarian and condescending way to other members, sometimes as a result of cultural attitudes. For example, young male doctors have found it very difficult to accept advice and guidance from a female senior midwife or nurse in charge, or even a female senior consultant and clinical tutor.

Leadership

It is now being recognized that doctors in training need education in leadership skills. Spurgeon[7] has recently suggested that this is now no longer an optional extra. NCAA[2] suggests that there is growing evidence of links between the qualities of leaders and the qualities of patient care. What we want are leaders who have the following characteristics. They are able, intelligent, warm and friendly, benevolent, emotionally stable, able to recognize limitations, have integrity and are able to delegate. They have good communication skills, are able to create a sense of justice, give people a sense of control themselves, and are able to predict and plan accordingly.

Health and sickness issues

Every doctor must be encouraged to register with a local general medical practitioner, and consult with their doctor in the first instance when ill. Under this broad heading we will consider disability, physical and mental illness, cognitive impairment, organizational culture and climate, workload issues, and adverse life events.

Disability

Disability may result from a congenital problem, or be acquired as the result of either long-term ill health, or of physical mental or sensory impairment. Many doctors may be able to function well with a disability or a long-term illness, but remember that there is a potential for problems to occur and not be recognized or dealt with appropriately. Such conditions include arthritis, diabetes, multiple sclerosis, inflammatory bowel disease, epilepsy, chronic respiratory problems, hepatitis B and C, and HIV/AIDS. Remember that depression is common with chronic physical illness. A full occupational health assessment will be needed, and guidance from such an occupational health physician must be followed in terms of protecting patient safety. Doctors with serious communicable diseased such as hepatitis B and C, and HIV/AIDS are able to practise medicine, but must follow guidance from an occupational health physician in relation to their area of practice.

Physical illness

Doctors are often reluctant to admit to illness, and to seek advice. In fact studies of junior doctors have shown that less than 50% of junior doctors have a GP. There is also considerable self-prescribing.[2]

Mental illness

Stress in doctors and nurses is high, compared with other workers. Depression is common, and as already stated, there is excess mortality from overdose of prescribed drugs, suicide, and cirrhosis of the liver. Drug addiction is also a problem for doctors who have easy access to opiates and other powerful drugs.[2] We have also seen problems with recreational drugs such as cannabis and cocaine in young doctors.

Depression is common, and up to 20% of UK doctors become depressed at some point. With increasing numbers of young women in the profession, postnatal depression is a particular difficulty. The author has personally seen and diagnosed several of these cases, when young doctors have returned to work after maternity leave, and have struggled to cope. Major psychiatric illness with psychotic illness such as schizophrenia, bipolar disorder, and severe postnatal depression is not common in my experience, but does occur from time to time.

Cognitive impairment

This is a term used to cover concerns about a doctor's memory, reasoning, or decision making. This is not common, but we have seen older doctors who have run into problems of underperformance and further investigations have revealed loss of short-term memory and even dementia. Also, remember that cognitive impairment may be the result of long-standing alcohol excess, which may produce alcoholic brain damage, and some neurological disorders such as multiple sclerosis, epilepsy, and parkinsonism may have similar effects on cognitive ability. In addition, severe head injury, stroke, and coronary heart disease may also be implicated as causes for cognitive impairment.

It is sometimes very difficult to diagnose cognitive impairment, and to differentiate cognitive impairment from depression, and expert referral and assessment will be necessary here.

Organizational culture and climate

Organizational climate is about staff perceptions of what it is like to work in the organization.[8] Organizational culture includes climate but also is about how to behave in the organization, about leadership style and values. Compared with educational climate where we have a variety of tools to use, and a growing literature summarized by Roff in 2005[9] there seems to be little research on organizational climate in the National Health Service (NHS).

Ideally, we would all like to work in an open, fair, friendly, sensitive, and supportive culture, where we feel appreciated and valued. Working in a culture of institutional bullying and intimidation, with scapegoating, and poor leadership is stressful, and should not be tolerated. Leaders who are ignorant, arrogant, dictatorial, hostile, boastful, and generally not up to the job cause many problems and result in less work being achieved, high staff absence and turnover, as people get fed up and look for opportunities to leave, and move to other jobs where they are appreciated.

We need to tackle the organizational culture where this is a problem, rather than just move the doctor in difficulty away from this situation; otherwise the situation recurs with the next trainee in that particular area of work. In many situations we have to do both. Giving the doctor in difficulty a fresh start is very important.

Workload

Although hours worked have declined since the 1970s, when junior doctors often worked 120 hours per week, the intensity and complexity of medical practice have greatly increased. Heavy workload, a 'long hours' culture, lack of sleep, and shift working can cause problems with poor performance, and can make worse existing problems with mental and physical health. Heavy workload may cause burnout. Sleep loss may affect performance adversely. Shift working may cause performance problems especially at times when sleepiness is high, such as between 1 a.m. and 6 a.m., as well as having adverse physiological effects on the individual. Ensuring proper timetabled breaks, as in the European Working Time Directive, will help here (see Chapter 21).

Adverse life events

When seeing doctors in difficulty one of the commonest areas of concern is in relation to adverse life events that have happened to the individual doctor. Often people will not volunteer such information, so if it is appropriate we will ask about bereavements, severe illness, problems with children, accidents, change of job, move of house, lack of family support, and so on. Often, as well as the problem of poor performance or behaviour, doctors may also have had the death of parents and close family members, financial difficulties, and a house move to cope with at the same time. One doctor seen by the author recently stated that she had been back and forth to India 17 times in the current year, often for a few days at a time, because of family illness and bereavement. Her performance had declined in terms of work; she was depressed and stressed, and very tired. She was given counselling through our stress counselling service, her depression was diagnosed and treated, and she had time off and a gradual return to work put in place once she was improving. She made a successful return to work.

To help matters with the young doctors we use the list produced by the University of Birmingham,[10] which details some of these main stressors and gives some measure of how severe each may be. This is freely available in the public domain from the University of Birmingham website on: http://www.as.bham.ac.uk/study/support/sscs/counsell/stress.shtml

A score of 50 in a 6-month period is considered to be stressful enough to cause illness. You might want to work out your own score for the past 6 months (see Table 7.1).

If you gain a high score on this quiz it does not mean that you will automatically become ill but it is an indication that you should look for ways of reducing and managing stress. Stress is cumulative and sometimes it may be a small event, which following after a series of major life events, tips the balance, hence the saying 'the straw that broke the camel's back'.

Table 17.1 Some stressors and their levels of severity.

Event	Score
Death of a parent	50
Death of a close relative	40
Loss of a parent through divorce	35
Death of a close friend	30
Parents having rows or in financial trouble	28
Serious health problems, surgery, pregnancy	25
Engagement or marriage	25
In trouble with the law	22
Unemployed, financial trouble	19
Break up with boy or girl friend	19
Interviews or starting a new job	18
Sexual difficulties	18
Not part of the crowd	16
Lack of privacy	15
Driving test	15
College pressures, exams, deadlines	14
Concern about appearance, weight, identity	13
Recent move, home, school, college	11
Lack of recognition	9
General feelings of frustration	6

However, in more senior doctors there may be problems with children. A disproportionate amount of domestic and child care falls on women, as well as that of elderly dependants. This all needs to be asked when discussing adverse life events.

Identifying the problems

Remember that in many cases the doctors will have multiple problems, not just one.

A study presented at the Association of Medical Education in Europe (AMEE) Conference in Trondheim in 2007 by O'Leary[11] of 123 consequential referrals of psychiatrists in difficulty to NCAS showed that most of them had multiple problems, not just one each. This is our personal experience as well. Often a doctor will have been referred with a performance or communication problem, but will turn out to have had several other adverse life events recently and also a major health problem as well. Often these are unknown to the referring body.

Is there a problem? The problem for the organization may be of underperformance, and how this manifests itself in the workplace. Unless we find out the cause, then we cannot address them and bring the performance back to an acceptable level. If there is, then the first step is to clarify things, to get both sides of the story, and not to jump to conclusions based only on one side of the story. Get on to the problem early. Do not leave it to the next appraisal or even the next year's annual assessment. It may be necessary to investigate the problem formally, with written statements from the various individuals involved, and records of what has happened. In order to sort things out, asking four simple questions may help you. These are:

- What is the real problem?
- Why has this happened?
- What can we do about it?
- Can we get back on course?

The six-step problem solving approach might help. The author has found this helpful in many situations over the years since first being introduced to it on my initial GP Trainers' Course at Keele University in 1977. It goes like this:

- problem presented
- problem discussed
- problem agreed
- solution presented

- solution discussed
- solution agreed

In addition, it is important to monitor the solution, to address progress and evaluate the results. So we could add to the model:

- solution monitored
- progress monitored
- results evaluated
- did it work?

Many problems can be resolved at local level, rather than involve all the processes described here. However, the principles of finding out the facts, using facts of the case and not opinions, constructive feedback and setting targets for improvement, and following these through, will hopefully work well in most cases.

Why has this happened?

Here are some possible points that you may with to consider.

- *Is it the trainee or is it the trainer? Is it the job?* It is important to define why we are in difficulties. Asking this basic question may be very useful in clarifying where we need to focus. Sometimes it is the trainer or the organization, and the poor unfortunate doctor in difficulty is a 'symptom' of greater and more fundamental difficulties in the organization.

  If it is the job, and not the trainee then the Deanery will need to sort this out. A visit to the place or work and a look at the post concerned will need to be done as a matter of urgency, and will attempt to put things right. Sometimes we will move the trainee to another post in a different practice or hospital, to enable a fresh start to be made, and to diffuse the situation. This is not punishing the victim, but trying to give the person a fresh start in a better environment. We do also need to address the causes of the underlying problem. However, for doctors in career grades this moving to another post will not usually be possible, so other measures to change and ameliorate the situation will be called for, including negotiations with the employing Trust or the PCO.

- *Does the doctor need career advice?* When all attempts to remedy the problem have failed, sometimes we find that the doctor is really in the wrong career? Here a detailed careers counselling approach may be needed, with advice and information about other career possibilities to be considered discussed in depth. At the West Midlands Deanery, for example, we do have detailed information on all careers in our Careers Information Pack – updated annually, and several of us have been trained in the giving of careers advice and even careers counselling. An approach to the local clinical tutor in the first instance, who may be able to help, or who may pass you on to a regional adviser or the deanery.

- *Does the doctor have other problems such as stress, physical or mental illness, etc?* Everyone should be registered with a GP, and this should be the first suggestion. Also, the employer is able to insist that the doctor sees an occupational health physician. This is especially important in terms of repeated absenteeism and prolonged sickness absence. This is built into trainees' contracts of employment, and occasionally we do have to insist on a consultant occupational health physician's opinion. In addition, where sickness absence or suspected illness does give cause for concern, or the individual has unfortunately developed a serious communicable disease or disability, then the views of a consultant physician in occupational medicine are essential in such cases. Remember the issues of patient confidentiality here (with the doctor in difficulty as the patient). Remember that such a referral must be labelled *private and confidential* and not sent round on the email with copies to all and sundry. This is confidential medical information that is being exchanged here.

We have found that working with senior consultants in occupational medicine who are experienced in dealing with doctors in difficulty, with time to meet, to discuss ideas and policies, has been immensely beneficial to us all, especially for the doctors in difficulty themselves.

Early diagnosis and tackling of problems

If you do start to run into problems, then some of the principles listed below will help.

- *Do it now.* Tackle the problem when it occurs, not at the end of the placement.
- *Find out the facts.* Do not jump to conclusions. Get information from all sides. However, there will in some circumstances be a patient safety issue, with patients at risk, and in such circumstances this calls for immediate action.
- *Share the problem.* Do not try to do it all on your own, but get advice from others – other trainers, educational supervisors, your speciality tutor, your clinical tutor, training programme director, chair of your STC, Regional Advisers, the Deanery, the Trust, and if appropriate the PCO. Expert assessments and opinions about occupational health and communication skills have proved really helpful.

◆ *Explain the problem*. Discuss the problem with the doctor in difficulty constructively, and plan how to get back on course. Sometimes you will find that no one has sat down with the doctor and explained what the difficulty is, and how this may be put right. Sometimes people will say that this was the first time that anyone has said to them that they have a communication skills or teamworking problem.

◆ *Give support*. Remember that encouragement does work. A regular review of progress is very important, with constructive feedback on performance. Access to stress counselling by telephone and/or face to face consultations are available in a confidential way, paid for by the Deanery, and outside of the workplace. A mentor, a wise senior colleague, will be offered. Follow up and assurance that we are here to help is also of great importance.

The role of the employer/contracting organization

The doctor in training will always have an employer. The employer may be the NHS Trust, the University, or the general practice trainer in the case of GP registrars. For doctors in the career grades, they may be employed by an NHS Trust, or be a self-employed contractor with a PCO. Legally, the employer must take the lead in all four areas of problems referred to earlier (personal conduct, professional conduct, competence and performance issues, and health and sickness issues). Employers will have procedures laid down for these areas.

It is very important that we in the Deanery know about problems when one of our trainees is involved. In order to deal with the issue of confidentiality, we oblige the Trust to inform the trainee that he/she may approach the Deanery for advice. The Deanery must be involved at the earliest stage in all cases. What happens next will depend on the types and seriousness of problems encountered.

This has been discussed above in greater detail above.

Back on Track Framework: a four-step model

In the publication by NCAS entitled *Back on Track: Restoring doctors and dentists to safe professional practice*[12] there were seven guiding principles for working in this area. These are:

1. *Clinical governance and patient safety*. Patient safety must come first.

2. *A single framework guiding individual programmes*. Use of a framework must encompass common principles, which are applicable in different specialties and for different grades on doctor, whether in the training grades or the career grades.

3. *A comprehensive approach.* We must identify and deal with the problems comprehensively, identifying all the issues and dealing with the needs of the doctor, the organization, and keeping the need to protect patient safety as a primary concern. Communication skills are often a problem and we work closely with our communication skills teachers within the university to help identify and improve communication skills in many of our doctors in difficulty.

4. *Fairness, transparency, confidentiality, and patient consent.* We need to be fair and open about what we do. The confidentiality of the doctor in difficulty needs protecting, although sometimes this may not be possible, with serious events that lead to a coroner's inquest, for example. Our usual policy is to copy letters we write only to the organizations involved and to occupational health, and to the doctor in difficulty so that they know exactly what we have said and why. However, there is a guiding principle here about the need to know, so such information should only be given to those helping in the process and not sent on email to all and sundry. Patients need to be properly informed if they are being seen by a doctor on a return to work programme.

   Fairness also involves being aware of and practising fairness in terms of the legislation on equality of opportunity regarding age, gender, ethnicity, religion, sexual orientation, and disability. Deanery staff and all trainers in both hospital practice and general practice do attend regular training and updating sessions on equality and diversity issues, provided by experts, and a record is kept of attendances and updating sessions.

5. *Ongoing and constant support.* This is essential. Support for some individual doctors in difficulty may be necessary for some years, sticking with it despite setbacks. Sometimes it is a long hard journey with considerable setbacks on the way. This is not to decide whether the doctors performance is acceptable or not, but to give support for a gradual and phased return to practice. Also the remedial training team that the doctor in difficulty is working in, and the organization, are also under considerable load. In the West Midlands we have 12 advanced training practices, who take doctors in difficulty for remedial training. We recognize that they need breaks from training after dealing with a doctor in difficulty. Sometimes this remedial training puts considerable stress on the whole practice, and we need to be aware of and recognize this is a considerable issue.

6. *Success and failure.* Although we all hope that dealing with the problems of doctors in difficulty will help them to succeed and get back on track, this is not always the case. It is useful to think of what to do if a programme of

return to work does not succeed, and to spell out what is to happen if objectives are not achieved. Sometimes with severe physical or mental illness, despite all measures to cope, the only solution may be an early retirement on medical grounds. Here obviously the continuing involvement and close collaboration of a senior consultant in occupational medicine is essential. On rare occasions, in other situations, where the doctor is felt to pose a danger to patients, a dismissal and a referral to the GMC will be appropriate. Again it is very important that we remember that patient safety is paramount.

It is important that those of us dealing with doctors in difficulty realize that we cannot succeed in every case. Career counselling will be used here, with the help of trained and skilled career counsellors. This is different from just giving careers information and careers advice. This is a difficult and complex situation, and calls for skilled work from an experienced and skilled careers counsellor. We also need support from our organizations here, such as the British Medical Association, the Medical Defence organizations and NCAS.

7. *Local resolution drawing on local and national expertise.* The final guiding principle is to use local procedures first, as has already been described above. A consistent approach at local level, using the principles derived and published by regional and nation bodies, such as the Deanery, the Strategic Health Authority, NCAS, and the GMC is essential. Sharing our experiences is also very valuables. We do this at meetings facilitated by NCAS, and should do the same at local and regional level. People need to be trained at local level in managing poor performance, so they know what to look out for, what to do and when and where to refer on for help if necessary.

Roles and responsibilities of different individuals and organizations

The individual doctor in difficulty

The individual doctor will need to cooperate with any investigation and assessment. They will need to cooperate with people trying to help then return to work. Unfortunately, one of our greatest difficulties is where the individual doctor has little or no insight into their problems, and thinks that all offers of help are part of the perceived underlying conspiracy to do them down or 'fit them up' as one put it to me. I think that lack of insight is the biggest problem faced in dealing with doctors in difficulty. We have to present them with good evidence of their performance using valid and reliable assessment tools, so that there can be no question about the rigour of the evidence. Repeated discussions need to be undertaken to reinforce what the problems are, how we need to address them, and that many problems are remediable.

The employing or contracting organization

There will be a policy of dealing with such issues, and this should be handled by a senior person within the organization. There is a need to deal with performance, funding issues for remedial training, and return to work programmes. There is also the consideration about continuing on the Performers' List of the local PCO (for those working in general practice, all doctors will need to be on the local Performers' List. Without it, a doctor will not be able to practice in a primary care setting), or referral to the GMC if there are serious concerns about the safety of patients or the doctor's fitness to be in practice.

The Postgraduate Deanery

For doctors in approved training posts, the deanery will have identified remedial training in well supervised posts, and be able to offer continued support, occupational health assessment, communication skills assessment and advice, and confidential psychological support for individuals.

It is more difficult to help doctors who are sent to us referred by the GMC or NCAS, who are not in approved training posts or who are unemployed, sometimes for considerable periods of time. Often the expectations of such doctors in difficulty are high. Some seem to think that we will give them a job, and when this is not forthcoming become even more disillusioned and antagonistic. With jobs in the medical profession now very tight, and open competition the rule, such doctors stand little or no chance of achieving a post in open competition with their peers, especially after periods of unemployment or conditions on their registration imposed by the GMC. I do believe that we need a national strategy to try to help this increasing group of desperate doctors in difficulty.

Medical Royal Colleges and Faculties

Regional advisers in the medical specialties may be able to help the Deanery in the design of retraining programmes and placement of individual trainees and possibly doctors in career grades.

The National Clinical Assessment Service

NCAS will provide advice to Trusts and PCOs (and occasionally to Postgraduate Deaneries) on doctors in difficulty. In some circumstance where local measures have not resolved the difficulty, NCAS will organize a full assessment of the individual doctor. NCAS will then issue a report and recommendations for further action.

In addition NCAS have produced some excellent policy documents[1,2,12] on their website[13] at http://www.ncas.npsa.nhs.uk/ to help guide us all in helping doctors in difficulty, and to help us develop policy at local level to fit in with these principles. These have already been referred to above. They are well worth getting a copy of each and reading them thoroughly.

The General Medical Council

The GMC is the regulatory body which maintains a register of medical practitioners, and issues standards for practice. Again, there are some excellent publications on areas about fitness to practice, health issues, consent and confidentiality, which are essential reading. The GMC will investigate concerns about an individual doctor's fitness to practise. The GMC may dismiss a concern, impose restrictions on practice, suspend the doctors for a period of time or erase the doctor's name from the medical register. Remember that the GMC will deal with a doctor's health problems as well as performance concerns.

A GMC referral is always a very serious and stressful event for an individual doctor. We always ask for a full occupational health assessment of such doctors, as they are often very depressed, if not at the start of such an investigation, they will often be so at the end. Sometimes such investigations will take a considerable period of time, sometimes years, to come to a conclusion.

The British Medical Association

For its members, the BMA will give advice and help on careers, on terms and conditions or service, and on employment issues, including assessment appeals for doctors in training. There is also a confidential advice and counselling service called *Doctors for Doctors*. It is advertised in the *British Medical Journal* weekly, with a telephone number for access to a doctor adviser (who are all volunteers) for advice. The BMA will not normally give advice in respect of a GMC referral. This is usually handled by the Medical Defence Organizations, for doctors who are members of such organizations. Membership is by subscription, and of course these organizations will only act for paid-up members. They will not take on non-members' cases.

Funding

Who pays for the doctor to be re-trained? This is a very difficult issue.

For those who are trainees and who are already in approved training programmes, it is easier, as the Deanery will keep some posts for such eventualities.

For doctors who are employed or contracted in career grades, some Trusts and PCOs have been willing to fund or part fund a return to work programme, including help with courses, for a specific period of time according to a programme of training and assessment. In fact the Chief Medical Officer[14] in his review of *Good Doctors, Safer Patients* in 2006 did make a recommendation about the need for a funding contribution from the employing Trust or PCO. In the author's experience this varies enormously in practice. Some organizations are very willing to fund one of their doctors in difficulty, but others have refused point blank and said that they have no funding for such eventualities. For GPs, there is also the considerable problem of locum costs for back-filling the work of the GP while they are away re-training.

We really do need to have a clear policy and ring-fenced funding if we are expected to help rehabilitate such desperate individuals. In addition we need to remember that not everyone is remediable, as will be discussed in the next section of this chapter.

Remediability

Here are some of the thoughts based on the NCAS Conference '*Back on Track*' which the author attended in 2005 (in particular, a keynote talk by Dr Jennifer King), and partly on his own experiences of seeing such doctors and dentists in difficulty over many years.

The problems

These may be divided into three areas, the individual, the team in which the individual works, and the organization. We tend to focus on the individual too much – and too little on the team and the organization.

Behavioural themes

Doctors and dentists are usually highly motivated, and may be too demanding of themselves and others. As a result, some good traits may become difficulties. For example, diligence may become obsessional behaviour, and confidence may become arrogance. Creativity may become maverick behaviour. Some may become overtly compliant, may take on more and more work and then may become overwhelmed.

Loss of power and control in a situation that rapidly escalates out of the doctor's control may lead to depression, poor self-esteem and more entrenched behaviour. There may be poor insight into the impact of such behaviour and denial of responsibility of one's own actions. This may be shown by feelings of victimization and alienation, and allegations of bullying, intimidation, racism, sexism, ageism, and so on. However, do remember that some of us may be working in hostile environments where bullying and intimidation do indeed occur, and may be the cause of such difficulties.[16] It is sometimes too easy to blame the individual when in fact the organizational culture is hostile to good working relationships.

Causes underlying such behaviours

Some of the causes of stress have already been discussed. In summary these may include illness, family problems, bereavement, financial problems, excessive workload, being bullied and harassed, training and education problems, the culture of the organization and the educational climate.

Factors leading to failure at work include several categories of problems:

Capacity to learn	may have reached limit	prognosis poor
Learning deficit	more training will often help	prognosis good
Arousal and motivation	too bored or too overwhelmed	prognosis good
Distraction	problems elsewhere (e.g. health)	prognosis good
Alienation	deep rooted feeling of injustice	prognosis very poor

Behaviours and their prognosis: Are they treatable?

Regarding personality, it may be almost impossible to change this. However, it may be able to change behaviours – but not in all cases. Feedback on performance (with good evidence to back it up – from 360 degree assessment, for example) is the key to behaviour change. For example, we have been able to help many individuals work better within a team, and understand how to relate to other team members. For this, we have used evidence from 360 degree assessment, from role play sessions with exerts on clinical communication within the university, and constitutive feedback on such behaviours. We have continued to monitor the doctor's performance using 360 degree assessment, and in many cases have produced an acceptable level of performance, which has been sustained.

There are pre-conditions for changing behaviours. The individual needs to be intelligent enough, stable enough, perceptive enough, and have insight into their problems. As we have noted before, lack of insight is a considerable problem in this area. Also a history of previous successful change, and being motivated to change are really important. Unless the individual sees a reason to change and really wants to change, achieving success is very difficult.

Considering the team: in trying to change things

What do we need to help change things for the better? We need a supportive educational climate, a culture of learning from mistakes and open communications within the team. We need clear leadership with clear tasks, roles, and objectives. We need a culture of handling conflict in a constructive way, with considerable trust within the team, Team meetings, open discussion of difficulties with a skilled facilitator, using principles of constructive feedback, and the use of significant event analysis will all help here.

Considering the organization: in trying to change things

The author believes that we place far too much emphasis on the individual and far too little on the organization. How many dysfunctional organizations have we all worked in within the NHS? How many of these have been reported to NCAS for advice on improvement, or reported to the GMC for poor practice?

So what do we need in a good organization? We need proper processes within the organization and a history of change attempted successfully. There needs to be efficient systems, clear leadership, and a realistic workload. There must be open communications within the organization, not a culture of fear and silence. Accountabilities must be clear and understood by all.

What do we do in practice?

We try to follow the procedure shown in Figure 17.1, which is explained below.

Phase 1: the referral

This may be by letter, by telephone, face to face contact or, email (which we discourage because of lack of confidentiality). Information is read, and a decision made to accept the referral or suggest other ways of dealing with the situation. For example, we in the deanery may say that the police or the GMC may be the more appropriate route for some situations.

Phase 2: meeting the doctor

We would meet with the doctor concerned at this stage. We offer confidential counselling, and ask the doctor to tell their story. Rather than have an

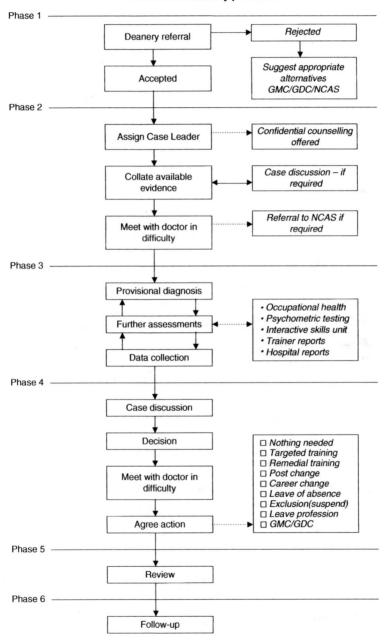

Fig. 17.1 Procedure for dealing with the doctor in difficulty.

unstructured and sometime rambling conversation, we would try to structure the conversation as follows.

- *Introductions*: including an explanation that this process is hopefully to help the doctor, and is *not* a telling off or disciplinary meeting.
- *Career history* from undergraduate medical school up to the present time.
- *The present problem* as the doctor perceives it.
- *Adverse life events*: see above.
- *Any other issues* we or the doctor might wish to raise.
- *Summarizing*.
- *Reflecting back to the individual.*
- *Putting a plan in place* and explaining what will happen next.

Phase 3: a provisional diagnosis

Here we would make a provisional diagnosis of what we think is the problem. Often we will ask for further information and other assessments in order to gather further information to clarify the situation further. For example, we might ask for an occupational health assessment, a communication skills assessment from our Interactive Skills Unit in the university, further trainer reports, and a further 360 degree assessment and so on. We would then arrange to meet again to review all of this.

Phase 4: a case discussion

We would then meet again with the doctor and discuss their case, with all this extra information available. We would explain all this to the doctor, including making a decision on what to do. Sometimes nothing is needed, but often we need to put in place a **development plan**, which may include further training of some sort, and sometimes move the doctor to another post, where hopefully things might be better for the doctor concerned. Career advice and sometimes career counselling may be necessary. Sometimes the problem may be addressed by flexible working, less than full time, so that pressures of illness, disability, or family problems may be helped. In this way a skilled and valuable member of the workforce may be retained in work. Rarely may we advise suspension, or even leaving the training programme altogether. Rarely will we need to refer to the GMC. Hopefully the doctor concerned will agree with our course of action, which is often a training package of some form or another. This needs to be clearly set out.

Phase 5: the review

It is essential to follow up and see the doctor again so that we may review the training package has been completed and improvement has occurred. It is essential that evidence is available (often including 360 degree assessment) to show that the training package has been completed satisfactorily. Usually this is the case.

Phase 6: follow-up

Sometimes we do need to keep a longer-term follow-up of some doctors in difficulty, in order to keep them back of track. Sometimes this is because of illness, or a GMC requirement or because they do not make the required levels of progress.

This process is presented diagrammatically in Figure 17.1. The author wishes to thank Dr Mike Clapham for providing the *Doctors in difficulty flowchart*.

Finally, the author wishes to conclude this chapter with two comments stemming from his work with doctors in difficulty. These comments are often reiterated at faculty development meetings. These are as follows:

... The biggest trainer problem is lack of documentation about the problem ...
... The most difficult trainee problem is lack of insight about the problem ...

References

1. National Clinical Assessment Service. *Handling concerns about the performance of healthcare professionals: principles of good practice*. London: National Clinical Assessment Service, 2006.
2. National Clinical Assessment Authority. *Understanding performance difficulties in doctors*. An NCAA Report. London: National Clinical Assessment Authority, 2004.
3. Whitehouse AB, Hassell A, Bullock A, Wood L, Wall D. 360 degree assessment (multisource feedback) of UK trainee doctors: field testing of TAB. *Med Teach* 2007; **29**: 171–6.
4. Bligh J. The first year of doctoring: still a survival exercise. *Med Educ* 2002; **36**: 2–3.
5. Wall D, Bolshaw A, Carolan J. From undergraduate medical education to pre-registration house officer year: how prepared are students? *Med Teach* 2006; **28**: 435–9.
6. Farrah K. Time to review prescribing in hospitals by pre-registration house officers. *Pharm J* 2002; **268**: 136.
7. Spurgeon, P. Leadership Education for all doctors: no longer an optional extra. Short presentation 7G/SC4 presented at AMEE Conference 2007 in Trondheim 27 August 2007. Abstract available on http://amee.org/.
8. Scott T, Mannion R, Marshall M, Davies H. Does organisational culture influence health care performance? A review of the evidence. *J Health Serv Res Policy* 2003; **8**: 105–17.
9. Roff S. Education environment: a bibliography, *Med Teach* 2005; **27**: 353–7.
10. Understanding Stress Life Events. http://www.as.bham.ac.uk/study/support/sscs/counsell/stress.shtml Accessed 14 September 2007.

11. O'Leary D. Performance Concerns in Psychiatrists. Poster 4P/P8 presented at AMEE Conference 2007 in Trondheim 27 August 2007. Abstract available on http://amee.org/.

12. National Clinical Assessment Service. *Back on track: restoring doctors and dentists to safe professional practice framework document.* London: National Clinical Assessment Service, 2006.

13. National Clinical Assessment Service at http://www.ncas.npsa.nhs.uk (accessed on 22 September 2007).

14. Chief Medical Officer. *Good doctors, safer patients.* London: Department of Health, 2006.

15. Oxford Dictionary of Quotations (6th edn). (Ed. Knowles E). Oxford: Oxford University Press, 2004.

16. BMA. *Bullying and harassment of doctors in the workplace.* Report – May 2006. London: British Medical Association, 2006.

Chapter 18

Fitness to practise

John Spencer

Introduction

As Sir Donald Irvine describes in Chapter 1 of this book, a major element of the implicit contract a profession holds with the society it serves is that it shall be self-regulating and accountable, at both individual and collective levels.[1] However, it is an understatement to say that, until as recently as the 1990s in the UK, the medical profession fell woefully short of fulfilling this contract. It has always carried within its ranks doctors who are simply not up to scratch, whether because of ill health, addiction, questionable attitudes and morals, or just plain incompetence. Indeed, as one author put it 'The exploits of difficult, eccentric or poorly performing doctors are a time honoured part of the library of war stories which are told late at night in the hospital residents' mess.'[2] Clinical colleagues turned a blind eye, compensating for any deficiencies and closing ranks; managers avoided confrontation because of the legal implications, potential disruption and costs involved; and patients either accepted their lot, or if they had any choice in the matter, avoided having to see the offending doctor. Similarly, most medical teachers will recall students with worrying behaviour or attitudes who were able to progress academically and graduate because traditional assessment methods rewarded only mastery of knowledge and technical skills and did not look, for example, at communication or ethical awareness (all the more alarming as there is evidence that a significant proportion of such students reappear later in the ranks of doctors about whom there is concern[3]). The situation was compounded by the fact that the procedures for dealing with poor performance operated by the profession's regulatory body, the General Medical Council (GMC), were simply not fit for purpose. They were effectively only adequate for handling doctors who were guilty of 'serious professional misconduct', with the emphasis on 'serious', which behaviour usually came to light through the courts.[4]

It took several major, high profile medical catastrophes in the 1990s to finally bring the issue of poorly performing doctors and how to deal with them into focus, not only in the UK but also in Canada, the USA, and New Zealand. This was against a backdrop of major changes in the relationship between the medicine and society, changes the profession failed to appreciate until it was too late.[4] These included challenges to the traditional paternalism of the doctor–patient relationship resulting from changing expectations, the rise of consumerism and the information explosion, and a demand for greater accountability. The Bristol paediatric heart surgery scandal, arguably the most significant of these events, revealed serious problems both at the level of the individual doctors involved (lack of insight, poor communication and teamwork, inadequate leadership, perpetuation of a 'club culture'), as well as the level of the organization (in short, systems failure in responding to concerns about doctors' professional attitudes and behaviour, and in monitoring quality of care). A broader 'cultural' issue was also exposed, namely that professional values were completely out of kilter with the needs and expectations of society as it approached the twenty-first century.

The inquiry, chaired by Ian Kennedy, took nearly 3 years to complete, exploring not only the events in Bristol itself, but also looking toward the future. It was far reaching in its conclusions. The final report made close to 200 recommendations, including the need to 'root out unsafe practices', introduce systems for monitoring clinical performance, promote greater openness, and support teamwork, the central focus being in the patient's interests.[5] The report sparked a series of major developments and policy changes, many of which are now part of everyday practice, including clinical governance; appraisal, revalidation and recertification; and, pertinent to this chapter, new procedures for dealing with poorly performing doctors. Richard Smith, then editor of the *British Medical Journal*, was indeed prophetic when, in a leader about Bristol, he quoted Yeats' words: 'All changed, changed utterly'.[6] The inquiry into the case of Harold 'Fred' Shipman, the serial killer, several years later, reiterated concerns about the regulation of doctors' performance. Dame Janet Smith's report, as with Kennedy's, catalysed a further series of major policy initiatives that are now embedded in professional practice, not least the emphasis on patient safety.[7]

What do we mean by 'fitness to practise'?

Although major lessons were learnt from the high profile cases, it is easy to focus on them, thus to lose sight of the fact that they actually represent the tip of an iceberg. Below the waterline lies a much larger group of doctors whose performance is under par, not in any way serious enough to trigger a 'scandal', but significant enough to be considered potentially harmful to, or disrespectful of patients, the kind of doctors referred to by Irvine in Chapter 1 as those one would not want to look after a member of one's family. It is important to emphasize that the majority of doctors, for most if not all of their working lives, are perfectly competent and professional in their behaviour and conduct. It is also worth reflecting on the fact that the majority of doctors whose performance is *not* acceptable, whether temporarily or permanently, almost certainly start off with the very best intentions of helping their patients.

But what do we mean by 'fitness to practise'? There are two aspects to this. First, the basic concept itself, and second, the way in which this is operationalized in policy. As with concepts such as 'quality' or 'love', everyone probably knows what they mean by 'fitness to practise', but might find it hard to actually define, let alone to agree on a definition – 'fitness to practise' to one individual may be borderline incompetence to another. However, without a description to 'anchor' it, it is rather nebulous concept and certainly too vague to use in practice.

Professional practice is highly complex, involving a range of cognitive, technical, and non-technical skills underpinned by particular attitudes and dispositions, grounded in a moral and ethical framework. Even in a routine clinical encounter an effective doctor will deploy clinical and communication skills, appraise evidence, exercise judgement and make decisions that take account of context. They will display ethical awareness, recognize their own limitations and know to call for help if the need arises. They will be self-aware, for example in respect of professional boundaries, and of their own state of physical and psychological health. Finally, they will function well in a team but be capable of autonomous practise. Inevitably a wide range of factors influence professional behaviour, some of which are discussed below.

Standards against which fitness to practise could be assessed were finally laid down in the GMC's document *Good Medical Practice*. First published in 1995, it has been updated several times, most recently in 2006,[8] and now forms the 'template', not only for judging standards of performance, but also for professional development, revalidation, and appraisal. Its strength lies in the fact that it puts the care and welfare of the patient at the centre of clinical practice. The key areas are shown in Box 18.1.

In relation to 'fitness to practise', the underlying philosophy, according to the GMC, is that:[8]

> To practise safely, doctors must be competent in what they do. They must establish and maintain effective relationships with patients, respect patients' autonomy and act responsibly and appropriately if they or a colleague fall ill and their performance suffers. But these attributes, while essential, are not enough. Doctors have a respected position in society and their work gives them privileged access to patients, some of whom may be very vulnerable. A doctor whose conduct has shown that he cannot justify the trust placed in him should not continue in unrestricted practice while that remains the case.

Box 18.1 Generic standards listed in *Good Medical Practice*[8]

Good clinical care

- Providing good clinical care
- Supporting self-care
- Avoiding treating those close to you
- Raising concerns about patient safety
- Decisions about access to medical care
- Treatment in emergencies

Maintaining good medical practice

- Keeping up to date
- Maintaining your performance

Teaching and training, appraising and assessing

- Making assessments and providing references
- Teaching and training

Relationships with patients

- The doctor–patient partnership
- Good communication
- Children and young people
- Relatives, carers, and partners
- Being open and honest with patients if things go wrong
- Maintaining trust in the profession
- Consent
- Confidentiality
- Ending professional relationships with patients

Working with colleagues

- Working in teams
- Conduct and performance of colleagues
- Respect for colleagues

> **Box 18.1** Generic standards listed in *Good Medical Practice*[8] (continued)
>
> - Arranging cover
> - Taking up and ending appointments
> - Sharing information with colleagues
> - Delegation and referral
>
> **Probity**
>
> - Being honest and trustworthy
> - Providing and publishing information about your services
> - Writing reports and CVs, giving evidence, and signing documents
> - Research
> - Financial and commercial dealings
> - Conflicts of interest
>
> **Health**
>
> - If your health may put patients at risk

A definition of a set of standards in this way enabled the development of procedures for assessing a doctor's fitness to practise. However, before considering these in detail, it is worth considering the scale of the problem, before reviewing what we know about factors that influence professional behaviour and performance.

The scale of the problem

How prevalent is poor performance among doctors? (see also Chapter 17 by David Wall). In the mid-1990s Liam Donaldson described the profile of 49 doctors in the North East of England who, over a 5-year period, had come to the notice of the regional health authority because their conduct, competence, or performance was 'sufficiently grave to warrant disciplinary or other formal action being considered as an option by the person raising the concern'.[2] This represented 6% of senior hospital staff in the region. Nearly 100 problems were encountered, and were categorized as: poor attitude and disruptive or irresponsible behaviour in relation to colleagues or patients (the largest category); lack of commitment, for example, refusing to share workload, or being unavailable for emergencies (half of these instances were linked to private practice); clinical incompetence, in the form of poor skills and knowledge; dishonesty, for example, submitting false claims for expenses; sexual impropriety; disorganized practice; and poor communication with colleagues. A postal survey was undertaken in the same region a couple of years later, its aims included being able to quantify the size of the pool of general practitioners considered to be underperforming.[9] The main areas of concern identified were communication and clinical skills, and management skills. Patients' representatives were concerned about the lack of power of patients and doctors' lack of accountability. There were also concerns about the mechanisms for identifying underperforming doctors, and doctors' professional loyalty. The number of doctors thought to be underperforming was small but significant, comprising a very small group whose performance was of such concern that they had been referred to the GMC (see below), but in addition a much larger pool of doctors who, it was felt, could fall into that category unless action was taken to help them.

What factors influence professional behaviour and performance?

Given the complexity of professional practice as outlined above, as well as complexity at organizational level within healthcare systems, it is not surprising that there are many factors that may influence professional behaviour. Factors may conveniently be divided into personal and organizational categories. Personal factors include personality and attitudes, the state of physical and psychological health, life-style issues, including substance use and misuse, whether or not the doctor is up to date, and ability to tolerate uncertainty, take appropriate risks, and so on. Organizational factors include climate and culture, team working, leadership, workload, sleep, and shift work.[10] Some of these factors may be active at the same time in an individual. It is recognized that doctors are more likely to suffer mental ill health than the rest of the population, and unsurprisingly mental health problems, including cognitive decline, along with substance misuse are common factors in poor performance. Further, in the words of a recently published book on the topic, doctor's health problems 'are classically underdiagnosed and poorly managed, not least when doctors choose to self-diagnose and self-treat'.[10] As the authors say, this raises the question as to whether doctors should receive regular health checks. There is almost always more than one factor at work. Early detection and intervention are crucial in helping prevent problems arising in the first place, ultimately protecting the public. One much neglected issue is that of general ongoing support and supervision for doctors. Most other caring professions have built supervision into their working practises, recognizing that the job can take its toll, both physically and psychologically. The culture in medicine has always been 'work hard, be tough, don't cry', which ultimately may not be a very helpful strategy, not just for the individual doctor, but also their patients due to a decline in empathy and compassion.

The GMC's 'Fitness to Practise' procedures

The Council started work on developing new procedures for dealing with doctors' fitness to practise in the mid-1980s, ironically well before the high profile cases hit the headlines, but the required legislation was not secured until 1997.[11] The procedures were carefully developed and meticulously piloted through the late 1990s and fully implemented by 2004, at last enabling identification of doctors whose performance is poor enough to possibly to call into question their registration, where previously, as mentioned above, the GMC's interventions had been limited to conduct or health-related matters.[12]

A key principle was that both the doctor's *competence* (i.e. what they do under test conditions) and their *performance* (what they do in the work place) should be investigated. There is a well documented gap between the two, first described in the literature by Miller, an American psychologist.[13] Put simply, competence does not predict performance. None the less it is still important to assess competence in its own right, but also to recognize that the relationship between competence and performance is highly complex and context-dependent, influenced as it is by factors at both individual and systems levels.[14]

A case may come to the notice of the Council from a range of sources: a clinical colleague, the doctor's employer, a service user or possibly through the courts. The referral may be made for several reasons: professional misconduct; deficient performance; a criminal conviction; or concerns about a doctor's physical or mental ill-health. If the case is considered to *potentially* raise serious questions about the doctor's fitness to practise (innocent until proven guilty!) the process will be set in motion. This is meant to be transparent, so the nature of the concerns, for example the specific details of a complaint, will be disclosed to both the doctor and their employer at the outset. A case that is *not* felt to fall within the remit of the Council will be referred back to the doctors' employer, at which point 'local procedures' will be invoked. If the case *is* taken on by the GMC, it is allocated to two senior GMC staff known as 'case examiners', one medical, the other a lay person.

Fitness to practise procedures are divided into two separate stages: 'Investigation' and 'Adjudication'. In the first stage cases are investigated to assess whether they need to be referred for adjudication. The adjudication stage consists of a hearing of those cases to a 'Fitness to Practise' panel.[15]

The investigation stage

The investigation will depend on the nature of the concerns, and may include obtaining further evidence from employers, the complainant or others; obtaining witness statements or external reports on clinical matters; an assessment of the doctor's performance; and if appropriate, an assessment of the doctor's health. It is important to emphasize that the purpose of this stage is not to explain *why* the doctor is underperforming but to *describe* the doctor's performance against GMC standards. At the end of the investigation the case is considered by the case examiners who have a number of options: to conclude the case with no further action, issue a warning, refer the case to a full Fitness to Practise panel, or agree so-called 'undertakings'. These are certain restrictions imposed on the doctor's practice or behaviour, as well as commitments to practise under medical supervision or to undergo retraining.

If one is required, a performance assessment will be carried out by an assessment team comprising at least one lay and two medical assessors. The assessment itself is tailored to the practitioner's circumstances, and to inform this process, they are asked to complete a portfolio describing their practice. The assessment will generally include a peer review (a visit to the practitioner's place of work, a review of his or her records and practice documents, and interviews with the practitioner and third parties – see below) and a test of competence to assess knowledge and skills. A health assessment, if required, involves examination of the practitioner's physical and/or mental condition by two separate doctors.

The peer review visit

The peer review visit is the most important part of the investigation as it attempts to assess 'performance'.[16] A visit is conducted over 2 days by three trained assessors, two medical and one non-medical. The doctor completes a portfolio describing their background, their practice and the problems they face, and a self-rating of clinical competence. The assessment includes a review of clinical records, case discussions, observation of consultations, a tour of the doctor's workplace, and interviews with both the doctor and 12 others. The observations use validated instruments, between 500 and 700 separate data items are usually amassed, and judgements are made in reference to the main headings of *Good Medical Practice*. The methods are based on best practice, and considered valid and reliable.

The competence tests

A doctor may be required to take the competence tests if the peer review visit does not allow the assessors to confidently rule out serious underperformance.

The purpose is to confirm and clarify findings from the visit, essentially to see if underperformance is based on incompetence.[17] As with the peer review visit, the three elements of the assessment process were based on internationally accepted approaches to assessing clinical competence. The detail of the tests is specialty-specific but equivalent across disciplines, and comprises: a written knowledge test; a structured viva voce in some specialities; observed interactions with real and simulated patients; and a test of practical skills and procedures using mannequins and simulators. Extensive field testing has shown the procedures to be valid, reliable, feasible, and acceptable.[17]

The adjudication stage

A Fitness to Practise Panel comprises three to five members, both medical and non-medical members (at least one of each) appointed by the Council; however, they are *not* GMC members. A legal assessor sits with each panel and advises on points of law and the procedure and powers of the panel. The Council is represented at the hearing by a barrister. The doctor usually attends and is also legally represented. Both parties may call witnesses who may be cross-examined by the other party or the panel. Hearings are usually held in public, except where they are considering confidential information, for example about the doctor's health.

Once the panel has heard the evidence, it must decide whether the allegations have been found proved, whether, on this basis the doctor's fitness to practise is affected, and if so, whether any action should be taken about the doctor's registration with the GMC. If the panel concludes that the doctor's fitness to practise *is* impaired, there a number of possible sanctions: no action; accept 'undertakings' (see above) offered by the doctor (provided the panel is satisfied that these are in the patients' interest); place conditions on or suspend the doctor's registration; or, the ultimate sanction, erase the doctor's name from the Medical Register, so they are no longer able to practise as a doctor.

If the panel decides the doctor's fitness to practise is *not* impaired, it can issue a warning to the doctor or may recommend further assessment of the problem, for example, by referral to the National Clinical Assessment Service (NCAS), see below. Doctors have a right of appeal to the High Court (Court of Session in Scotland) against any decision by a panel to restrict or remove their registration.

Procedures for dealing with sick doctors

Most doctors who are sick and whose performance is affected never come to the GMC's attention, and rightly so, provided they take and follow independent advice about their situation. However, when local arrangements are not working effectively, referral to the GMC may be appropriate, especially when the illness is impacting (or may impact) on performance and, in addition, one or more of the following also applies: their ill health poses a risk to patients; they refuse to follow advice and guidance from their own doctor, occupational health adviser or employer; and/or their conduct has led to the involvement of the courts. In these instances, the doctor will undergo an independent medical assessment by two doctors. If this establishes that their fitness to practise is impaired due to their illness, arrangements will be made for their medical supervision for the entire period of their restricted registration, however long that might be, taking into account the nature of the health problem(s). If the doctor fails to comply with the assessment or the undertakings they will normally be referred to a Fitness to Practise panel for a hearing.[18]

The National Clinical Assessment Service

NCAS was set up in 2001 following recommendations made in a report by the Chief Medical Officer in England.[19] The aim of NCAS is to promote 'patient safety by providing confidential advice and support to the NHS in situations where the performance of doctors and dentists is giving cause for concern.'[19] It is a division of the National Patient Safety Agency. There were concerns that the expertise required to tackle problems with medical performance that were not serious enough to refer to the GMC was not always available in individual NHS trusts. NCAS uses similar assessment methods to those used by the GMC, for example on peer visits. However, the aim is different, namely to try and *explain* the reasons for poor performance in order to help remedy them, thus the process is developmental. Occupational health and psychological and behavioural assessments are an important component. A new framework called 'Back on Track' was launched in 2006 to try and standardize approaches to supporting practitioners in getting back to work (while ensuring patients or services are not put risk).[20]

Medical students

It was inevitable that pressure would come to bear upon medical schools to look at fitness to practise procedures for students. Graduates from UK medical schools attain automatic provisional registration with the GMC on graduation, and thus there was an imperative to achieve some kind of congruence with mechanisms that apply to qualified practitioners (see also Chapter 3 by Yvonne Carter and Neil Jackson). As mentioned earlier, until relatively recently it was the norm for a medical student to be able to graduate, and perfectly possible for them to win all the class prizes to boot, on the basis of academic merit alone. Communication, ethical awareness, and general professional attitudes, if assessed at all, were at best considered relatively unimportant aspects of the qualifying examination – the graduate's professionalism was taken for granted. However, over the past couple of decades, as the profession itself has been reflecting on and revisiting the nature of medical professionalism,[4,21,22] so too medical educators have started to tackle the challenges of teaching and assessing professionalism, all this in the context of major reforms in medical education.[23] The challenge is formidable, however, particularly in respect of assessing professionalism (see also Chapter 2 by Richard Hays), but there is consensus that it must be done.[24] Thus schools have developed curricular strands on personal and professional development,[25] and in parallel, mechanisms for addressing fitness to practise.

A huge 'industry' has been dedicated over the past decade to developing measures of professionalism that are reliable, authentic, valid, and practicable. At the present time, based on several comprehensive literature reviews,[25–31] the consensus is that there is no single, 'all singing all dancing' tool, indeed there is a need for 'triangulation' of findings using multiple methods (the more observations and observers across the full range of settings, the more reliable will be the judgements). A combination of quantitative and qualitative approaches should be used, judgements should be based as much as possible on direct observation rather than recall, and should preferably be carried out in the workplace (i.e. looking at 'performance' rather than 'competence'). Some aspects of professionalism should be assessed over time (recognizing that professionalism is developmental and not an end-point). Finally, there should be symmetry of approaches at all levels in the system. Interestingly, it has been suggested that exploration of a student's reflections about lapses in behaviour and value conflicts and their resolution may give valuable insight into elements of students' professionalism and may therefore be an important adjunct.[28]

Typically, a medical school, in addition to traditional assessments of clinical competence, knowledge, and technical skills, will also assess professionalism across a range of domains, using a variety of methods. For example: clinical exams to assess communication; portfolios to explore reflection, ethical reasoning, and self-awareness; reports from teachers about a range of professional behaviours and attitudes; assessment by peers (and possibly patients) using multisource feedback methods, and so on. Professional behaviour (for example honesty and integrity, relationships with staff, peers, and patients, punctuality and motivation) is commonly monitored using an 'exception report' system, i.e. a report is only made if there are lapses in professionalism, analogous to the yellow card system in soccer. There may also be a parallel 'cause for concern' or critical incident reporting mechanisms, partly to make sure that such lapses are captured and documented, also to get round a common problem whereby teachers seem reluctant to fail a student on the basis of their professionalism, but none the less have serious concerns. Such an assessment schedule will link with the medical school's fitness to practise procedures, and will also have strong links with pastoral support systems and occupational health.

The GMC published guidance on the matter of fitness to practise in medical students in 2007, noting that it was intended to be 'advisory rather than mandatory', but adding 'it would be surprising if a medical school thought it sensible to disregard this advice'.[32] It outlines the professional behaviour expected of medical students, discusses areas of misconduct and the sanctions available, lists the kinds of behaviours that might cause concern and thresholds of acceptable behaviour, and outlines possible outcomes. Key elements of fitness to practise arrangements for students, including raising awareness among both students and staff, being explicit about the process, ensuring communication is effective and confidentiality respected, and establishing support systems for students under investigation, along with practical advice about systems are also outlined. There is more work to do to identify specifically which kinds of behaviours in students predict later lapses in professionalism,[3,33,34] and to further develop reliable and valid measures.

Remediation

Whereas procedures for assessment of poorly performing doctors are now relatively well established, models of remediation are still evolving.[10] Nevertheless broad principles have been described to guide good practice.[35] First, remediation needs to be flexible and customized, not standardized, as each case is unique. Secondly, an holistic approach is desirable, one in which the services of a range of professionals are available (e.g. occupational health, psychologists, educationalists) according to need. This begs the need for good communication between all concerned to ensure continuity. Such a multidisciplinary strategy has resource implications that need to be taken into account. Thirdly, engaging the individual is crucial as this is the only way of helping them overcome the considerable stigma and negative emotion associated with referral for help. It is also the key to reaching a mutual understanding of the issues and ultimately to motivating them to embrace change. Lastly, the remediation process must be acceptable to all 'stakeholders' (i.e. doctors, patients, and employers) and must be rigorous, transparent, and documented.

As in most areas of clinical practice, effective and sensitive communication is crucial. The analogy with patient-centred medical communication is strong; at least the same micro-skills will be relevant, particularly early in the remediation process. Thus active listening, appropriate use of silence, responding to verbal and non-verbal cues, reflecting, and summarizing are all likely to be called into play. Motivational interviewing techniques also have a role.[35] The remediator's role is facilitatory not prescriptive. Enabling the doctor to describe and reflect on significant events will help them understand the root problems (for example, relationships with staff, attitudes to patients, recognising their own limitations, and so on). A framework for evaluating significant events is helpful: What happened? What led up to the event? How did you handle the situation? How did you feel, what did you think? Could you have handled the situation any differently? Role play may be another useful approach. Exploring the problems in this way may point to patterns of behaviour and associated factors that provide insight into solutions. A language problem in an international medical graduate will need specific assessment. Underlying health problems, in particular mental health problems or maladaptive behaviours such as substance misuse, may also come to light. Here referral for an occupational health assessment is essential. These discussions will also give an impression of the doctor's insight, lack of which is a common underlying factor in poor performance. Personality assessment may also be appropriate. Having fully assessed and evaluated the problems, it is then be possible to draw up a plan of action for remediation.

Conclusions

Despite the fact that it took a series of disasters to jolt the profession into action on fitness to practise, significant progress has been made in developing robust but fair procedures for dealing with both medical students and practising doctors. At the time of writing there are a number of developments in the UK that have a significant bearing on the issue of fitness to practise. First, revalidation and its components re-certification and re-licensure – will these processes be sensitive enough to pick up poorly performing doctors, particularly those operating just below the threshold of acceptability? Secondly, there is a debate about whether medical students should be provisionally registered with the GMC from the start of their training. Thirdly, although not discussed in this chapter, there is the question of selection and admission to medical school – might we be able to screen out individuals who are likely to run into problems?

References

1. Irvine D. Professionalism and professional regulation. In: *Medical Education and Training: from theory to delivery*. Carter Y, and Jackson N (Eds). Oxford: Oxford University Press, 2009.

2. Donaldson LJ. Sick doctors. *BMJ* 1994; **309**: 557–8.

3. Papadakis MA, Teherani A, Banach MA, Knettler TR, Rattner SL, Stern DT, Veloski JJ, Hodgson CS. Disciplinary action by Medical Boards and prior behavior in medical school. *N Engl J Med* 2005; **353(25)**: 2673–82.

4. Irvine D. *The doctors' tale. Professionalism and public trust*. Oxford: Radcliffe Medical Press, 2003.

5. Bristol Royal Infirmary Inquiry. *Learning from Bristol: the report of the public inquiry into children's heart surgery at the Bristol Royal Infirmary, 1984–1995*. London: Stationery Office, 2001.

6. Smith R. All changed, changed utterly. *BMJ* 1998; **316**: 1917–18.

7. The Shipman Inquiry. *Safeguarding patients: lessons from the past—proposals for the future. Fifth report*. http://www.the-shipman-inquiry.org.uk/fifthreport.asp (accessed March 2008).

8. General Medical Council. *Good medical practice*, 4th edn. London: GMC, 2006. http://www.gmc-uk.org/guidance/good_medical_practice (accessed February 2008).

9. Taylor G. Underperforming doctors: a postal survey of the Northern Deanery. *BMJ* 1998; **316**: 1705–8.

10. Cox J, King J, Hutchinson A, McAvoy P (Eds). *Understanding doctors' performance*. Oxford: Radcliffe Medical Press, 2006.

11. General Medical Council. http://www.gmc-uk.org/about/legislation/index.asp (accessed March 2008).

12. Southgate L, Cox J, David T, *et al*. The assessment of poorly performing doctors: the development of the assessment programmes for the General Medical Council's Performance Procedures. *Med Educ* 2001; **35** (Suppl. 1): 2–8.

13. Miller GE. The assessment of clinical skills/competence/performance. *Acad Med* 1990; **65** (Suppl.): S63–7.

14. Rethans J-J, Norcini JJ, Baron-Maldonado M, *et al*. The relationship between competence and performance: implications for assessing practice performance. *Med Educ* 2002; **36**: 901–9.

15. General Medical Council. *A guide for doctors referred to the GMC*. http://www.gmc-uk.org/concerns/doctors_under_investigation/a_guide_for_referred_doctors.asp (accessed March 2008).

16. Southgate L, Cox J, David T, *et al*. The General Medical Council's Performance Procedures: peer review of performance in the workplace. *Med Educ* 2001; **35** (Suppl. 1): 9–19.

17. Southgate L, Campbell M, Cox J, *et al*. The General Medical Council's Performance Procedures: the development and implementation of tests of competence with examples from general practice. *Med Educ* 2001; **35** (Suppl. 1): 20–8.

18. General Medical Council. *Hearings and decisions*. http://www.gmc-uk.org/concerns/hearings_and_decisions/index.asp (accessed March 2008).

19. Department of Health. *Assuring the quality of medical practice: implementing supporting doctors protecting patients.* 2001. http://www.dh.gov.uk/en/Publicationsandstatistics/Publications/PublicationsPolicy AndGuidance/DH_4006753 (accessed March 2008). http://www.ncas.npsa.nhs.uk (accessed March 2008).

20. http:// www.ncas.npsa.nhs.uk/aboutus/whatwedo/ (accessed 23 September 2008).

21. Rosen R, Dewar S. *On being a doctor. Redefining medical professionalism for better patient care.* London: King's Fund, 2004.

22. Royal College of Physicians. *Doctors in society. Medical professionalism in a changing world.* Report of a Working Party of the RCP. London: RCP, 2005.

23. General Medical Council. *Tomorrow's doctors.* London: GMC, 2003.

24. Cruess SR, Cruess SL. Professionalism must be taught. *BMJ* 1997; **315**: 1674–5.

25. Thistlethwaite J, Spencer J. Teaching about professionalism. In *Professionalism*. Oxford: Radcliffe Medical Press, 2008.

26. Lynch DC, Surdyk PM, Esier AR. Assessing professionalism: a review of the literature. *Med Teach* 2004; **26**: 366–73.

27. Stern DT (Ed.). *Measuring medical professionalism.* Oxford: Oxford University Press, 2006.

28. Ginsburg S, Regehr G, Hatala R, McNaughton N, Frohna A, Hodges B, Lorelei L, Stern D. Context, conflict and resolution: a new conceptual framework for evaluating professionalism. *Acad Med* 2000; **75**: S6–11.

29. Arnold L. Assessing professional behaviour: yesterday, today, and tomorrow. *Acad Med* 2002; **77**: 502–15.

30. Veloski JJ, Fields SK, Boex JR, Blank LL. Measuring professionalism: a review of studies with instruments reported in the literature between 1982 and 2002. *Acad Med* 2005; **80**: 366–70.

31. Epstein RE, Hundert EM. Defining and assessing professional competence. *JAMA* 2002; **287**: 226–35.

32. General Medical Council. *Medical students: professional behavior and fitness to practice.* 2007. Available at: http://www.gmc-uk.org/education/undergraduate/undergraduate_ policy/ professional_behaviour.asp (accessed March 2008).

33. Papadakis MA, Hodgson CS, Teherani A, Kohatsu ND. Unprofessional behaviour in medical schools is associated with subsequent disciplinary action by a state medical board. *Acad Med* 2004; **79**: 244–9.

34. Teherani A, Hodgson CS, Banach M, *et al.* Domains of unprofessional behaviour during medical school associated with future disciplinary action by a state medical board. *Acad Med* 2005; **80** (10 Suppl.):S17–20.

35. Cohen D, Rhydderch M, Cooper I. *Managing remediation. Understanding medical education.* Edinburgh: Association for the Study of Medical Education, 2007.

Chapter 19

Interprofessional learning and working in medical education and training

Sue Morrison

Introduction

A series of policy changes in the UK over the last two decades has urged health and social care professionals to adopt new ways of working to break down barriers and work more effectively in multiprofessional teams. The most recent of these, *A Framework for Action*[1] recommends 'truly integrated care and partnership working, maximizing the contribution of the entire workforce'. Many healthcare needs now involve more than one healthcare professional and new integrated approaches to case management and care plans require new integrated ways of working:[2] for example, avoiding separate records, separate management, jargon, and interprofessional prejudice. The burgeoning of clinical advances has also contributed to more complex clinical situations that require more complicated solutions,[3] often involving several different professionals. Even when working alone, professionals still need to understand something of the work and language of related colleagues. These changes in the ways we work expose a raft of underlying interprofessional issues that need to be understood and addressed before effective professional networking can be achieved. Collaborative working has become a key quality issue.

This chapter is divided into four sections:

1. The case for interprofessional learning (IPL) and working: policy, context, and evidence.

2. Interprofessional education (IPE)and curriculum development.

3. Evaluating IPE.

4. The next steps: education for collaboration.

The case for interprofessional learning and working

The terminology in this field confuses many of us.[4] According to the Centre for the Advancement of Interprofessional Education (CAIPE), IPL occurs when two or more professionals learn with, from and about each other to improve collaboration and the quality of care.[5] I have used multiprofessional to mean where professionals from different groups learn along side each other, but unlike IPL, do not significantly interact to produce and learn new knowledge. (I am including colleagues who work in related disciplines not usually accorded professional status, such as practice administrative staff.) I have used the term collaborative to encompass both inter- and multi-interprofessional ways of working and learning. *Collaboration* is the concept of 'working with'; literally, it is 'co-labor-ation'[6] and describes working together to achieve a shared outcome.

IPE can help professionals learn new vocabularies and skills to work together in groups and teams in order to enhance patient outcomes.[7] According to Freeth *et al.*, IPE is 'an initiative to secure IPL and through this to promote interprofessional collaboration and enhance professional practice in public services'. However, it can be tricky: collaboration does not just happen because several professionals from different disciplines are grouped together and called a team; it is essential to have both the skills and the intention to work together.[8] There is widespread agreement about the perceived benefits for both users and workers of effective collaborative working (see Box 19.1), but increased quality of care for patients is the most persuasive. There is evidence for this from a wide range of clinical contexts across both primary and secondary care, for example, reduced adverse patient incidents, reduced mortality and morbidity and improved functional outcomes.[2,9] This improved quality follows the breaking down of stereotypes through understanding and respect for different professional roles and responsibilities within well functioning teams,[10] which can result in improved staff morale[11] and enhanced professional development.

Barr *et al.* have proposed a 'chain reaction'[12] conceptual framework for the linkage of enhanced professional development and improved patient outcomes (see Figure 19.1).

The study of 400 primary healthcare teams by Borrill *et al.*[13] confirms this model. Those teams where objectives related to new ways of quality working and were agreed cooperatively, achieved better levels of patient care and greater staff satisfaction.

It is difficult to know the extent to which we work collaboratively in health and social care. My experience on the ground in primary care is that we can do

Box 19.1 Perceived benefits of interprofessional education

- Understanding profess roles and responsibilities
- Developing skills for effective teamwork
- Increasing knowledge of clinical skills or subjects
- Collaborative learning leading to collaborative care
- Breaking down stereotypes
- Cost-effective training and care
- More patient choice
- Improved staff morale and support
- Enhanced personal confidence
- Enhanced professional development
- Enhanced respect between professions
- Encouragement of reflective practice

(From Holland & Fielding, 2004)

it well, but not surprisingly, some still have misgivings and patchy implementation of initiatives is documented in some areas.[14] Working together does not happen easily and needs appropriate preparation and training. Young doctors are now being taught about collaborative IPL within the foundation years and are required to show collaborative competencies in their subsequent training.[15] But we do need to want to work together and have particular skills in knowing how to in order for it to be successful.

In general, groups that work well have been shown to have a clear shared aim, clear processes to underpin the aim and flexible structures to support the processes (Box 19.2).

Hine et al.[16] has set out more detailed characteristics associated with effective collaborative working in teams (Box 19.3):

But while multiprofessional groupings might make potentially effective teams on paper, there are hurdles to be overcome. Things don't always run effortlessly: the object of a team may inadvertently become the smooth functioning of the group rather than the original outcome related to patient care. Differences in expertise, value systems and organizational hierarchies may challenge as well as enrich collaborative working. GPs have been reluctant to

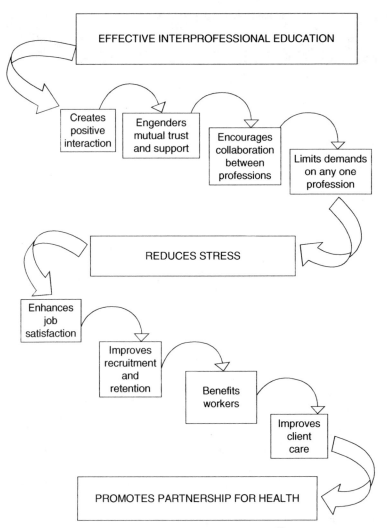

Fig. 19.1 Barr's chain reaction. Reproduced with permission.[12]

Box 19.2 Key characteristics of groups that work well

1. clear and shared aim

2. clear processes

3. flexible structures to support processes

(After McPherson *et al.*, 2001)

Box 19.3 Characteristics of effective teams

- Members must consider their roles in the team to be essential and rewarding, working towards clear goals
- Team size should enable preservation of communication and autonomy
- Attention to structures (e.g. allocated meeting times, communal meeting places) can facilitate positive attitudes and effective teamworking
- Policy should promote opportunities for teamworking
- Aspirations for teams need to be adequately resourced to maintain motivation
- Workforce changes constantly shape training and the opportunities for teams to deliver successful outcomes
- Some teamworking can happen electronically

(From Hine, 2000)

become members of multidisciplinary teams, only 'involving themselves with new aspects of collaboration where congruent with their own value systems'[17] and competitive medical educations have provided unconscious training in anti-team working for doctors.[18]

Doctors are considered to have very high autonomy needs, but do carry a very high level of personal responsibility supported by a very long training. Care needs to be taken not to let power, rivalry, and control attempt to derail the collaborative process.[19,20] Authoritative leadership, 'holding the ring', provided not only by doctors, but also by management and nursing partners can provide a safe arena for development between professions so that collaboration can take place.

Meads and Ashcroft (p. 33)[21] have considered 'working together in the face of both commonality and difference' and posed some process questions for professionals interested in effective collaborative working (see Box 19.4).

Interprofessional education and curriculum development

Despite its relatively simple definition, IPE is complex and multilayered.It is underpinned by the essential principles of collaboration and equal opportunity and is a reflective and experiential process. It is not a theoretical activity, but an application for practice, which when implemented properly, can be a useful tool for work-based learning. It builds on the principles of adult learning,[22] where the learning is actively driven by the need to solve a problem,[23]

Box 19.4 Questions to support the planning of interprofessional working

- Who and what do I need to work with?
- What kind of relationship do we want?
- How do we expect the relationship to operate?
- Is our experience of the relationship satisfactory?
- Do organizational factors support the relationship?
- Do people factors support the relationship?
- Is the relationship delivering the required outcomes?

(From Meades and Ashcroft, 2005)

is self-directed[24] and often collaborative.[25] It tends to be more effective when it is work-based[26] and therefore possible to make links between doing and learning.[27] These characteristics favour the development of practitioners with an interprofessional awareness, rather than a melting pot of generic workers, with acknowledgement and respect for the usefulness of difference.

Selection of the educational approach from the uni- to multi- and interprofessional continuum should match the goals and curriculum for a particular context and add to the richness of the learning. Similarly, the location of programmes in either a college- or work-based setting needs to be considered. Learning together in joint educational programmes can help us learn the skills necessary for effective collaboration in formal and informal settings, according to different tasks. For example, an IPL activity relating to Child Protection issues may be appropriate for a group of school nurses, GPs, and health visitors but a uni-professional educational focus may be more appropriate for GPs learning about congenital heart disease. While formal programmes of IPE and MPE are most often considered and researched, much unplanned informal learning goes on in practice where blurred clinical boundaries create opportunities for shared learning.[28] There is some debate about ideal times for effective IPL: some believe that new professionals need to feel secure in their uniprofessional identity before embarking on formal IPE. Others think that in preparation for professional collaboration and the avoidance of stereotypes[29] so-called 'silo mentality', it is good to have elements of IPE throughout undergraduate training.[30]

Many now favour IPE as a continuum of learning throughout all stages of education and training, where integrating curricula can address the

Box 19.5 Interprofessional competencies (after Barr *et al.* 1998)

- Ability to communicate roles and responsibilities to other professionals
- Recognizing constraints of one's role
- Respecting the roles of others

development of interprofessional competencies. There are still insufficient data to know what combination of professions in the teacher and student cohort is most effective for competency development and most teachers of IPE have little or no formal experience of training.

Barr *et al.* have distilled core IP competencies (see Box 19.5), and highlighted some benefits of the integration of learning curricula (see Box 19.6). But whichever model is pursued, academic, clinical, or mixed,there are some fundamental requirements for the organization of IPE activities (see Box 19.7).

However, the difficulty in implementing all types of IPE should not be underestimated, especially in undergraduate education where resistance has been described.[11,31] Within some of these more traditional educational frameworks in health and social care,[15,32] uniprofessional orientations can foster norms and attitudes that interfere with collaboration.

Enablers and barriers to interprofessional education

Hewstone and Brown[33] among others, have considered factors that enhance IPL. Not surprisingly, they are largely to do with secure institutional support that generates a cooperative ethos and confers equal status on its participants. But history and culture get in the way, contributing to long-standing interprofessional

Box 19.6 Integrating curricula

- Counters compartmentalism of knowledge
- Counters proliferation of health professions
- Makes connections to enhance practice
- Enhanced cognitive development of students
- Transcends tribalilsm; promotes teamwork, collaboration, partnership
- Reframes professional into interprofessional knowledge
- Promotes new type of worker and skill mix

(After Barr *et al.* 2005)

Box 19.7 Prerequisites for interprofessional education activities

- champions
- killed programme manager
- pre-training for faculty staff and teachers
- creation of long-term benefits for clinical partners and educational institutions
- inclusion of a work-based project
- provision of booster doses of team training

(After Barr *et al.*, 2005)

rivalries that relate mostly to power and competition and symbolized by differences in pay and status.[34] These attitudinal dynamics are often reinforced by structural factors such as schedules, regulation, and accreditation policies.

So the task of IPE is to transform these competitive attitudinal barriers through the building of cooperative trust and respect that foster a secure sense of interprofessional identity and autonomy. While barriers can be managed and overcome, it is important to remember that professional differences can be sometimes be understood and exploited for patient gain. Development of an inclusive model will be sufficiently flexible to accommodate diversity and difference, and to respond to the prevailing societal and political climate.[35]

Evaluating interprofessional education

The aims of IPE are to improve patient outcomes and experience and enhance the working lives of professionals. However, effectiveness is a complex concept and the best hope of a meaningful measure is when outcomes are viewed in their practical contexts in the real world. Koppel *et al.* reviewed the main factors contributing to the effectiveness of IPE, citing the maturity and receptivity of the learner, the importance of a work-based context and input of longer duration.

Freeth *et al.*[36] have conceptualized what it is we intend to achieve from IPL in terms of attitudes and behaviours that will ultimately affect patient outcomes (see Box 19.8), while Barr *et al.*[11] has considered quality in IPE programmes that intend to deliver this learning (see Box 19.9).

Box 19.8 Outcome measures for interprofessional learning (Freeth *et al.*[36])

- *Level 1:* learners' reaction-participants' satisfaction and view of the experience
- *Level 2a:* modification of attitudes/perceptions towards other professions or clients
- *Level 2b:* acquisition of knowledge/skills
- *Level 3:* change in behaviour – transfer of skills/attitudes from the classroom to the workplace
- *Level 4a:* change in organization practice – attributable to the multiprofessional learning
- *Level 4b:* benefits to clients

Supporting evidence

Methodological challenges have contributed to the lack of evidence for IPE. Much of the literature is qualitative description of short-term projects and biased towards uni-professional norms. A Cochrane report in 2001[35] failed to find any evaluation of IPE initiatives that met required criteria. The JET critical review of 53 evaluations of IPE,[37] mostly from the USA, found a preponderance of post-registration short courses that were not generalizable.

The next steps: education for collaboration

Collaborative learning between professions is key to quality care for patients and IPE strategies may well contribute to this agenda, but only if:

1. the goals of IPE agreed between stakeholders (nature of the student and the initiative);
2. the desired outcomes are clearly specified;
3. the most effective methods of delivery are determined at different stages of training (including the need for faculty development);
4. there is robust evaluation and external accreditation.

While some believe that a focus on IP relations is unlikely to improve teamwork, it is a minority view and most observers consider it is essential to recognize and value the contribution of other professionals.[38]

IPL has the capacity to improve patient care and professional satisfaction.

Box 19.9 Checking quality in interprofessional education provision (from Barr *et al.*[11])

- Do the aims as stated promote collaboration?
- How do the objectives contribute towards collaboration?
- Do the A+I contribute to the improving quality of care?
- Are the A+I compatible?
- How is IPE built into the programme?
- Is the programme informed by a theoretical rationale?
- Is the programme evidence based?
- Is the programme informed by IP values?
- Does comparative learning complement common learning?
- Are the learning methods interactive?
- Is small group learning included?
- Will the numbers from the participant professions be reasonably balanced?
- Are all the professions involved in planning and teaching?
- Are clients and carers involved?
- Will the IPL be assessed?
- Will it count towards qualification?
- How will the programme be evaluated?
- Will findings be disseminated?

IPE should be a continuing intervention along the professional educational continuum that seeks to maintain a core interprofessional competency through post-education experience and lifelong Continuing Professional Development.

References

1. Darzi A. *A framework for London.* 2007. Available at: http://www.healthcare-forlondon.nhs.uk/pdf/.
2. McPherson K, Headrick L, Moss F. Working and learning together: good quality care depends on it, but how can we achieve it? *Qual Healthcare* 2001; **10**: 1146–53.
3. Plsek P, Greenhalgh T. Complexity science: Coping with complexity: educating for capability. *BMJ* 2001; **323**: 799–803.
4. Kenny G. Interprofessional working: opportunities and challenges. *Nurs Stand* 2002; **17**: 33–5.

5. UK Centre for the Advancement of Interprofessional Education. CAIPE Bulletin No. 26 Autumn 2006.

6. Wikipedia. Available at http://en.wikipedia.org/wiki/Collaboration (accessed 14 December 2006).

7. Freeth D, Hammick M *et al*. *Effective IPE: development, delivery and evaluation*. Oxford: Radcliffe, 2005.

8. Morrison, S. A case study of interprofessional learning and working at Marylebone Health Centre. *Work Based Learn Prim Care* 2006; **4**: 116–29.

9. Smith B, Hopton, Chambers W. Chronic pain in primary care. *Fam Pract* 1999; **16**: 475–82.

10. Tunstall-Pedoe S, Rink E & Hilton S. Student attitudes to undergraduate interprofessional education. *J Interprof Care* 2003; **17**: 162–72.

11. Barr H, Gower S, McGruer C, Whiteman J, O'Connell J. *Interprofessional Learning in Primary care: developments in North West London*. London: Department of Postgraduate General Practice, Imperial College School of Medicine, 1998.

12. Barr, H, Koppel I, Reeves S, Hammick M, Freeth D. *Effective interprofessional education*. CAIPE. Oxford: Blackwell, 2005.

13. Borrill C, West M *et al*. Teamworking and effectiveness in healthcare. *Br J Healthcare Manage* 200X; **6**: 364–71.

14. Elston S, Holloway I. The impact of recent primary care reforms in the UK on interpprofessional working in primary care. *J Interprof Care* 2001; **15**: 19–27.

15. RCGP. *Core competencies for GP*. London: RCGP, 2007.

16. Hine D *et al*. *Teamworking in primary healthcare*. London: Royal Pharmaceutical Society and British Medical Association, 2000.

17. Pratt J. *Practitioners and practices: a conflict of values?* Oxford: Radcliffe Medical Press, 1995.

18. Payne M. *Teamwork in multiprofessional care*. London: Macmillan, 2000.

19. Eraut M. *Developing professional knowledge and competence*. London: Falmer Press, 1994.

20. Pietroni P. Teamwork, ownership and power. *Med World* 1992; 22–3.

21. Meades G, Ashcroft J. *The case for interprofessional collaboration*. CAIPE. London: Blackwell, 2005.

22. Knowles M. *The modern practice of adult education: from pedagogy to andragogy*. NJ: Cambridge Adult Education, 1980.

23. Kolb D, Fry R. Toward an applied theory of experiential learning. *Theories of group process*. London: John Wiley, 1975.

24. Brookfield S. *Understanding and facilitating adult learning*. Milton Keynes, Open University Press, 1986.

25. Argyris C, Schon D. *Organisational learning*. Reading, MA: Addison-Wesley, 1978.

26. Lave J, Wenger E. *Situated learning; legitimate peripheral participation*. Cambridge: Cambridge University Press, 1991.

27. Cable S. *Clinical experience: preparation of medical and nursing students for collaborative practice*. Dundee: University of Dundee, 2000. (Cited in Barr 2005.)

28. Holland M, Fielding E. Interprofessional learning – the way forward? *Geriatr Med* 2004; 11–18.

29. Pietroni P. Streotypes or archetypes? A study of perceptions amongst healthcare professionals. *J Soc Work Pract* 1991; **5**: 61–9.

30. Humphris D, Hean S. Educating the future workforce: building the evidence about IPL. *J Health Serv Res Policy* 2004; **9** (Suppl. 1): 24–7.

31. Wakefield A, Boggis C, Holland M. Team working but no blurring thankyou! The importance of teamwork as part of a teaching ward experience. *Learn Health Soc Care* YEAR; **5**: 142–54.

32. Ahluwalia S, Clarke R, Brennan M. Transforming learning: the challenge of interprofessi onal education. *Hosp Med* 2005; **66**: 236–8.

33. Hewstone M, Brown R. Contact is not enough: an intergroup perspective on the 'contact hypothesis'. *Contact and conflict in intergroup encounters* (Eds Hewstone M, Brown R). Oxford: Blackwell, 1986; 1–44.

34. Menzies-Lyth I. A personal review of group experiences. *The Dynamics of the Social*. I. Menzies-Lyth. London: Free Association Press, 1989.

35. Zwarenstein M, Reeves S *et al*. Interprofessional education: effects on professional practice and healthcare outcomes. *Cochrane Review*. Oxford, 2001.

36. Freeth D, Reeves S, Koppel I, Hammick M, Barr H. *Evaluating interprofessional education: a self-help guide*. London: Higher Education Academy, Health Sciences and Practice Network, 2005.

37. Freeth D, Reeves S, Koppel I, Hammick M, Barr H. *A critical review of evaluations of IPE*. London: LTSN for Health Sciences and Practice, 2002.

38. Covey S. *The seven habits of highly effective people*. London: Simon and Schuster, 1992.

Chapter 20

Work-based learning and the development of the NHS workforce

Neil Jackson and Jonathan Burton

Introduction

The needs of patients and local communities are paramount in the new NHS and must be supported by an appropriate system of planning, educating, and developing a multiprofessional/multidisciplinary workforce of healthcare professionals at national and local levels. Along with modernization in the NHS comes a greater need for lifelong learning to ensure that NHS staff continue to develop and enhance their knowledge and skills throughout their working lives.

Work-based learning (WBL) as a model of lifelong learning enables healthcare professionals working as individuals and in teams in the NHS to participate in regular and systematic educational activity. This in turn will contribute to the maintenance and development of clinical competence and performance and promote quality service provision for patients. When applied effectively, WBL may also raise staff morale and increase their sense of purpose, while enhancing job satisfaction and retention in the NHS workforce.

Theoretical background

Those who think about and research on the subject of WBL enter the debate from a variety of different standpoints. The majority of writers see WBL as a formalized process, organized by colleges or universities.[1,2] They show how educational institutions can integrate traditional academic learning with learning that can come from the work experience. They propose that WBL can be formalized, assessed, and given academic credits. This is the main dialectic in the thinking about WBL. Very many universities now have departments of WBL or similar commitments to this 'new field.'

A second view of WBL is close to this first view. Those who are committed to this view are less interested in incorporating WBL into a formalized academic process, but propose WBL as part of an occupational training programme, such as that undertaken by the nurses training for NHS24.[3]

The third view of WBL is different. Proponents of this view see WBL as being in the ownership of the learner, occurring in a relatively unstructured way, and existing, in theory, throughout a person's working life in response to the experiences and needs of work. Such is the view that we proposed in our book.[4] Anne McKee and myself (JB) have described these three viewpoints as the three dimensions of WBL[5] and this topic is dealt with later in this chapter in further detail. But first we must move on to the policy background, under which lifelong learning and WBL are to be promoted within the NHS.

Policy background

The principles and values behind modernizing the NHS workforce were set out in the consultation document published in April 2000 *A health service of all the talents: developing the NHS workforce.*[6] These included:

- Team working across professional and organizational boundaries.
- Flexible working to make the best use of the range of skills and knowledge that staff have.
- Streamlined workforce planning and development, which stems from the needs of patients not of professionals.
- Maximizing the contribution of all staff to patient care and doing away with barriers that say only doctors or nurses can provide particular types of care.
- Modernizing education and training to ensure that staff are equipped with the skills they need to work in a complex changing NHS.
- Developing new, more flexible careers for all staff.
- Expanding the workforce to meet future demands.

The results of the consultation and plans for implementation were subsequently analysed and grouped under the headings of:

- Modernizing education and training
- Changing working patterns
- New systems of workforce planning
- Modernizing funding arrangements
- Further reviews

Further details can be found online at the Department of Health website as follows: http://www.doh.gov.uk/wfprconsult/results.htm/.

Various NHS stakeholder organizations and healthcare professionals were already actively addressing the workforce development agenda at the time of publication of *A health service of all the talents*. In London, for example, the NHS Executive (London regional office) published a document of good practice for workforce and development in July 2000, which highlighted the kind of NHS workforce needed in London, i.e. one that:[7]

- is equipped to recognize and meet the needs of the communities it services, and to reflect the nature of these communities;
- is fit for practice and purpose, now and in the future;
- is able to work in teams within and across professional and organizational boundaries;
- is capable of sustained learning and development;
- has easy access to appropriate knowledge and the facility to put this into practice.

The *Human resources in the NHS plan* policy document[8] takes forward the human resource commitment set out in *The NHS plan*[9] to ensure that the NHS becomes a model employer offering model careers to NHS staff. *Human resources in the NHS plan* highlights four main objectives:

- making the NHS a model employer;
- ensuring the NHS provides a model career through offering a 'skills escalator';
- improving staff morale;
- building people management skills.

The 'skills escalator' is designed to offer NHS staff at all levels a means of career development and progression through a strategy of lifelong learning to develop and extend their knowledge and skills. As an example, by using the 'escalator' model the primary care workforce can be developed as follows:[10]

- previously untrained people employed to work in administrative or supporting roles, e.g. training for receptionists;
- existing non-clinical staff in primary care taking on new roles and responsibilities, e.g. healthcare assistants, practice management;
- developing the nursing role e.g. nurse practitioners and nurses with special interests;
- developing the general practitioners (GP) role, e.g. GPs with special interests.

The principles of retaining and developing the NHS workforce

Although the recruitment of healthcare professionals is crucial to the NHS as an employer in terms of adequate numbers and skill-mix across various professional groups, so too is the retention and development of staff. This applies to both the primary and secondary care sectors of the NHS.

There are many principles that influence the retention and development of NHS staff. Some of these are employer – or employee-specific, and some are shared between employer and employee, as summarized below.

- ◆ Employer-specific principles:
  - staff loyalty and commitment to the employing organization and the NHS as a whole;
  - quality of working life for staff, particularly during 'out of hours' service provision;
  - regular appraisal and feedback on performance to encourage personal and professional development;
  - 'family friendly policies' within the employing organization to support flexible working for staff members, mothers with young children, etc.;
  - fair rates of pay for employees and incentive schemes where appropriate.
- ◆ Shared principles:
  - shared values, aims, and objectives between employers and employees at all levels within the NHS employing organization;
  - corporate responsibility for retaining and developing staff to include input at board level and throughout the organization, including individual employees/employee representatives;
  - learning together across professional/disciplinary boundaries at organizational, team, and individual healthcare professional levels;
  - maintaining an appropriate balance between personal and professional development and employability in the NHS, i.e. continuing professional development for healthcare professionals that links personal and professional development needs to the wider needs of the employing organization and the NHS as a whole.

Work-based learning and the development of the NHS workforce

WBL in the NHS is central to lifelong learning and by its very nature it can profoundly influence the retention and development of NHS staff.[4]

Various definitions of WBL exist. One useful definition from Seagraves et al.[11] describes WBL as linking learning to work through three different processes:

+ learning *for* work
+ learning *at* work
+ learning *from* work

Barr[12] has defined WBL as 'work located (at work)' or 'work related (away from work)'and Burton and Jackson[13] have defined WBL as 'what and how healthcare professionals learn at work (as individual professionals and within teams) and how they effectively turn that learning into improving their performance'.

In the pursuit of lifelong learning in the NHS, models of education and development are required to give NHS staff a clear understanding of how their own roles integrate with those of others in the healthcare system. In addition, the emphasis on delivering quality standards in the NHS has been frequently highlighted within its various policy documents (e.g. *A first class service – quality in the new NHS*).[14] To deliver the quality agenda in the NHS, lifelong learning for all healthcare professionals is required to meet the challenge of a fast changing world, medical advances, new technologies, and new approaches to patient care. WBL as a model of lifelong learning in the NHS can contribute towards delivering the quality agenda and provide benefits for employers, employees (possibly also enhancing their retention and development in the workforce) and patients in the NHS. These benefits include the promotion of individual and team development within NHS organizations; the enhancement of self-motivation, critical thinking, and reflective practice: a greater understanding of working within the complex environment of the new NHS; and enabling a balance to be achieved between personal fulfilment for individual healthcare professionals and the wider needs of the employing organization and the NHS as a whole.[10]

Case scenarios to illustrate work-based learning in the NHS

Each case scenario illustrates various aspects of WBL based on the definition of: learning for work, learning at work, and learning from work.[15]

Case scenario 1

A 30-year-old mother of two children aged 2 and 5 months presents to a family planning nurse in a community based family planning clinic for contraceptive advice. She has suffered a deep vein thrombosis in the past and feels her family is now complete. This case scenario illustrates the following aspects of WBL.

- ◆ Learning for work:
  - knowledge base/awareness of the range of methods of contraception;
  - awareness of side-effects/contraindications of each method of contraception;
  - risks of unwanted pregnancy/efficacy of each method of contraception.
- ◆ Learning at work:
  - the importance of good record-keeping and the use of patient records as a tool for quality patient care;
  - learning from patients by a patient-centred approach (addressing the patients' ideas, concerns, and expectations);
  - the various aspects of patient management, e.g. what investigations are appropriate in this consultation?
- ◆ Learning from work:
  - shared learning between family planning doctors and nurses in respect of their professional roles in patient management;
  - managing risk in a primary care setting;
  - developing management protocols for family planning.

Case scenario 2

A male patient aged 18 presents to a general practitioner with a sore throat of 3 days' duration and he requests a prescription for antibiotics. This case scenario illustrates the following aspects of WBL.

- ◆ Learning for work:
  - background knowledge of the likely causes of sore throats;
  - the evidence base for the use of antibiotics;
  - possible side-effects of antibiotics.
- ◆ Learning at work:
  - practice audit meetings to review antibiotic prescribing;
  - checking the appropriate dosage of specific antibiotics as necessary;
  - assessing the patient's ability to cope with minor illness.
- ◆ Learning from work:
  - teaching trainee general practitioners about the appropriate use of antibiotic prescribing;

- reviewing the cost of antibiotic prescribing in primary care;
- the pros and cons of nurse prescribing/developing nurse prescribing protocols.

Case scenario 3

An 8-year-old boy presents to a practice nurse with a history of a persistent night cough and increasing shortness of breath on exercise.

- ◆ Learning for work:
  - knowledge of the anatomy, physiology, and pathology of obstructive airways disease;
  - awareness of national evidence-based guidelines;
  - education in methods of diagnosing asthma/treatment options;
  - regular updating by resourcing journals, Internet, etc.
- ◆ Learning at work:
  - development of accurate history-taking skills and the use of a systematic approach;
  - utilization of practice guidelines and protocols;
  - the use of patient care plans thus ensuring safe and consistent practice.
- ◆ Learning from work:
  - the value of patient/parent education in both the disease and treatment in order to promote medication compliance;
  - case review with colleagues;
  - cohort asthma therapy review;
  - the importance of audit as a learning tool for the primary healthcare team.

Case scenario 4

A woman in her twenties presents at an accident and emergency department with abdominal pain.

- ◆ Learning for work:
  - updating knowledge of anatomy, physiology and pathology;
  - importance of an organized and systematic approach;
  - differential diagnoses to cover presenting problem;
  - prioritization of diagnostic possibilities;
  - confirmation of adequacy of clinical examination skills.

- ◆ Learning at work:
  - ethical considerations, e.g. consent and confidentiality;
  - rapport with patient;
  - appreciation of cultural and social setting;
  - history-taking skills;
  - examination skills/use of chaperones;
  - reaching provisional diagnoses;
  - appropriate confirmatory investigations;
  - taking responsibility and planning disposal;
  - giving uncertain diagnoses or bad news;
  - referral versus temporization – concept of risk minimization;
  - immediate requirements, e.g. analgesia;
  - importance of good record-keeping.
- ◆ Learning from work:
  - opportunity for case discussion;
  - did we get it right? – diagnostic/management review;
  - looking at deficiencies and planning accordingly;
  - audit;
  - consideration of development of protocols and use of flow charts.

The three dimensions of work-based learning

We wish now to enlarge this discussion of WBL within the NHS by referring to what McKee and Burton have called three dimensions of WBL:[5]

- ◆ WBL as part of an academically accredited course;
- ◆ WBL as part of a managed and structured occupational learning programme, which is obligatory or highly recommended for certain jobs;
- ◆ WBL as an individual and/or collective responsibility within a work setting.

Understanding the cultures of these three dimensions is critical to understanding what and how each dimension can contribute to learning from and for the workplace. Preparation for working roles varies widely. For example, a consultant surgeon will prepare for his or her role over a period of some 15 years (including 5 or 6 years at medical school). Surgical training has elements of all three dimensions of WBL.

On the other hand, a receptionist may start his or her working life with no prior preparation. Some receptionists may then participate in in-house training, perhaps linked to a structured occupational learning programme, with elements of the learning being work-based.

Some healthcare workers may already have basic, professional qualifications but need to undergo significant 'upskilling' in order to take on new roles. For such individuals, a university- or institution-linked programme may provide opportunities for developing new skills and may open up new horizons, both personally and professionally. For example, Linda Chapman has described how healthcare workers (mainly nurses) learn, in a modular, WBL programme, to perform literature searches, plan healthcare interventions based on the literature, and introduce changes to practice – in a way in which they had not been able to do previously.[16]

Others come from different working backgrounds, perhaps switching careers within the NHS, and for such people the need is often about reorientation, in order to build on their existing knowledge and skills, so that they are able to deliver health services in a different setting. In this situation, individual learners can benefit from structured opportunities to develop themselves. An example of such structured training is the training provided by NHS 24. NHS 24 is a Scottish telephone advice service for the general public and is staffed by advisors who have a general nursing background. The advisors need to be trained to work on the phone and follow computer-based algorithms. The programme of preparatory and continuing learning, which has been devised in collaboration with a local university, has been designed to prepare them for the realities of their jobs. It uses simulations, feedback, preceptorship, and other sorts of work-related learning.[17]

Finally, there is the third dimension of WBL. This is largely self-directed, and has been historically relatively unstructured. It is often incremental – bit by bit, extra knowledge and skills are added to pre-existing ones. Though skills can decay and knowledge when not used is forgotten, the sense of development implied by the incremental approach roughly reflects how work-based experience forms part of professional development. Learning by doing the job is essential for those whose practice is independent, for example GPs and community physiotherapists. Simulations and theory prepare but do not substitute for the real thing where a practitioner must decide autonomously what to do and take responsibility for that judgement. There have been many attempts to describe and formalize this essentially informal approach to learning, for example, by encouraging the use of portfolios as evidence of reflective practice and of learning achieved.[18] By using portfolios and personal development plans and by the discussion of these in an educational setting we give structure to that which has been unstructured.

Learning and experience

In speaking about learning and experience we need to have an understanding of how everyday experiences shape professional judgement and practice. It is this reality that makes the learner centredness of education critical. Whatever the environment, learning begins with the individual and their own experiences. Learning must be contemporary, taking account of present realities and present experiences. Somehow these experiences have to dovetail with the major interests of the health service – its policies, its views of good practice and its managerialism driven by the need for accountability.

Individuals cannot learn as though each were still living in a distant comfort zone, before such and such a change occurred in the way that healthcare was delivered. Learning has to occur in a way that is sensitive to the demands of external reality.

Over a lifetime, learners should be able to devise ways of personal and collaborative learning that are appropriate for their working situations and can become appropriately rigorous. But does this happen and does it happen over the long term? Characteristics of self-directed learning, common among several professional groups in healthcare, suggest that WBL based on day to day needs forms a critical part of the professional passage from novice to retirement.[19] Burton and Perkins have written about the learning habits of nurses, GPs, and practice managers, and how these habits are conditioned by events in their every day working lives.[20] McKee and Watts have shown how practice teams are capable of becoming competent in self-directed learning.[21]

For many individuals and teams the culture of self-deliberation is strong enough to enable successful, team-based, and self-directed learning to occur. It is something about resting responsibility for learning on those who are already carrying through wide-ranging responsibilities in their adult and working lives. It is the opposite of expecting learners to fail and reflects a liberal educational philosophy. Readers are directed to Dewey and Stenhouse for further reading in this important area.[22,23] The changing philosophy of our times now means, however, that liberalism has to find its place alongside accountability. Healthcare workers must show that they can both sustain appropriate learning throughout a lifetime and transmit their learning into practice.

Informal and incremental learning

If we look in more detail at how we learn, we will begin to realize that our lives are divided into formal learning and informal learning. People usually associate the concept of learning with their formal experiences of learning; for example, being at school or undertaking professional training. But much of our learning comes, as already discussed, through our exposure to the experiences of work – what has been called, variously, incremental learning, experiential learning, or self-directed learning.

Informal learning occurs in unstructured, unassessed, and unaccredited ways. Formal learning, on the other hand, occurs in institutional settings, is accredited and assessed. For those who want to read widely around the subject of informal education and informal learning, there is an excellent website – http://www.infed.org.uk – which carries a wealth of information on the subject.

Many writers on informal learning[24,25] draw attention to the fact that we ourselves do not recognize our own learning.

Michael Eraut[19] has written about the difficulties of doing research into informal learning. Those who are being researched upon usually do not recognize, acknowledge, or understand that they have been involved in something called informal learning and this makes the researcher's task difficult. Eraut says that the knowledge that has been acquired from informal learning may be regarded 'as part of a person's general capability rather than something that has been learned'. To illustrate this point, Burton and Launer wrote descriptively about the working and learning progress of young GPs.[26] They noted that GPs constantly have to adapt their practice as the context of practice changes. The primary adaptation occurs when they change from hospital practice to their general practice apprenticeship. They have to relearn practice for a completely new context. Here are patients without labels round their necks, saying I have arrived here with the following diagnosis. The skill of history taking has to change so that the transaction can be completed within 10 minutes, and the range of diagnoses to be entertained changes out of all proportion. No longer are the patients ill enough to be in hospital. Many are not ill at all, and the young GP is faced with the enormity of the task of re-adapting previous learning to new situations. Burton and Launer suggest that this re-adaptation occurs 'on the job', through exposure to experience. Other writers have detailed how life experience has endowed them with specific skills for healthcare jobs: we have published a number of autobiographical accounts in the journal we have edited (*Work Based Learning in Primary Care*). In one such account a practice receptionist described how nursing her husband through a terminal illness had made her more sensitive to patients who were having similar experiences,[27] and we have published numerous similar accounts in the journal.

Throughout a working life all those working in the caring occupations have to learn the social dimensions of caring, the social situated-ness of caring.

In this respect, much of what is learned can only be learned from reflection on experience and can hardly be learned at all outside the context of personal or team experience.

As every half decade passes, the context of work changes. External changes such as those associated with the advances of science, the development of the role of healthcare, consumerism, evidence-based practice, and professional accountability all demand further adaptations. There is the need to integrate new trends into working practice. The science of healthcare and the practice of healthcare become context (workplace) bound.

Conclusions

The idea that we can learn from experience is not new. Aristotle examined it when he wrote about practical wisdom and more recently writers such as Knowles, Kolb, Schon, and Eraut have written about what kind of knowledge is learned from experience and how it can be supported. Others, on the other hand, argue that we do not necessarily learn from experience. Paul Alinsky suggested that for many people experience can be a 'series of happenings which pass through their system undigested.'[28] Learning happens, it is argued, only when experiences are reflected upon, patterns recognized and synthesized. Experience needs to be integrated, systematically, into the learner's previous knowledge and awareness. And, the learner needs, then, to match their actions or capabilities against accepted practice, as set out in all four of the case scenarios in this chapter.

It is perhaps not a coincidence that the cloudiness of practice, the unexplored learning from experience, has come under scrutiny in recent years. Much of the educational research in this area identifies the moving from novice to expert. Capability, competence, and professional judgement are a few of the dimensions of professional practice, that have been examined. In this age of accountability, a more rigorous approach to WBL is bound to supplant some of the more haphazard approaches that have been referred to in the latter part of this chapter.

References

1. Brennan J, Little B (Eds). *A review of work based learning in higher education.* London: Quality Support Centre, The Open University, 1996.
2. Boud D, Solomon N (Eds). *Work-based learning – a new higher education.* Buckingham: The Society for Research into Higher Education and the Open University Press, 2001.
3. Begg S, Alexander L. The development of a work based induction programme for nurses undertaking telephone conversations. In *Work-based learning in health care* (Eds Rounce K, Workman B). Chichester: Kingsham Press, 2005.

4. Burton J, Jackson N (Eds). Theory and practice of work based learning and why work based learning in the new NHS. In *Work based learning in primary care*. Oxford: Radcliffe Medical Press, 2003; pp. 5–12.

5. McKee A, Burton J. Recognising and valuing work based learning in primary care. In *Work-based learning in health care* (Eds Rounce K, Workman B). Chichester: Kingsham Press, 2005.

6. Secretary of State for Health. *A health service of all the talents: developing the NHS workforce*. London: Department of Health, 2000.

7. NHS Executive. *Workforce and development: getting people on board*. London: NHS Executive, 2000.

8. Secretary of State for Health. Human resources in the NHS plan. Department of Health: London, 2002.

9. Secretary of state for Health. The NHS plan: a plan for investment, a plan for reform. Department of Health: London, 2000.

10. Bowler I. The 'Skills escalator' in primary care: developing new roles for the primary care health team. *Work Based Learn Prim Care* 2003; **1**: 12–18.

11. Seagraves L, Osborne N, Neal P, Dockrell R, Hartshorn C, Boyd A. *Learning in smaller companies, final report*. Stirling: University of Stirling, 1996.

12. Barr H. Interprofessional issues and work based learning. In *Work based learning in primary care* (Eds Burton J, Jackson N). Oxford: Radcliffe Medical Press, 2003; pp. 73–85.

13. Burton J, Jackson N (Eds). *Work based learning in primary care*. Oxford: Radcliffe Medical Press, 2003.

14. Secretary of State for Health. *A first class service: quality in the new NHS*. London: Department of Health, 1998.

15. Jackson N, Jackson P, MacCarthy P, MacCarthy D. Work based learning and overseas development. In *Work Based Learning in Primary Care* (Eds Burton J, Jackson N). Oxford: Radcliffe Medical Press, 2003; pp. 145–153.

16. Chapman L. Advancing practice through work based learning. *Work Based Learn Prim Care* 2004; **2**: 90–6.

17. Health Information and Self Care Advice for Scotland. http://www.nhs24.com

18. Cole M. Capture and measurement of work-based and informal learning: a discussion of the issues in regard to contemporary health care practice. *Work Based Learn Prim Care* 2004; **2**: 118–25.

19. Eraut M. Information learning in the workplace. Studies in Continuing Education. 2004; **26**: pp. 247–73.

20. Burton J, Perkins J. Accounts of personal learning in primary care. *Work Based Learn Prim Care* 2003; **1**: 19–32.

21. McKee A, Watts M. Practice and professional development plans in East Anglia: a case of politics, policy and practice. *Work Based Learn Prim Care* 2003; **1**: 33–47.

22. Dewey J. *Democracy and education*. New York: Free Press, 1916.

23. Stenhouse L. *An introduction to curriculum research and development*. London: Heinemann, 1975.

24. Cole M. The practice of developing practice. *Work Based Learn Prim Care* 2004; **2**: 1–5.

25. Eraut M. Informal learning in the workplace. *Stud Continuing Educ* 2004; **26**: 247–3.

26. Burton J, Launer J (Eds). Raising the profile of supervision and support in primary care. In *Supervision and support in primary care*. Abingdon: Radcliffe Medical Press, 2003; pp. 29–38.

27. Jackson N. Work and learning: interviews. *Work Based Learn Prim Care* 2004; **2**: 285–7.

28. Alinsky SD. *Rules for radicals*. New York: Random House, 1972.

Chapter 21

Leadership and management in education and training

Sue Morrison and Neil Jackson

Introduction

Leadership is concerned with achieving results through people and historically has been placed in the context of warfare. More recently, leadership has been identified as an important function within the wider spectrum of management and the concept has been welcomed enthusiastically throughout business, industry, and the public sector. The term strategic leadership has also become fashionable, but here again is an implied reference to the military model as illustrated by the following dictionary definition strategy: *strategy* n. the art of science of the planning or conduct of war.[1]

This chapter is divided into six sections:

1. Leadership through the ages: three role models.

2. Educational management and leadership.

3. Leading in organizations.

4. Leadership in a culture of change.

5. Values, vision, and setting strategic direction.

6. Educational leadership in practice.

Leadership through the ages: three role models

The hero

Throughout the centuries, men and women have emerged as leaders for many different or circumstantial reasons, and often at times of crises, democratic election, or by dint of birthright. What is a leader and how does he or she exemplify leadership? Many of us when asked to bring a prominent leader to mind would evoke an image of a romantic hero, perhaps blessed with striking physical attributes, who is charismatic and capable of influencing and inspiring large numbers of people to follow or to fight 'the good cause'. Such an individual might also command total respect and unquestioning loyalty from his or her band of followers. The 'Warrior King' Richard Cœur-de-Lion (1157–99) was one such romantic hero, renowned for his exploits as a crusading knight and accomplished warlord. It is said that he achieved fame at home and abroad both as a chivalrous knight and a brilliant but cautious general. In terms of leadership he combined both the inspiration to energize the troops around him with the ability to set strategic direction, make appropriate decisions, and to plan warfare in great detail.

It might also be argued that Richard Cœur-de-Lion was an exemplar of 'knowledge in leadership', whereby in any given situation a man or woman who knows what do and how to do it is willingly obeyed and followed by other people.

The strategist

Some 15 centuries before Richard's crusade, the great military hero Sun Tzu wrote the Art of War,[2] a magnificent military treatise in which he embodied the core principles for achieving success over all opposing forces. In his treatise, Sun Tzu described the five fundamentals of strategy that act as the great work of the organization:

1. Tao: inspiring people to share in the same ideals and expectations, sharing life and death.
2. Nature: the dark or light, the cold or hot, the systems of time.
3. Situation: the distant or immediate, the obstructed or easy, the broad or narrow, the chances of life and death.
4. Leadership: intelligence, credibility, humanity, courage, and discipline.
5. Art: a flexible system wherein the 'master' or 'sovereign' and its officials employ the Tao.

Here there is an emphasis not just on leadership alone but on strategy. Sun Tzu further emphasized the need for leaders to be familiar with all five fundamentals, because the triumphant would be those who understood them, and the defeated would be those who did not.

The facilitator

Contrast the above with a definition of leadership coined in more recent times. Senge[3] places his leader at the developmental heart of the learning organization: 'In a learning organisation, leaders are designers, stewards and teachers. They are responsible for building organisations where people continually expand their capabilities to understand complexity, clarify vision and improve shared mental models – that is they are responsible for learning.'

Educational management and leadership

Appreciation of the different perspectives and discourses regarding themes of management and leadership within an educational setting

'Herding cats' – how often have we heard this unfortunate analogy for attempts to lead and manage a group of doctors? We are a group with high autonomy needs, whose undergraduate training, on the whole, prepares us to be leaders rather than followers. However, high-quality leadership is central to the survival and success of healthcare organizations in which we work: we need to understand the basic principles of both leading and following so that we can respond effectively in complex and changing medical environments. In NHS teams, this includes responding to the demands of successive policy change as well as complex medical scenarios.

There is a vast and often contradictory literature in the field of educational leadership and management, but there is agreement that the end-point is to produce well rounded healthcare professionals able to deliver sustainable high-quality patient care. Although there is little evidence for the effectiveness of leadership interventions[5] it is widely considered that the best chance of achieving it is by developing a vision of an ideal educational scenario,[6] setting a direction for a work plan to be rolled out[7] and creating an environment in which people can learn effectively. Bennis and Nanus[8] added a sense of 'doing the right thing' to these requirements.

Three main leadership attributes and behaviours have been encapsulated in the NHS Leadership Quality Framework (NHSLQF) (see Figure 21.1). and we will return to this framework in more depth later in the chapter.

Our situation in medical education is unusual, in that as doctors, and to some extent, medical students, we are not only consumers (of learning) within our organizations, but are also part of the workforce.[9] How we are led and managed in regard to our learning will have a profound influence on the way we deliver services to patients and the quality of patient care.

Leading is everyone's business. Although individual leaders and managers are identified by their formal roles, leadership is a quality that is found in people at all levels of an organization:[3] it is a quality as well as a role. We can all recognize colleagues who are not in designated leadership roles but who exert influence and who often indirectly interact with the nominated leaders. Kouses and Posner articulate this universality in their Leadership Challenge:[10] 'Leadership is

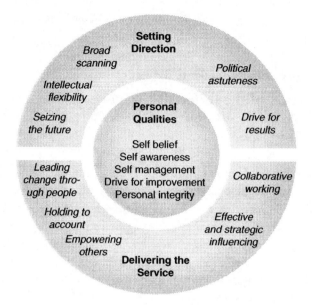

Fig. 21.1 The NHS Leadership Framework (copyright 2002, NHS Leadership Centre).

an observable, learnable set of practices. Leadership is not something mystical and ethereal that cannot be understood by ordinary people. Given the opportunity for feedback and practice, those with the desire and persistence to lead – to make a difference – can substantially improve their abilities to do so.'

It is no surprise that favourable conditions for successful leadership and management parallel those for a good learning experience or a successful consultation, where the learner or patient reaches shared meaning with the professional. This type of good communication and appropriate inclusivity facilitates development, motivation, and achievement of the aims of an organization. It also encourages reciprocity, where leaders are valued and respected by their colleagues and true commitment to a vision, rather than compliance, follows.

Dialectic between educational management and leadership

So far, we have been talking about leadership and management in the same breath, but they are clearly not the same thing.[11] Leadership tends to be about establishing values and creating a long-term vision for people to follow. Management tends to be about the structured use of resources,

Table 21.1 Different emphasis in leadership and management functions.

	Leadership function	Management function
Creating an agenda	Establishing a direction	Plans and budgets
Developing people	Aligning people	Organizing and staffing
Delivery	Motivating and inspiring	Controlling and problem solving
Outcomes	Produces change	Order, consistency, and predictability

From Buchanan and Huczinski.[18]

human and other, to deliver aspects of the overall vision in the shorter term[12–14] (see Table 21.1). There is a constant tension, or dialectic between the two, both in the literature and in the workplace. I find it helpful to remember that we are talking about leadership and management functions, rather than formal roles. There are numerous views about this relationship, deriving mainly from the business literature, but most agree on their inextricable linkage, as expressed by Bennis and Nanus:[8] 'Managers are people that do things right ... leaders are people that do the right thing'. Similarly, Mintzberg[15] expresses that 'management without leadership is sterile; leadership without management is disconnected and encourages hubris'. Managers are generally expected to lead[16] and many designated leaders spend considerable time with administrative tasks.[17]

Leading is sometimes seen as an aspect of management[19] although leadership tends to attract the more kudos.[8] As we have considered, leadership functions are not exclusively invested in designated leaders, but also found in those who have power through access to resources, for example in finance and human resource departments.[17]

Identification of concepts and taxonomies of leadership

There is no one definition of educational leadership, although there is a high degree of agreement about the main interacting themes, as considered in the introduction. Northouse's model, as in Figure 21.2, resonates with these consensus themes, namely, developing a vision of an ideal educational scenario[6] (the process towards goal attainment), setting a direction for a plan to be rolled out[7] (influence) and creating an environment in which people can learn (group context). His definition of leadership is 'a process whereby an individual influences a group of individuals to achieve a common goal'.

Similarly, there is no one type of leadership and organizations are enriched by a variety of leadership input as we considered earlier. It can be a useful

Leadership themes
(Northouse 2004)

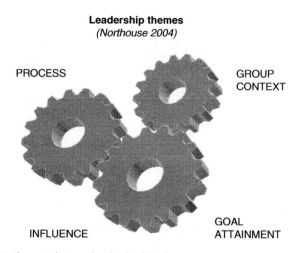

Fig. 21.2 Northouse's interacting leadership themes.

exercise to think about a leader you admire: this may or may not be someone with a formal leadership role in your organization (Figure 21.3).

There are multiple overlapping ways of thinking about educational leadership and management. A review of the chronological emergence of the major theoretical models will provide a framework to take a look at some relevant ideas and ideologies.(see Figure 21.4).

Lewin, from the early American business tradition, may have captured the moment in 1935 with his seeming oxymoron: 'there is nothing as practical as a good theory'.[20]

The early leadership theories, including those of Weber,[21] centred on the belief that a constellation of appropriate traits in a charismatic man

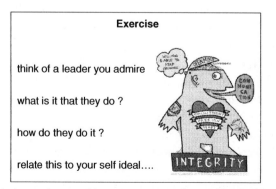

Fig. 21.3 Reader's exercise: consider your own experience of leadership.

Concepts of leadership

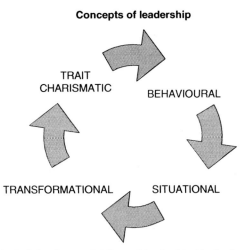

Fig. 21.4 Chronological developmental flow of leadership ideologies.

(and it was invariably male at this time) would make good leadership material: a so-called 'born leader'.

This approach gave way to a focus on leadership behaviours as researchers such as McGregor[22] and Blake and Mouton[23] began to take note of what visible leaders were actually doing: leaders were noticed to be relatively task-focused or people-focused.

This was followed by attention to the context in which leadership takes place, the Situational approach, where leaders were noticed (Fiedler,[24] Hersey and Blanchard,[25] Adair[26]) to be variously affected by contextual aspects such as people, the task, organizational concerns, or external variables. We will look at some of these models in greater depth later in the chapter.

These three takes on leadership analysis; trait, behavioural, and situational are known as transactional approaches and are considered by some to be somewhat inflexible and uninspiring and tend to be allied with concepts of management. Transformational approaches on the other hand are aligned with leadership behaviours. They have been widely developed, as they are believed to 'transcend[ing] organisational and human limitations and deal[ing] with change'.[5]

Bass and Alvolio[27] have been particular exponents of the transformative approach: 'the goal of transformational leadership is to transform people and organisations in a literal sense – to change them in mind and heart: enlarge vision, insight and understanding: clarify purposes; make behaviour congruent with beliefs, principles or values; and bring about changes that are permanent, self-perpetuating and momentum-building'.

Their 'Four I' framework for thinking about transformational approaches has been widely quoted:[28]

♦ Idealized influence

♦ Inspirational motivation

♦ Intellectual stimulation

♦ Individualized consideration

The main differences in emphasis between transactional and transformative approaches are outlined in Table 21.2.

Identification of challenges for practitioner in a leadership role

There is one other significant aspect to management and leadership in a medical context, in both educational and clinical domains. This is the challenge to a healthcare professional who, through promotion through the organization, finds themselves moving from a specialist practitioner to a management and or leadership role. Many practitioners in this position do not have any formal management training, and the change of focus and allegiance from one's profession to one's organization can be challenging. Some of these themes are briefly outlined in Table 21.3.

Leading in organizations

Definitions of organizations

We are all likely to have a sense of what we mean by an organization; a description of operational processes or the institutional entities in which we work.

Table 21.2 Transactional versus transformational leadership.

	Transactional	**Transformational**
Motivation	Need to get job done	Need for meaning
Preoccupation	Power and politics	Purposes and values
Focus	In the moment	Long-term aspirations
Behaviour	Tactical	Strategic
Operational	Current system	New designs and ideas
Values	Infrastructure and systems	Overarching goals

After Covey.[13]

Table 21.3 Motivational shifts from technical specialist to manager.

Specialist medical value/ motivation	Management value/motivation
Issues understood in the logic of own discipline	Open to wide variety of new ideas
High degree of specialization	Generalist skills
Low need for social interaction to succeed	High need for social interaction to form alliances
Loyalty to profession	Loyalty to organization
Good communication with other professionals	Good communication with both professionals and non-professionals
Intellectual freedom to discuss discoveries openly	Regard discoveries as proprietary information
Responsibility for own work	Responsibility for work of others

A simple definition is: 'a social arrangement which pursues collective goals, which controls its own performance, and which has a boundary separating it from its environment'.[29]

Hanna[30] has defined characteristics we readily recognize in organizations, namely boundaries, purposes and goals, inputs and outputs, transformations, feedback, and an environmental context in which they operate and Swanwick[31] has applied these to postgraduate medical education. These frameworks are very useful because they attempt to simplify the highly complex and often disorganized nature of the organizations in which we may be attempting to manage and lead.

Another term to consider here is that of a learning organization, one that facilitates the learning of all its members and continuously transforms itself. We cannot assume that educational organizations are necessarily learning organizations: they may be bound up by their internal bureaucracy and in focusing of educational provision for others, ignore the educational needs of their own organization. We have a responsibility to be aware of this as leaders in an educational environment. In the words of Peter Senge, who coined the learning organization term, 'organisations that will truly excel in the future will be the organisations that discover how to tap people's commitment and capacity to learn at all levels in an the organisation.'[3]

Ways of viewing organizations

As we have seen, organizations may be virtual, are usually complex and can be viewed from many different perspectives. This notion of 'conceptual pluralism' has been advanced by several theorists, including Bush,[32] Boleman and Deal,[11] and Mintzberg.[33]

Bush's framework examines organizational structure through the lenses of:

- bureaucracy
- collegiality
- micro politics
- subjective theories
- ambiguity theories
- organizational culture

and we will look at each in turn.

Many medical educational organizations, have a **bureaucratic** structure[31] that is familiar to us as both consumers and professionals. This is characterized by a hierarchical authority structure that is goal oriented and guided by rules and regulations. There is a clear division of labour, rational decision making, and public accountability.

In some organizations, there is a will to be more **collegial**, where staff wish to be involved in decision making, ownership, and consensus. Sometimes, however, only 'contrived collegiality'[34] is achieved where staff may be consulted but have no real decision-making power.

Examining the micro politics (or who has the power) at work is always fascinating. Different interest groups vie for power through negotiation, bargaining, and their access to resources. We saw earlier that leadership functions may be invested in or assumed by those who are not nominated leaders, but who derive power from other sources, e.g. resource allocation. (?egs here).

The lens of **subjective** theories moves the focus to the individuals within organizations, putting the emphasis on meanings and individual purposes. So the organization is seen to be made up of human interactions.

The uncertainty, unpredictability, and complexity of real (as opposed to theoretical) institutional life is expressed in **ambiguity** theories. In these situations there is a lack of clarity regarding the aims of the organization. The structure is regarded as a hindrance and the decision making may be erratic.

Boleman and Deal suggest alternative frameworks to analyse an **organization**; structural, human resource, political, and symbolic. They believe skilled management and leadership can maximize organizational effectiveness by using these frames as tools and matching the frame to the situation. Re-framing enables problem solving via different interpretations of a situation and sometimes involves the use of multiple frames. The frames are explained by the use of everyday metaphor as in Table 21.4.

Table 21.4 Frames as tools.

Frame	Metaphor	Organizational characteristics
Structural	Factory	Rules, policies, and procedures
Human resource	Family	Relationships
Political	Jungle	Bargaining, negotiation, and coercion
Symbolic	Theatre	Ritual and ceremony

From Bolman and Deal.

Mintzberg has similarly likened organizations to everyday concepts (see also Table 21.5), namely:

- Machine bureaucracy
- Professional organization
- Entrepreneurial start-up
- Ad-hocracy

Most medical education institutions are run as one of Mintzberg's professional organizations, where the professional operating core have considerable power and influence in the organization. They tend to work to standards set outside the organization by their professional bodies and the structure then tends to be inflexible and resistant to change, because of the professional constraints. It is interesting to consider this in conjunction with issues raised for the healthcare professional in the management role that we considered earlier.

Organizational culture

We can now return to the concept of organizational culture, cited as a way of viewing organizations by Bush and others. A cultural perspective emphasizes

Table 21.5 Mintzberg's linkage of organizational cultures with everyday concepts.

Organizational concept	Characteristics
Machine bureaucracy	Factory with managed production line
Professional organization	Small strategic executive management, small middle line management and large operating core of professionals, with technical support
Entrepreneurial start-up	Owner-manager who is also hands – on in the business
Ad-hocracy	Structures constantly change in response to varying situations

From Mintzberg.[33]

informal aspects of organizations that focus on shared values and beliefs of their members. It might involve rituals and ceremonies and heroes and heroines from Bolman and Deal's symbolic frame. Prosser[35] sees these aspects as a system of related subsystems that comprise a total culture.

Organizational culture is one of the main determinants of effective leadership. A strong organizational culture and communication enables members to align their vision and values with those of the organization's. This can promote a feeling of coherence and stability and contribute to the organization's overall strength.

But while we have seen that organizational culture can provide a channel for effective leadership and change, some aspects need to be actively managed. Hall[36] has suggested attention to 'Eight C's':

1. Commitment
2. Conditions of service
3. Communication
4. Consultation
5. Creativity
6. Collaboration
7. Conflict
8. Control

By harnessing this organizational culture and matching with the appropriate conceptual structure the aims and objectives can be achieved.

Values, vision, and setting strategic direction

To explore our educational values

Individual behaviour in organizations is a blend of the personal beliefs we bring into the workplace[37] and how we can express them within the organizational structure and culture. In medical education, many of our attitudes and beliefs are formed through our previous educational experience. Value is a central issue in the development of an organizational culture; people's behaviour at work is enhanced when they feel valued. Outstanding leaders secure commitment by consulting and communicating with their workforce so that a shared vision based on collective values can be developed. In a professional medical educational system, leaders also need to be aware of the potential conflict between values that underpinning the management aspects and those derived from a specialist medical ethos (considered in Table 21.3). The culture of an organization will determine whether the workforce is motivated by task, i.e. they are a means to an end, or people-driven, an end in themselves.

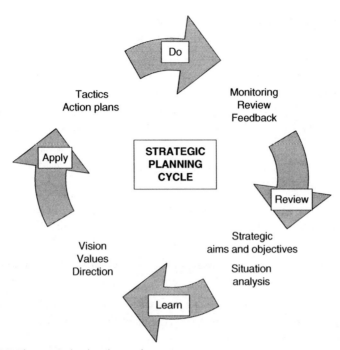

Fig. 21.5 The strategic planning cycle.

Returning to Bass's 'Four I's', an ideal transformational leadership approach will invoke several elements along this motivational spectrum. Having secured the trust and influence of the workforce, the leader will inspire individuals to be creative with their ideas and values in the construction of the overall vision. If the transformational approach is successful, the leadership will share the goals concerning professional culture, professional development, and specific problem solving.

The professional development strand is central and needs to constantly refined by reflecting on professional practice. The vision can then be implemented be implemented through a strategic planning process.

The main aspects of strategic planning are encapsulated in the NHSLQF 'Setting Direction' area (see Figure 21.1), which is comprised of five domains:

1. Seizing the future
2. Intellectual flexibility
3. Broad scanning
4. Political astuteness
5. Drive for results

As with all aspects of leadership, strategic planning can become restricted and inflexible if it is viewed as a linear activity rather than a constant action–reflection cycle, as in Figure 21.5.

There are several tools that are useful in the analysis of an organizational situation, some of which we will briefly consider here.

- The most familiar is a SWOT analysis[38] where organizational **strengths** and **weaknesses** are identified alongside **opportunities** and **threats** posed by the operating context.
- A Gap analysis identifies the gap between where an organization wants to be and where it is.
- A PEST analysis takes account of wide ranging potential influences on organizational development: **political**, **economic**, **social**, and **technological**.
- A stakeholder analysis explores how the views of stakeholders might advance or hinder a proposed strategy.
- Finally, scenario planning[39] is a way of envisioning a series of hypothetical scenarios and their outcomes that can help in the developing of a strategy; a sort of organizational role play.

Leadership in a culture of change

The strategic dimension in leadership is paramount: the power and capability of a leader to set direction underpins an organization's capacity to achieve change. And change we must if we are to respond to ever changing policy directives in health and Social care. However, it is worth remembering that organizations are comprised of people and people both create and resist change: many of us will recognize these opposing factors in our work behaviours. As Machiavelli put it: 'there is nothing more difficult to plan, more doubtful of success, nor more dangerous to manage than the creation of a new system. For the initiator has the enmity of all who would profit by the preservation of the old institutions, and merely lukewarm defenders in those who should gain by the new ones.'

So effective leadership has to understand people management, as well as strategic and organizational processes. Fullan has written extensively on leadership in a culture of change,[40] describing a framework for leadership that incorporates:

- moral purpose
- understanding change
- coherence making

- building relationships
- knowledge creation and sharing.

He stresses the need to lead and learn in a context that is changing so that the individual and the organization are changed together. He believes that mutual respect and partnership in organizations can foster the safety to 'disturb the future', akin to one of Bass's 'Four I's', 'Intellectual stimulation'.

This idea is supported by Cockerill[41] who has found that leadership and management competencies exert a greater influence on performance in dynamic rather than static environments, confirming that leadership and management are especially useful in times of change.

Educational leadership in practice

Leadership competencies and performance

Despite the lack of evidence for a standard set of leadership characteristics, the competence notion (derived largely from American management literature (of which Goleman's Emotional Intelligence[42] is one) has been widely adopted in UK.

Bolden's review[5] found that some version of transformational leadership is the most popular approach in most frameworks, although there is little evidence that this is the best way to achieve high organizational performance.

Generally, leadership attributes are seen as a set of values, behaviours, and skills. Skills can be viewed as hard (e.g. project management) and soft (e.g. communication) skills. An example of this way of conceiving leadership qualities is demonstrated in the NHSLQF, where 15 key qualities (personal, cognitive, and social) are distributed across three broad clusters; personal qualities setting direction, and delivering the service (see Figure 21.1). This is a framework rates perceptions of behaviours thought to underpin leadership competence; it is a useful professional development tool, rather than an assessment of competency or performance.

Alimo-Metcalfe and Alban-Metcalfe[43] have developed a similar 360 feedback instrument with attention to inclusivity of gender and ethnic minority dimensions, based on transformational leadership attributes. Again, key qualities are itemized within three broad domains of leading and developing others, personal qualities, and leading the organization.

Bolden and Gosling[44] similarly brought together senior leaders from a wide range of backgrounds to consider key leadership qualities thought to be relevant for the next 10 years:

- integrity and moral courage
- self-awareness and humility

- empathy and emotional engagement
- transparency and openness
- clarity of vision
- adaptability and flexibility
- energy and resilience
- decisiveness in the face of uncertainty
- judgement, consistency, and fairness
- ability to inspire, motivate, and listen
- respect and trust
- knowledge and expertise
- delivering results

Leadership and performance

However, as we know, having competencies does not ensure competent practice and again, there is little evidence in the literature of linkage between effective leadership and organizational performance. Some believe that management and learning development activities (MLD), such as the NHSLQF, will lead to enhanced management and leadership capability(MLC), but the interactions are very complex.

Bolden's review found that the most useful development tools are exchange of detailed feedback, goal setting, and action planning. What is clear though, is that leadership and management do have a range of effects (both 'hard' and 'soft') on the individual, the group, and the organization as a whole, although there is likely to be a time lag before these are revealed.

It is perhaps worth mentioning that leadership and management are not always the organizational holy grail; there can be a downside. Adverse personality factors or situations in organizational structures where leadership is mostly invested in a single leader can allow inappropriate personal ambition or greed or subtle psycho-social undermining. And, in parallel with a doctor-centred consultation, there is the potential for employees to become creatively de-skilled and dependent, although some may seek this out as a defence against their own involvement.

Conger[45] describes three main areas in which an overly controlling or dominating leader can undermine their organization:

- rigid strategic vision;
- distort presentation of information to enhance message;
- unconventional practices that become a liability.

Conclusions

Medical education is undergoing an unprecedented period of policy change and reorganization. This is coupled with changing work patterns: increase in part-time, home-based, and portfolio careers. At the same time, there is a rise in consumerism so that both the users and employees of the NHS are wanting more of a say in how things are run. In the light of these factors, leadership needs to become increasingly adaptable.

We have seen that leadership processes are more useful than the concept of an individual leader and the benefits of shared responsibility in organizations where everyone feels entitled to make a contribution. This is a win–win situation as organizational potential can be maximized by tapping into the creative qualities of all employees and avoiding overdependence on leaders.

We began this overview by seeing that to be effective, leadership needs to form a central part of an integrated strategic, management, and human resources process. Promoting leadership without management and without followership will not be successful and is a false divide.

The who, the what and the how in a leadership process will differ in different local contexts; it is socially constructed. So the most useful way forward as leaders and managers in medical education, as with most things in medicine, is to hone our situational awareness of people and organizational structures. We need to carefully consider how the process of leadership occurs within our organizations and our role within it and be prepared to be responsive and adaptable.

So for our final encouragement, we return to Kouses and Posner: 'Leadership is an observable, learnable set of practices. Leadership is not something mystical and ethereal that cannot be understood by ordinary people. Given the opportunity for feedback and practice, those with the desire and persistence to lead – to make a difference – can substantially improve their abilities to do so.'

References

1. Jackson N. Leadership. In *The management handbook for primary care* (Ed. Swanwick T). London: Royal College of General Practitioners, 2004; pp. 197–206.
2. Wing RL. *The art of strategy: the leading modern translation of Sun Tzu's classic the Art of War.* London: Thorsons 1997.
3. Senge PM. *The fifth discipline: the art and practice of the learning organisations.* London: Century Business, 1992.
4. Payne M. *Teamwork in multiprofessional Care.* London: Lyceum Books, 2000.
5. Bolden, R. *What is leadership?* University of Exeter, 2004; 35.
6. Bryman A. *Leadership and organisations.* London: Routledge and Kegan Paul, 1986.

7. Hodgson P. Management can be taught but leaders have to learn. *ICT* 1987; **November/December**.

8. Bennis W, Nanus N. *Leaders: the strategies for taking charge*. New York, 1985.

9. Kydd L, Anderson A *et al*. *Leading people and teams in education*. London: Sage, 2003.

10. Kouzes JK, Posner BZ. *An instructor's guide to the leadership challenge*. Santa Clara, CA: Jossey Bass, 1995; p. 93.

11. Boleman L, Deal T. *Reframing organisations: artistry, choice and leadership*. San Francisco, CA: Jossey Bass, 1997.

12. Kotter J. *A force for change: how leadership differs from management*. New York: Free Press, 1990.

13. Covey S. *Principle-centred leadership*. New York: Summit Books, 1992.

14. Northouse P. *Leadership: theory and practice*. London: Sage, 2004.

15. Mintzberg H. *Managers not MBAs*. San Francisco, CA: Berrett-Koehler, 2004.

16. Schon D. *Educating the reflective practitioner*. San Francisco, CA: Jossey Bass, 1987.

17. Bush T, Coleman M. *Leadership and strategic management in education*. Leicester: Paul Chapman, 2000.

18. Buchanan D, Huczynski A. *Organisational Behaviour: an introductory text*. Harlow: Pearson Education, 2004.

19. Law SGD. *Educational leadership and learning: practice, policy and research*. Philadelphia PA: Open University Press, 2000.

20. Lewin K. *A dynamic theory of personality*. New York: McGraw Book Co., 1935.

21. Weber M. *The Theory of social and economic organisations*. New York: Free Press, 1947.

22. McGregor D. *The human side of enterprise*. New York: McGraw-Hill, 1960.

23. Blake RR, Mouton JS. *The managerial grid*. Houston, TX: Gulf, 1964.

24. Fiedler F. *A theory of leadership effectiveness*. New York: McGraw-Hill, 1967.

25. Hersey P, Blanchard K. Life-cycle theory of leadership. *Train Dev J* 1969; **23**: 26–34.

26. Adair J. *Effective strategic leadership*. London: Macmillan, 2002.

27. Bass B, Avolio B, *Improving organisational effectiveness through transformational leadership*. CA: Thousand Oaks, 1984.

28. Bass B. *Leadership and performance beyond expectations*. New York: Free Press, 1985.

29. Wikipedia accessed 28 August 2007.

30. Hanna D. The organisation as an open sytem. In *Organisational effectiveness and improvement in education* (Eds Harris A, Bennett N, Preedy M). Buckingham: OUP, 1997.

31. Swanwick T. Organisational structure and culture in postgraduate general practice education: implications for the management and leadership of change. *Educ Prim Care* 2005; **16**: 115–28.

32. Bush T. Educational management: theory and practice. In *The principles and practice of educational management* (Eds Bush T, Bell L). London: Paul Chapman Publishing, 2002; pp. 15–33.

33. Mintzberg H. *Structure in fives: designing effective organisations*. Harlow: Prentice Hall, 1992.

34. Hargreaves A. *Changing teachers, changing times: teachers' work and culture in a post modern age*. London: Cassell, 1994.

35. Prosser MTK. *Understanding learning and teaching: the experience in higher education*. Philadelphia PA: Open University Press, 1999.

36. Hall V. Managing staff. *Choices for self-managing schools* (Eds Fidler B *et al.*). London: Paul Chapman, 1997; p. 154.

37. Riches in Kydd, L., A. Anderson, et al. (2003). *Leading people and teams in education*. London: Sage, 2003; p. 18.

38. Chapman A. *The origins of the SWOT analysis*. 2004. Available at: http://www.businessballs.com (accessed 19 December 2007).

39. Ringland G. *Scenario planning: managing for the future*. London: Wiley, 2006.

40. Fullan M. *Leading in a culture of change*. San Francisco, CA: Jossey Bass, 2001.

41. Cockerill AP. *Validation study into the high performance managerial competencies*. London: London Business School, 1993.

42. Goleman D. Leadership that gets results. *Harvard Business Review* (March-April): 78–90.

43. Alimo-Metcalfe B, Alban-Metcalfe J. Leadership: time for a new direction. *Leadership* 2005; 1: 51–71.

44. Bolden R, Gosling J. Leadership, society and the next ten years. Report for the Windsor Leadership Trust, Centre for Leadership Studies, University of Exeter, 2003.

45. Conger JA. The dark side of leadership. *Organisational Dynamics* 1990; **19**: 44–5.

Chapter 22

Flexible working and training

Anne Hastie

Introduction

The history of higher professions, including medicine, has been one of male domination but women now have equal access to medical career opportunities. The number of women working in medicine has increased every decade since the introduction of the National Health Service (NHS) in 1948 and it is predicted that women doctors will out number men by 2012.[1]

Most female doctors continue to work but many are seeking a better work life balance and traditional patterns of work are no longer acceptable. Forty-eight per cent of doctors (24% male and 74% female) who qualified in 1995 indicated they might wish to work part-time at some point in their career.[2] Full-time work is still the norm and there remains a higher degree of status in comparison with some part-time arrangements. However, working patterns are beginning to change with increasing opportunities to work and train part-time.

The demand for part-time and flexible ways of working and training have been supported and encouraged by the Department of Health through their *Improving working lives* initiative.[3] In 2000 *The NHS plan*[4] was closely followed by a consultation document *A health service of all the talents: developing the NHS workforce*,[5] which identified the need for investment and reform. The Department of Health acknowledged the need to develop the NHS workforce with an emphasis on flexible training and working in order to make the best use of the wide range of skills and knowledge available.

Employment rights

Flexible working law[6] enables parents with a child under 6 or a disabled child who is younger than 18 years to make a request for flexible working. The law extended the right to request flexible working to carers of adults from 6 August 2007. To be eligible to make a request for flexible working the doctor must be an employee and have worked for the employer continuously for 26 weeks at the date of application. The employee has the right to apply to work flexibly and the employer must consider the application properly but can reject an application when the desired working pattern cannot be accommodated within the needs of the organization.

It is important that doctors are able to balance professionalism against their employment rights and this is particularly important for doctors who want to work flexibly as changes in their working patterns may have implications for their colleagues and patient care. This is a two-way process and requires negotiation between employer and employee so discussion and planning in advance is essential. If everyone benefits there is a win–win situation, which is always better than a negative effect on the employer and colleagues.

Flexible training

Flexible training in the UK has been a success and is envied by many other countries. Flexible trainees must meet the same training requirements as those doctors who are doing full-time training and a better title is 'less than full-time training', which is used in Scotland and has now been adapted by the rest of the UK. Trainees must work at least 50% of full-time and this should reflect all activities carried out by their full-time colleagues, including on-call duties in the evenings and weekends, on a pro rata basis. Part-time trainees may be required to swap their working days during a post to gain the full training experience of the post. Child care needs to fit round the job and not the other way round, which is often difficult for flexible trainees to understand. Flexible training is not an easy option and needs time to organize. Postgraduate deaneries will give advice but it is up to the individual flexible trainee to organize their placements.

Flexible training is available to doctors at the outset or at any point during foundation and specialty training programmes. All flexible trainees must be appointed to a training programme through the same competitive process under equal opportunities as full-time applicants and only those who are successful can organize a flexible placement. Trainees can apply for flexible training at any time during their training and can return to full-time training providing a suitable post is available. The UK deaneries complete a bi-annual survey of flexible training and for the period November 2005 until April 2006 there were 2143 flexible trainees, which equated to 5% of all doctors in training posts.

Eligibility

Doctors are eligible for flexible training if they have a well-founded reason for being unable to work full-time. Category 1 doctors are automatically eligible and take priority for funding over category 2. In recent years most deaneries have been unable to support category 2 applicants because they have had insufficient funding.

Category 1 includes:

◆ Doctors with young children who wish to spend part of the week at home.

◆ Doctors who are carers for sick or dependent relatives.

◆ Doctors with illness or disability who are unable to work full-time.

Category 2 includes:

◆ Doctors wishing to train part-time, while in other paid employment for the remainder of the week.

◆ Doctors wishing to train part-time in order to follow non-medical interests.

Training in secondary care specialties

The length of full-time training varies from specialty to specialty. The minimum is 5 years and the maximum can be seven of more years, particularly in some surgical specialties. In addition the opportunities for family friendly work on completion of training can vary and this may affect the choice of speciality. The 2005/06 flexible training survey showed the following breakdown of chosen specialty by registrars who were working flexibly:

◆ medicine: 32%

◆ paediatrics: 17%

◆ anaesthetics: 11%

◆ psychiatry: 9%

◆ obstetrics and gynaecology: 8%

◆ surgery: 5%

◆ accident and emergency: 2%

◆ other: 16%

In 2005,[7,8] NHS Employers published new guidance on the pay arrangements for flexible training in hospital and community Trusts. Pay is proportional to full-time doctors working at the same grade in the same department. The deanery pays an amount towards the basic daytime educational sessions but the Trust has to pay for any additional hours of actual work and any supplement. The deanery gives approval for flexible training funding but it is up to the Trust whether they will agree to employ the doctor as a flexible trainee. The deanery cannot force a Trust to employ a doctor on a part-time basis.

Although the deanery gives advice it is up to the flexible trainee to organize their posts. There are three ways of organizing a flexible training post in a hospital or community Trust:

1. training in a full-time post on reduced sessions;
2. slot sharing a full-time post;
3. supernumerary post.

Training part-time in a full-time post is rarely possible because of problems covering the remaining sessions. Slot sharing a substantive full-time post usually provides a better educational experience than being supernumerary as the slot sharers are participating in mainstream training. It is the preferred option of deaneries as it is more cost-effective than supernumerary posts and more flexible trainees can be funded. Slot sharing differs from job sharing as each flexible trainee is paid as an individual depending on their annual increments and each can work more than 50%, subject to agreement with the employing Trust. The posts will already have educational approval and deaneries will try and help match flexible trainees.

If it is not possible to organize a slot share then a supernumerary post may be the only alternative to working full-time. However, it is up to the Trust whether they are willing to employ a trainee on a supernumerary basis. The average salary would be approximately two-thirds deanery funded and one-third Trust, but there will be extremes at both ends. Some Trusts may be reluctant to pay their proportion, which may prevent the supernumerary flexible training post being implemented. If a trainee is unable to organize a flexible training post it could result in a period of unemployment. Trainees must also obtain educational approval for their supernumerary post before starting in post.

Training as a general practitioner

Specialty training for general practice normally takes 3 years or the equivalent part-time and this is less than other specialties, which makes it an attractive option for doctors with domestic commitments. At least 12 months training must be completed in hospital and/or community specialties and 12 months in general practice, with the remaining 12 months in either general practice or other specialties. The preferred option is 18 months in general practice and 18 months in hospital and/or community specialties.

It can be difficult to organize flexible training during the hospital or community placements because the trainees rotate through several specialties. There isn't always another flexible trainee who can slot share and Trusts may be unwilling to support a supernumerary post because of the cost of out of hours. One option is to choose specialties where full-time trainees don't have to work out of hours, such as dermatology or public health.

Working part-time as a specialty registrar in general practice is relatively easy to organize because most GP trainers are happy to employ a flexible trainee. The trainee's pay is pro rata, in contrast to training in secondary care where the pay is proportional. However, the trainer still receives a full trainer's grant even if their trainee is part-time. Specialty registrars should work at least 50% and the timetable should be based on the training of a full-time specialty registrar in the same practice with the same percentage of clinical sessions, educational sessions, and out of hours. The specialty registrar cannot reduce the number of clinical sessions but continue with 100% of educational activities. At the end of their part-time training they should have completed the same amount of training as a full-time specialty registrar.

Flexible working

Once a doctor has completed their specialty training they are in an open job market. It is relatively easy to find flexible work in general practice but hospital specialties have been traditionally more difficult. The NHS needs to provide a workforce that serves the needs of its community and hospital Trusts are increasingly developing more flexible ways of working to ensure they attract the most appropriate staff.

Consultants

An increasing number of consultants are choosing to work part-time for a variety of reasons, including carer responsibilities or a wish to combine medicine with a non-medical career. In addition some consultants spend part of their week undertaking other work within the NHS, such as a medical director, clinical tutor, or associate postgraduate dean.

A hospital or community Trust may need an additional or replacement consultant but do not require a full-time post, resulting in an increasing number of part-time posts being advertised. Alternatively, some doctors have accepted a full-time consultant post and then negotiated a reduction in sessions. Job sharing is another possibility where two doctors can apply 'as a pair' for a full-time consultant post. If one of the job sharers leaves or retires then their half of the post can be advertised by the Trust.

The current consultant contract, introduced in 2003, applies to all newly appointed consultants and is based on 10 programmed activities (PAs) per week. Each PA is 4 hours in duration, so the basic working full-time week is 40 hours. There are two types of PAs, one for direct clinical care and a second for supporting professional activities such as audit, appraisal, and continuing professional development (CPD). The new contract has increased the ability to work part-time,[9] although there are some restrictions if the consultant wants to undertake private practice. Flexible working can include annualized hours and this may helpful for a consultant with young children who wants to work less in the school holidays but is willing to increase their hours during term time.

Non-consultant career grades

Doctors who have GMC registration can work in hospital or community trusts in posts that are neither training nor consultant grade. The more junior posts tend to be short term, full-time, and fill gaps in service, which are not covered by doctors in training. Opportunities to work part-time are often available for more experienced doctors who do not wish to work as a consultant, or have not obtained the appropriate certification to enable them to be on the specialist register. Trusts may want an experienced doctor to provide a limited number of sessions in a department but do not require, or cannot afford, a full-time post. Associate specialists are senior career-grade doctors who work with a named consultant and these may be advertised as part-time posts. Some flexibility in working patterns may be possible and need to be discussed with the employing Trust.

General practice

Doctors who want to work in general practice must have the appropriate general practice specialty certification and be on a primary care organization (PCO) GP Performer List. This is in contrast to secondary care where doctors can work without being on the specialist register. It has always been relatively easy to work part-time in general practice and opportunities have increased in recent years with more flexibility. This trend has in part been due to male GPs wanting increased flexibility to pursue other interests within and outside general practice.

There are two main ways of working in a substantive post in general practice. One is to be self-employed, either in partnership or single-handed (previously know as principals). The alternative is to be salaried, which normally means being employed by a GP partnership or single handed GP, although other providers are beginning to employ GPs. A third way of working is as a locum but this is not guaranteed work and has many disadvantages.

In the past most GPs became principals on completion of their training and there were fewer options to work in other ways. Principal posts were often full-time, with on-call and out of hour's responsibilities. Traditional ways of working have changed and there are now partnerships where all the GPs work part-time. During a GP's career within a partnership it may be possible to increase or decrease their workload and profit share. A GP with young children or an older doctor approaching retirement may want to reduce their workload but any change must be with the agreement of the other partners.

General practice is a business and the partners' income is dependent on the partnership profits, which will be higher in an efficiently run practice. GP partners do not just undertake clinical work but also have to be involved in the smooth running of the practice. Partners will vary in the additional duties they cover but part-time partners should do their share. For example, one partner may lead on practice management and another on staff development. Some partners prefer to develop additional clinical skills as a GP with special interest (GPwSI) while others choose to become involved in teaching. Partners may also be involved in activities outside the practice, such as working as a hospital practitioner, member of the Local Medical Committee (LMC) or a medical education appointment. Providing the income generated goes into the partnership account the time should count towards their share of profit.

When GPs initially become partners they can find it difficult to understand the implications of no longer being employed. They no longer have the entitlements and protection of an employee and have to negotiate the terms and conditions in the partnership contract. Although partners are not employees it is still unlawful for a partnership to discriminate on grounds such as sex, disability, and ethnic origin when appointing a new partner. This also applies to the way partnership benefits are shared.

Salaried GPs may be employed on a part-time basis by a GP practice, a PCO or an alternative provider of medical services (APMS). There are advantages over a partnership as the hours are defined and there are no management responsibilities. However, the terms and conditions of the post are dependent on the contract and salaried GPs are recommended to use the BMA salaried GP contract.[10]

The new GP retainer scheme was introduced in 1998[11] and is unique to general practice. The original retainer scheme included hospital doctors but is no longer available. The scheme is designed to allow GPs, who can only undertake a limited amount of paid professional work, to keep in touch with general practice and includes clinical and educational components. It helps members retain their skills with a view to returning to a substantive NHS general practice post at some point in the future. The retainee can work between one and four sessions per week and receives regular support from a named GP who acts as their educational and clinical supervisor. The role of the retainee is supernumerary but the practice benefit from the input of a well-motivated doctor who keeps up to date with current practice.

Locum GPs are self-employed and have the freedom to work when they choose, providing locum work is available. However, there are many disadvantages, including lack of employment rights, loss of NHS continuity of service, and no protected time for continuing professional development. Working as a locum can be isolating and it may be difficult in the future for locums to meet the criteria for revalidation.

Portfolio careers

Doctors with a portfolio career have more than one job and sometimes several, which may all be medical or involve alternative careers. Handy[12] suggests portfolio working has developed as a response to changing social patterns. Whatever the reason for this change, there are now a wide variety of job opportunities available for GPs. Some hospital doctors also have portfolio careers, although this is less common.

A typical part-time portfolio working week for a GP might include:

- three sessions as a salaried GP;
- one session teaching undergraduate medical students;
- one family planning session.

It is important that GPs maintain their 'core' medical skills, which include managing complexity, comorbidity, and uncertainty; otherwise they may find their future as a GP is at risk.

Returning to clinical practice

There is a significant loss of trained doctors from the NHS[13] for a variety of reasons, but some may wish to return at a later date. In November 2002 the Department of Health introduced the Flexible Career Scheme (FCS)[14] in England, which contained a returner option for hospital doctors including those who wanted to re-enter training.

At the same time the Department of Health also introduced the GP Returner Scheme[15] to facilitate a re-entry programme into general practice through refresher training. The campaign was aimed at qualified GPs in the following circumstances:

- GPs who were working as locums rather than substantive NHS posts.
- GPs who were not working.
- GPs who were working but not in general practice.

The scheme allowed a period of refresher training of up to 6 months full-time or 12 months part-time. This was usually undertaken in a training practice, although placements in other practices could be approved with suitable educational support.

Both the hospital and general practice schemes were successful and popular but after 3 years the funding was withdrawn by the Department of Health. Some postgraduate deaneries have continued to fund GP returners but there are very few opportunities for hospital doctors. Many Primary Care Trusts refuse to allow GPs on to their performer list if they have been out of general practice for more than 2 years unless they undertake a period of induction and refresher training.

Conclusions

Opportunities for doctors to train and work flexibly in primary and secondary care have become a reality in recent years and are essential to maintain and develop the future workforce of the NHS. However, doctors should try and avoid career breaks of more that 2 years as it is becoming increasingly difficult to return to a medical career. The NHS will need to develop schemes similar to the GP retainer scheme and allow other doctors to retain their skills. Currently, doctors who are in training or working in secondary care may be lost to the profession if they are only able to work a very limited amount of time for a number of years.

As more women qualify as doctors and both sexes want a better work life balance there will be an increasing demand for flexible ways of working. It is essential that employers are creative in changing working patterns and do not make financial constraints an excuse to stick to historical ways of working. When funding is limited, new ways of working may be more cost-effective.

References

1. Griffiths E. Just who are tomorrow's doctors? *BMJ Careers* 2003; **326**: 4.
2. British Medical Association. *BMA Cohort Study of 1995 Medical Graduates, Sixth Report*. London: BMA, 2001.
3. Department of Health. *Improving working lives standard*. London: Department of Health, 2001.
4. Secretary of State for Health. *The NHS plan – a plan for investment, a plan for reform*. London: Department of Health, 2000.
5. NHS Executive. *A health service of all the talents: developing the NHS workforce*. London: Department of Health, 2000.
6. http://www.dti.gov.uk/employment/workandfamilies/flexible-working/faq/page21642.html (accessed 17 July 2007).

7. NHS Employers. *Doctors in flexible training: equitable pay for flexible medical training.* Leeds: NHS Employers, 2005.

8. NHS Employers. *Doctors in flexible training: principles underpinning the new arrangements for flexible training.* Leeds: NHS Employers, 2005.

9. British Medical Association and Department of Health. *Part-time and flexible working for consultants.* London: British Medical Association, 2003.

10. British Medical Association. *Model terms and conditions of service for a salaried general practitioner employed by a GMS practice.* London: BMA, 2003.

11. NHS Executive. *GP retainer scheme.* Health Service Circular 1998/101. Leeds: Department of Health, 1998.

12. Handy C. *The age of unreason.* London: Random House, 1995.

13. Goldacre JM, Lambert TW, Davidson JM. Loss of British-trained doctors from the medical workforce in Great Britain. *Med Educ* 2001; **35**: 337–44.

14. Department of Health. *Flexible careers scheme for hospital doctors.* Leeds: Department of Health, 2002.

15. Department of Health. *GP returners and flexible career scheme for GPs.* Leeds: Department of Health, 2002.

Chapter 23

Equality and diversity

Rex Bird

Introduction

The mention of equal opportunities can raise a host of fears and misapprehensions in individuals. This is understandable in a climate of populist headlines that speak of 'political correctness gone mad'. Many suspect that equal opportunities and diversity training and policies are in some way designed to make them think differently, a form of brain washing. Another reaction that emerges frequently in the health service is 'What do we need it for? We already have a diverse work force.' This chapter is designed to allay those fears and dispel some of that complacency. It will provide a rationale for why quality frameworks in medical training and education require providers to strive for best practice in equality, diversity, and opportunity practice and policy. This will be located within the context of the Post Graduate Medical Education Training Board (PMETB) domain as currently detailed.

It is informed by my experience as a lay visitor inspecting deaneries. During my visits equality, diversity, and opportunity were the domains that were consistently underdeveloped. That is not to say that deaneries were discriminating or acting in anyway prejudicially or illegally but just that they did not have the systems to demonstrate that they were striving for best practice in this area. It is hoped that this chapter will also prove to be informative for providers of training and education and those with an interest in developing medical education and training.

I must emphasize that this is a personal view, developed over many years of working in and managing a wide variety of organizations. It is not endorsed by PMETB and does not necessarily represent their views or opinions.

The business case

You may be thinking that the first area for discussion is the legal framework that governs equal opportunities issues. However, I take the view, and will hopefully demonstrate that, irrespective of the legislation, adopting sound policies and practices in equality, diversity, and opportunity is good business sense. A by-product of this approach is that an organization will also be legally compliant.

It has been demonstrated repeatedly that having effective and well monitored equality and diversity policies is good for business.[1,2] For any business or organization its biggest overhead, often 70% or more of its outgoings, is the cost of staff. Investment in staff is essential for any organization but it can be expensive. Therefore, anything that reduces the rate of return on the investment needs to be at least reduced if not eliminated. An organization needs to try and ensure that it maximizes the return on its investment in staff. The NHS is wholly dependent on the quality of staff it employs. To train a consultant in the NHS costs at least £265 000[3] so the NHS needs to ensure there is a good return on its investment. Practices and procedures that hinder the recoupment of that investment do not make good business sense.

Good personnel practice is designed to ensure that the most competent person gets the job. This simple theory is dependent on the ability, first, to accurately define the job – the job specification – and then define the full set of competencies and knowledge that are necessary to fulfil the specification. This is easier said than done because roles change and so do people. It also ignores much of the past experience that people bring with them to a job. It is this wider experience that can be vital to an organization that deals with people. Take any workforce and probe their backgrounds and experience and one often uncovers a wealth of skills and knowledge, which, while not immediately relevant to a specific role, may be of significant value to an organization. The ability to speak a foreign language is a good example. Many organizations and businesses undertake skills audits on existing staff to gauge the full range of skills and experience its workforce have, and that can be drawn on. This is a simple step towards understanding the value of diversity within an organization.

When an organization takes an interest in its staff and their well-being there are demonstrable improvements in organizational performance (this is known as the Hawthorne effect).[4] Having effective policies that value a diverse work force and strive for equality of opportunity sends important messages to the workforce contributing to the overall morale and motivation of staff. All of us thrive in environments where we know we are valued. This in turn helps reduce wastage of investment in people through improving retention. People are less likely to leave if they know they are valued and have an equal chance to develop their full potential. This can be an enormous cost saving for an organization or business.

Having good equal opportunities policies also reinforces a stable and healthy corporate image of an organization. This is good for stakeholders and customers alike giving them confidence in an organization that is maximizing its potential.

However, the most important aspect of this approach is that it must be transparent – an organization must be seen to be doing it by its staff and stakeholders, as well as the outside world. And not just doing it once but as a continued part of its business cycle, assessing, reviewing, and improving its performance to ensure that it is effective.

This is where the PMETB standards play a crucial role in providing a clear framework for deaneries and training providers to operate within. But more of this later.

The legal case

The other pressing reason for an organization to ensure that it has effective policies and procedures in place is that there is a legal requirement to do so. Current legislation that relates to equality and diversity are covered by at least 15 different acts of Parliament, and these are constantly being amended or revised.[5] There are also some variations in different parts of the UK, thus Northern Ireland has had legislation that deals with religious discrimination for some time and does not apply in the rest of the UK, although this is likely to change.

It is not the remit of this essay to explain each of these in any detail suffice to say in all of them it is the employer's responsibility to demonstrate that they have not discriminated on the basis of gender, race, disability, etc. Thus it is essential that an organization has transparent policies, and knows that they are effective.

The costs of failing to ensure can be dramatic. The total cost to employers for 2006 is £1.7 billion in compensation and legal fees.[6] It has been calculated that during 2006 the legal cost of discrimination was £320 million.[7] The Employment Tribunal Service reported that it dealt with 176 000 claims during 2006 and that the figure is rising due to the 'no-win, no-fee' approach of lawyers.

And it is not sufficient to blame staff's lack of knowledge or awareness of policies and procedures. In a recent tribunal case against a university, staff on an interview panel admitted they had not read the equal opportunities policies. This factor was significant in the findings of the Industrial Tribunal and led to a hefty fine for the university.[8] Thus the economic argument for ensuring that policies are in place and followed is overwhelming.

Recent changes to discrimination legislation (Equality Act 2006) have introduced new obligations on employers to not only ensure that discrimination does not take place but also to promote equality of opportunity between men and women. (The Equality Act 2006 also has changed the governing structure for equality bringing into being The Commission for Equality and Human Rights bringing together several other agencies dealing with discrimination.) This is particularly aimed at the public sector, which obviously includes the NHS. The requirement to promote equality of opportunity underlines the importance of the PMETB standards and the need to comply with them fully.

The Post Graduate Medical Education Training Board standards

It should be noted that, PMETB are currently reviewing the Generic Standards for Training and that the standards may be changed or amended. It is unlikely that the general principles embodied in the existing standards will be altered.

The opening sentence of the document detailing the generic standards for training states: 'This domain deals with equality and diversity matters pervading the *whole* of training …' (author's emphasis). This encapsulates the crucial importance of this domain and how it underpins all the other domains. The standard specifies the key elements that are encompassed: widening access and participation, fair recruitment, the provision of information, programme design, and job adjustment.

Currently, there are four mandatory standards and one standard is deemed to be developmental. It should be noted that developmental standards tend to evolve into mandatory standards very quickly. Let's look at these standards individually.

> 3.1 At all stages training programmes must comply with employment law. The Disability Discrimination Act, Race Relations (Amendment) Act, Sex Discrimination Act, Equal Pay Acts, The Human Rights Act and other equal opportunity legislation that may be enacted in the future, and be working towards best practice. This will include compliance with any public duties to promote equality.

Here is the clear statement of the need to comply with legislation. Note also that this is future proofed by its reference to future legislation. It also references the imminent change that will require public bodies to promote equality. (This duty has been in existence for sometime in Northern Ireland.) But it is the tag line '… and be working towards best practice.' that is critical here. From my limited experience of inspection, all too frequently deaneries and Trusts have a static view of equal opportunities and there is no dynamic that requires regular review, amendment, and change. This is vital because as the legislative requirements change so does the environment in which medical training takes place. An example of this, to which I will refer later, is the changing profile of medical training intake; the majority of new entrants to medical school are women. Best practice requires systems to be flexible, responsive, and dynamic. Effective systems change because they are prompted from within rather than being forced to due to external events and circumstances.

> 3.2 Information about training programmes, their content and purpose must be publicly accessible either on or via links on Deanery and PMETB websites.

This is straightforward: tell people what you do, and preferably give as much detail as possible. This is the first step in being an equal opportunity compliant organization. PMETB requires the information to be available via websites. The rush to develop websites has sometimes ended up with poorly designed websites that are not user friendly or easy to navigate to find the relevant information. When commissioning websites it is important to consider how people use websites and to pilot them prior to launch.

> 3.3 Deaneries must take all reasonable steps to ensure that programmes can be adjusted for trainees with well founded individual reasons for being unable to work full time to work flexibly within the requirements of PMETB Standards' Rules. Deaneries must take appropriate action to encourage trusts and other training providers to accept their fair share of doctors training flexibly.

The issue of flexible working has become more important in recent years due to the changing profile of the workforce but also due to changing social demands. I have already outlined the business case in general terms – it is very expensive to lose trainees midway through their training due to inflexible rules and procedures that do not take account of an individual's particular needs. While the driver for increased flexible working has been the increasing number of women in the workforce and the consequent demand for time off for childbirth and child care, it is important to remember that these issues also affect men. And it may not be just parental issues that require flexibility in training plans; sometimes it can be social issues or health issues that require the opportunity to work more flexibly rather than lose a valued member of staff.

This standard also urges deaneries to be proactive in encouraging Trusts and other training providers to accommodate requests for flexible working and training patterns. This is easier said than done but is becoming easier due to the legislative framework changing. Deaneries may need to begin to specify minimum standards to providers of training.

> 3.4 Appropriate reasonable adjustment must be made for trainees with, disabilities, special educational or other needs.

This is a catch-all standard to ensure compliance with the Disability Discrimination Act. However, the standard is qualified, as is the Act, by the words 'appropriate reasonable'. This allows for a common sense judgement on the part of the employing organization. With medical trainees, where their competence and aptitude have been rigorously assessed, the necessary adjustments required to facilitate full participation are usually small. Where there is a demand prior to commencement of training this will be made known and the simplest way to assess what is required is to ask the trainee. Most people with a disability are well aware of what their requirements are to ensure that they fully participate. Areas that often get overlooked are non-visible disabilities such as hearing or visual impairment. So, for example it may be necessary to ensure that your website can be viewed in larger font sizes or that teaching facilities carry an induction loop.

> 3.5 Trainees should have access to appropriate evidence on trainee recruitment, appointment, and satisfaction, and on RITA panel results analysed by ethnicity, place of qualification, disability, gender and part-time training/working.

This is a developmental standard but developmental standards usually translate into mandatory standards quite quickly. Behind this standard is the need for policies and practices to be transparent. A current survey of deaneries indicates that none of them provide this full range of information for trainees and the wider public to view. At first it may seem a major task to gather all this information, and first time round it is, but with good recording systems established, each year this becomes a simpler routine. These data will also form the basis of an action plan because it will identify areas where improvements can be made. It will also inform longer-term strategic planning, as the profile of the trainee intake is established, it enables manager to plan for changes.

Managing equality, diversity, and opportunity

Most, if not all, public organizations have an equal opportunities policy although its value is not always recognized. It has been compared with a bidet: adds a touch of class but no one knows what it is for. The problem is that most policies are static; the organization has it as a statement of good intent but does little to see if it is working and doing the job it was designed for. Similarly, many organizations do collect data for equal opportunities monitoring – at least that is what it says on the form. The results of such monitoring are rarely published or cited in reports. Thus there is a need for proactive management of the equality and diversity function within an organization.

Good management requires good leadership and that starts at the top; therefore it is vital that senior management teams make their commitment to an equal and diverse organization clear at the outset. This commitment needs communicating to all levels of staff and requires a 'whole organization' approach. That means equality and diversity appears regularly on agendas, are topics that are regularly reviewed with regards to trainee intake, on course progression and outcomes. There is no one model that works for every organization but there are plenty of effective means to ensure that an organization is dynamic and continually improving.

Some organizations, especially those embarking on implementing changes to their equality policies, have found it helpful to convene a specialist committee or task force who have been charged with overseeing the implementation and continued monitoring of the policies. Membership needs to be drawn widely from staff in the organization and its reporting line needs to be directly into senior management team. One deanery has designated a member of staff as an equality and diversity champion, tasked with ensuring that the policy is monitored as well as being a point of contact for trainees and staff if there is a relevant issue that needs investigation or action. However, this approach needs some caution – equality and diversity are 'whole organization' issues and managers need to ensure that if a champion is appointed they don't become a dumping ground for issues to do with equality and diversity.

To ensure that the dynamic is sustained it is useful to develop a calendar that indicates when meetings will take place and when actions need to be taken. This will form part of a regular planning cycle: audit, analysis, development and action planning, implementation, leading to audit again. At each stage it is important to make known to all stakeholders and audiences where you are and what you are trying to do. Regular document review is required to ensure that polices and procedures are fit for purpose. It is also useful for organizations to assess the impact of polices over time. (In Northern Ireland Impact assessments, at least every 5 years, are a legal requirement for public bodies. It is likely that the rest of the UK will follow this practice.) This will demonstrate distance travelled for an organization and this can be a vital tool for maintaining the momentum and assisting change within organizations. It also helps an organization anticipate change and become proactive in reviewing policies and procedures.

As with any new system or improvements there will be a requirement to train staff that will need to operate the revised procedures. My experience tends to suggest that there is a wide variation in the quality of training provided in equality and diversity. In organizing any training it is essential that the training fits the needs of the organization, that is, it is not an 'off the shelf' course. Its purpose is for the organization to operate more effectively and therefore must be tailored to the requirements of the organization. The context and purpose need to be explicit: training should be about changing behaviour, not attitudes, so that everyone is clear about what is expected from them in the performance of their roles. A good training organization will be constantly updating its basic training as well as providing training that extends and grows its staff. Training in equality and diversity is not a 'one-off' either. Staff will need regular refresher training as legislation changes, but also systems and procedures will change.

Managers may be daunted by the size of the task but organizations that have implemented effective systems have found that it becomes easier year on year. It is also important to continually remind oneself that the purpose is to maximize the efficiency and effectiveness of the organization by recruiting, developing, and retaining the best possible workforce and maximizing their contribution.

Conclusions

At a time of massive change in the NHS and particularly in postgraduate training and education managers need to be alert to issues concerning diversity and equality. The recent Medical Training Application Service (MTAS) events indicated that almost a third, approximately 10 000, of the applicants for posts were from overseas.[9] With this volume of applicants it is essential that equality and diversity polices are in place and robustly monitored – failure to do so could be very expensive. But rather than be concerned managers should see it as a sign of optimism as this allows organizations to have a choice of some of the best medical talent in the world. To take full advantage of this opportunity it is essential that managers take equality and diversity issues as seriously as any other aspect of their organization's operation. The reward will be a rich and dynamic organization with confident and motivated staff.

References

1. Department of Trade & Industry. *Changing Job Quality in Great Britain*. London: Stationary Office, 2006.
2. *The 100 Best Companies to Work for. The Sunday Times*, 2007 June.
   Both the above sources emphasise that companies that are praised by their employees have robust policies on equality and diversity.
3. Personal Social Services Research Unit: *Unit Costs of Health and Social Care*. University of Kent, 2006.
4. Mayo E. *The Human Problems of an Industrial Civilisation*. Harvard, 1933.
   Mayo's research at the Hawthorne plant in Chicago into factors affecting productivity failed to take account of the effect of the research itself. Mayo's experiments showed an increase in worker productivity was produced by the psychological stimulus of being singled out, involved, and made to feel important.
5. Improvement and Development Agency for Local Government (IDeA) website, available at: http://www.idea.gov.uk, flags up forthcoming changes to equality and diversity legislation that will encourage organisations and businesses to adopt a 'single equality policy'.
6. Ward Lucy. Gender Equality. A Society Guardian Supplement. *The Guardian*, 28 March 2007.
7. Reid A. quoted in *Management Today* article Diversity in the Workforce. 24th June 2007.
8. Dyer C. University Agress to pay £35,000 after losing discrimination case. *The Guardian*, 23 April 2007.
9. Genes S: Training overhaul blamed for junior doctors fiasco. *The Guardian*, 8 October 2007.

Chapter 24

Ethical and legal issues

Anne Slowther and John Spicer

Introduction

In considering the ethical and legal issues arising in medical education and training we need to acknowledge two distinct but interlinked domains. The first domain encompasses the ethical and legal content of a medical education or training programme; including questions of what should be included in a medical ethics and law curriculum, how best to deliver such a curriculum effectively and what we are trying to achieve with the teaching of medical ethics and law to medical students and trainee doctors. The second domain is more concerned with what can be described as the ethical and legal context of medical education and training. This includes issues that are common to most if not all education and training programmes such as probity of students and teachers, dealing with failing students, conflicts of interests, and students as research participants. However, some ethical and legal issues that arise in medical education and training are more specific to the context of medicine (although not exclusive to it). Broadly speaking in education and training generally the central ethical relationship is between student and teacher but in medical training there is a third party in this central relationship, the patient. Many of the ethical and legal issues specific to the context of medical education and training arise from this essential tripartite relationship and range from obligations of patients to participate in medical education through avoidance of harm to patients from inexperienced trainees, to selection of medical school entrants based on their ethical disposition. In this chapter we will consider briefly the ethical and legal content of medical education and training and then focus on the ethical and legal context of medical education, which has received less attention in the literature but we would argue is of equal importance.

The ethical and legal content of medical education and training

Ethics has in some way been a part of medical education for as long as there have been physicians. This has been either explicit, with reference to professional codes such as the Hippocratic Oath,[1] or more recently the codes of practice issued by Professional Organizations, such as the General Medical Council (GMC) in the UK[2] and the American Medical Association[3] or implicit through role modelling and mentoring during a doctor's training. Formal recognition of the need for specific education and training in ethics and law in the context of medicine is a relatively recent phenomenon. In the UK, publication of *Tomorrow's doctors* by the GMC in 1993 heralded a shift in medical under-graduate education, which included recognition of the importance of developing in students' attitudes appropriate to their future responsibilities to patients, colleagues, and society.[4] The reference to ethical knowledge, skills, and attitudes was made more explicit in the 2003 revision[5] and this together with the publication of a consensus paper on a core curriculum in 1998[6] led to the development of formal teaching of medical ethics and law in UK medical schools. The incorporation of ethics into the undergraduate curriculum has been accompanied by a similar move in postgraduate medical training with ethics forming part of the assessment for membership of some profes-sional organizations. The more recent focus on the teaching and assessment of professionalism during medical training, which is discussed elsewhere in this book, reflects a further development of the ethical content of medical educa-tion and training.

The core curriculum suggested in the consensus statement specified topics that ranged from key ethical elements of the doctor–patient relationship, such as confidentiality and consent to broader subject areas, including the ethics of using genetic technology and the ethics of conducting medical research. While there has been some debate about the curriculum content discussion in the ethics and education literature has focused more on the aims and method of ethics teaching in medical training. In a review of the literature on ethics edu-cation for medical students Eckles *et al.* identified two different views on the purpose of teaching medical ethics.[7] On one view the aim was to provide future physicians with the skills to analyse and resolve ethical dilemmas, on the other view the aim was to produce virtuous doctors. Rhodes suggests that this disagreement on the aim of ethics education stems from two distinct conceptions of medical ethics as either a subject in applied ethics or as the professional moral commitment of health professionals.[8] It is likely that both conceptions of medical ethics are important for medical education and stu-dents need to develop both specific ethical reasoning skills and professional moral attitudes to become a good doctor. Whether we follow one or both of the identified aims in medical ethics education the method required to achieve these aims is likely to involve the integration of ethics at all levels within the medical curriculum rather than ethics being taught as a theoretical subject in a series of lectures. The small amount of research in this area suggests that small group teaching, case based, and drawing on student's experience of ethical dilemmas in practice is the most effective method for changing knowledge levels, reasoning skills and ethical awareness among medical students.[9–11] The advantages of demonstrating to students that ethics is a fundamental part of the day to day experience of practising clinicians are clear. The implications for medical educators, both clinical and non-clinical, are significant. As students relate their ethics learning to their experience in clinical practice (including their experience of clinical teaching) their clinical teachers will need to be aware of and respond to this dimension of the student's work. This will require of clinical teachers skills in dealing with the ethical issues arising in the context of both patient care and medical education so they can provide ethical role models and respond to students' ethical concerns.

Doctors as teachers

Doctors, in one definition, are teachers, and concerned as much with education as the traditional practice of medicine. Though it is an old descriptor, it is consistent with the role of the doctor as a teacher of 'healthy living'. Quite clearly, that applies to work with patients. However, it also applies to the work of doctors as teachers. As the GMC has said 'all doctors should be willing to contribute to the education of students'. With this phraseology, the GMC imply a duty, obligation, or responsibility to teach. The Hippocratic Oath for all its historical inexactitudes elegantly describes the duty of the physician to teach, as well as the student physician to learn. Hippocrates attached importance to a duty to teach, as the GMC does today. However, it is worth trying to define what the scope of such a duty may be. Not all doctors are natural or intuitive teachers, despite the transferability of skills between teaching and clinical practice, so those of limited teaching aptitude or skill may do their students little good. Things have moved on since Hippocrates.

None the less, the modern trend is that doctors who do teach should in some manner professionalize their skills as teachers, as well their clinical skills. The tension clearly is between a putative duty to teach as set out by the GMC and an aptitude, or lack of aptitude, to teach. Professionalization as a doctor–teacher might therefore mean a formal course of study in teaching and learning, of which there is now no lack of opportunity. That may be through a graded academic progress at postgraduate level (Certificate, Diploma, Masters) or a less stratified, more local, achievement of skills and knowledge. Arguably by accomplishing such a course, doctors are skilling themselves up to teach in a way that traditionally has not been done hitherto. Other chapters in this book consider such a preparation in more detail. Recently, 344

Sir Kenneth Calman, erstwhile UK Chief Medical Officer beautifully summarized the role of the doctor–teacher in a pair of participles as follows: 'Handing on Learning'.[12]

Much has been written of the ethics of teaching.[13] Like any other professional activity, the ethical duties to perform to the best of one's ability, to update, to practise lawfully, and to conform to professional bodies' rules apply in teaching too. That this is so hardly needs to be supported or argued: doctors would have little difficulty accepting that, for example, sexual relationships between students and teachers are (almost) as unacceptable as between doctors and patients. A recent review found no evidence of sexual contact between student doctors and their supervisors in the USA, but did note other problematic boundary issues going on (inappropriate social contact, relationships with peers, etc.).[14] However, these sorts of boundary issues can be more complicated. Could it be argued that plagiarism, an activity held to be requiring of ruthless extirpation in academic circles, is a pointer to untrustworthy clinical practice in a doctor? Or differently stated, that it is an unprofessional academic activity marking an unprofessional doctor?[15] One author has taken this a stage further and suggested that there are student behaviours outside of the institution that would suggest medicine as an inappropriate career. Excessive substance misuse, drug theft, and document falsification *inter alia* are suggested as examples.[16] The GMC documents *Good medical practice*[2] (for qualified doctors) and *Medical students: professional behaviour and fitness to practise*[17] provide clear guidelines on behavioural standards that medical schools and professional organizations will follow in making decisions about a student's eligibility to continue training. However, the specific circumstances in individual cases will require judgements to be made based on ethical considerations, including the seriousness of the breach of professional conduct, the consequences for the student and for patients, and the duty owed by the teaching organization to the student and to society.

The tripartite relationship in medical education: teacher, student, and patient

The usual relationship between teacher and learner entails a duty of care on the part of the teacher in relation to the education of the student. The student also has a duty to engage in the learning process, and together student and teacher work towards a shared aim of the student acquiring certain agreed knowledge and skills, often including a qualification in the subject. In medical education and training both the teacher and student also have responsibilities in relation to both current patients who are participating in the educational process and to future patients who will be treated by the doctor who has undergone training.

Duty of care to future patients

In common with other vocational teachers, clinical teachers are preparing students to perform a particular job, which can entail risks to patient safety. Teachers and assessors must satisfy themselves that future patients will not be placed at risk of harm by permitting students who have not achieved a minimum standard of knowledge and skill to obtain a license to practice. This can place a different emphasis on the assessment criteria compared with other academic subjects where the consequences of allowing some flexibility in the pass/fail threshold do not include risk of harm to third parties. This area is clearly ethically complex. A putative duty on behalf of the clinical teacher to the future patients of his or her learners is not exactly a proximate relationship between them. This can be in conflict with the teacher's duty to learners (which is proximate). It is important for clinical teachers (and training bodies) to be honest with students about this potential conflict and the impact it may have on the teacher/learner relationship. This may be particularly important in graduate entry medical courses where students will have a different experience of the teacher/learner relationship and its associated duties from their previous undergraduate courses. This duty to protect future patients also has implications for the educational model of student-centred learning and its place in medical education. While it is important that students contribute to the development of learning objectives and appropriate methods of learning within the curriculum, this will be within an externally set framework of professional requirements that are non-negotiable, for example non-attendance or poor commitment to work can be seen as evidence of unprofessional behaviour in the GMC guidance on medical student fitness to practise.[18]

Assessments of the knowledge deemed necessary to the practice of medicine are fairly straightforward; and the assessment of skills though more complicated still achievable. The identification of attitudinal problems in students is more difficult[19] but could well have more impact on the future care of patients; therefore, it should be identified and remedied to a greater extent than it is. That is not to underestimate the difficulty of remediation of attitudinal or professional values problems, even more so than their identification. The increasing examination of poor performance in trained doctors leads to the conclusion that some negative traits were observable in undergraduate training, and perhaps should have been acted on at the time. Such individuals may not have, or been able to develop, the virtues of clinical practice.

The identification of attitudinal problems requires teachers and regulators to answer the question: 'What should physicians do, what do good physicians do?'.[20] This links with consideration of professionalism (Chapter 2) and fitness to practise (Chapter 18). There is also a legal dimension to a clinical teacher's duty. When poor performance is identified, by whatever route, in a practising clinician, the education and training of that clinician can be examined within a legal or investigative process that may follow. The aim here is to see whether there may have been deficiencies in the education process. This may result in restitutive justice for the poorly performing clinician, but it also emphasizes the legal duty of care to future patients owed by the clinical teacher or educational institution.

Duty of care to current patients

A fundamental characteristic of medical education and training is the involvement of patients in the learning process. Without the contribution of patients, either in providing their stories for case discussions or in permitting students and trainees to practise their skills in examination, investigation, and treatment it would be impossible for effective training to occur. The benefit that patients' bring to the medical education setting is the very fact that they are patients with potential or actual disease, and as such they are primarily owed a duty of care by the health professionals caring for them. This duty of care, and the ethical duties flowing from it such as maintaining confidentiality, respecting patients' wishes, and protecting them from harm, encompasses all aspects of the clinician–patient relationship, including involvement in education and training. It is the manifestation of this clinical duty of care within the educational setting that raises particular ethical issues for medical education and training that may not be so apparent in other educational fields.

The spectrum of patient involvement in medical education stretches from simple tasks such as history taking and examination at an undergraduate level, to the experiential aspects of patient care within postgraduate apprenticeship.[21] At one level we can question whether it can ever be in a patient's best interests to be treated by a medical student or doctor in training. If I am to have a surgical procedure or an invasive investigation surely my best interests are served by having the most experienced and competent person available perform it. Le Morvan and Stock have suggested that the Kantian imperative to treat people never only as a means to an end but always also as an end in themselves is inconsistent with medical training where inexperienced doctors and students practise their skills on live patients.[22] However, this view of the Kantian ideal in medical education has been challenged on the grounds both that a rational moral person would take account of the wider social context, including his or her own future interests,[23] and that patients do not expect to be treated by the best clinician in the field but only be a competent and qualified doctor.[24] Thus patients, as moral agents, agree to participate in medical education and training as participants in a shared enterprise of providing medical care to everyone who needs it both now and in the future. The duty of care owed to the patient by the clinical teacher (and the trainee) is then enacted by ensuring that the trainee is properly supervised and is competent to be learning the procedure (for example having practised on models previously) and that the patient is informed that the procedure will be carried out by a learner under supervision.

Providing patients with information about the participation of medical students in clinical activities or about doctors in training being involved in their care, and giving them the opportunity to decide, for example, if they are prepared to let a medical student examine them while they are anaesthetized, demonstrates respect for patients' autonomy and their right to decide to what extent they are prepared to participate in the educational process. The argument, alluded to above, that patients have an obligation to contribute to the education of future doctors and thus benefit future patients is an important one but does not justify the deception of patients. There is no evidence to suggest that patients, when asked to permit students or doctors in training to practise on them, refuse to be involved in medical education. Unless this was found to be the case in the majority of cases there would be little justification on consequentialist grounds for not asking them. Both the law and professional guidance emphasize the importance of patients being informed of the involvement of medical students and doctors in training in their care. For example, the GMC guidance on consent states that 'The information which patients want or ought to know, before deciding whether to consent to treatment or an investigation, may include: ... whether doctors in training will be involved, and the extent to which students may be involved in an investigation or treatment;' (Seeking patients' consent: the ethical considerations section 5).[25]

Most medical schools in the UK now have policies on consent for the examination of patients under anaesthesia by medical students. Hope *et al.* have described guidance for medical students in Oxford in obtaining consent from parents for the examination of children.[26] However, consent to examination under anaesthesia was still being debated in the literature as recently as 2005[27,28] and it is not clear that policies on consent with regard to medical education extend to other types of examination. Other issues for the medical educator to consider relate to the use of human tissue in medical education (see the Human Tissue Act 2005),[29] the use of medical records for educational purposes (see the *Data Protection Act 1984*)[30] and medical procedures on the recently dead.[31,32]

What of patients who cannot consent to participate in medical education and training? Clearly, if consent cannot be obtained there is an even more stringent duty to ensure that patients are not significantly harmed by students or doctors in training practising on them. The recently implemented *Mental Capacity Act* sets out the legal framework for treating patients who lack capacity and includes a section on medical research, although it does not refer specifically to medical education.[33] Those involved in education and training involving patients who lack capacity will need to be aware of the principles set out in the Act and ensure that their practice is consistent with them.

Ethical dilemmas for students in medical education and training

Occasionally students, in the course of their clinical attachments, encounter clinical practice that is not only ethically contestable, but clinically problematic or even dangerous. All clinical teachers will have heard reports of this sort when debriefing or reviewing such attachments with individual students. Surveys of medical students in North America have shown that students both identify ethical concerns about the behaviour of practising clinicians and experience ethical difficulties in their own role as student.[34,35] These difficulties include how to respond to observation of poor clinical or ethical practise in clinicians as well as conflicts between their own wish to learn and avoiding harm to patients. A key finding from these studies was a student's concern about speaking up when they observed or experienced ethically inappropriate behaviour; for example, witnessing deliberate deception of patients, or being asked to do things for which they did not feel competent or for which patients had not consented. The pressure on students to fit in with the team and to obtain good reports on their work can create ethical conflict that they feel unable to deal with. How this problem is handled will be vary between institutions, in the same way that there will be a variety of ways of responding to poor clinical performance, identified in every day clinical practice. It seems that the paramount aspect is that the student does not deal with it alone, and has a clear series of actions available to deal with his or her observations. Generally that will be access to whoever in the faculty is appropriate to take it further. While practical support for students with clear processes for reporting concerns in a safe environment is essential, there are other lessons to be learned by medical educators in this area. Ethics education in medical school and postgraduate training should explicitly address these issues and provide students with the skills to resolve these dilemmas, and development of a faculty should include an ethics component so that clinical teachers are aware of their ethical responsibilities to both their patients and their students, and the responsibility that they have as a role model both as a clinician and a teacher.[36]

Students as research participants

Both undergraduate and postgraduate medical training has undergone major changes in the last decade and this has been associated with an increasing amount of research into curricula, teaching methods, and assessments. While rigorous research is to be welcomed, it is important to ensure that appropriate ethical procedures are in place for both the conduct and oversight of research projects. There have been some concerns expressed in the medical education literature about the ethics of educational research, including the question of informed consent from student participants and ensuring the scientific quality is sufficient to warrant enrolling students in the project[37,38] A dual role of teacher and researcher can lead to conflicts of interest and care should be taken to ensure that coercion of students to participate in research does not occur. The development of robust research governance processes in universities and the requirement for university research ethics committees provides a framework within which high-quality educational research can develop.

Governance and law

All medical education exists in a professional and legal framework. The guiding documents in the UK emanate from the GMC at a undergraduate level and the Postgraduate Medical Education and Training Board (PMETB) at a postgraduate level. These bodies are statutory, and control medical education at all levels.[39] They have a strong professional input. Hence, in ethics teaching the importance of implementing the aims of *Tomorrow's doctors* is acknowledged by all institutions. Funding for the universities, within which undergraduate medical teaching takes place, is of key importance and is given by the Higher Education Funding Council for England (HEFCE), the Scottish Funding Council, and the Higher Education Funding Council for Wales. These are also statutory bodies. In fact the very fact of being a university (a form of Higher Education Institution) is subject to law as well: previously this was a common law definition, including the requirement to teach at least one subject of law, medicine, or theology.[40] This has been superseded by a definition under statute requiring:

- at least 300 full-time students in five of HEFCE's nine subject areas
- at least 4000 full-time students

- at least 300 full-time students doing degrees
- degree awarding powers.[41]

Medical, as other, students' relationships with their University invoke many aspects of law, the details of which are beyond the scope of this chapter, but will include aspects of contract law, landlord and tenant law, administrative and public law, disability discrimination law, and torts (for an overview see reference 42).

Conclusions

Medical education and training raises a number of ethical and legal issues, some of which are generic to adult education and others that are specifically related to the content and context of medical education. As awareness of the ethical difficulties inherent in the practice of medicine increases so the need for ethics education and training within the medical undergraduate and post-graduate curriculum has become apparent. The introduction of ethics teaching into the medical curriculum has to some extent illuminated the ethical issues inherent in medical education and training. In this chapter we have attempted to briefly sketch some of the key areas of ethical concern that medical educators need to consider in developing and delivering a training programme that addresses the needs of students, patients, and society.

References

1. Hippocrates. *Hippocratic oath*. In *The Hippocratic oath: text, translation, and interpretation* (Ed. Edelstein L). Baltimore, MD: Johns Hopkins Press, 1943. http://www.intute.ac.uk/healthandlifesciences/cgi-bin/ search.pl?term1=hippocratic+oath&gateway=medhist&limit=0
2. General Medical Council. *Good medical practice*. London: GMC, 2006.
3. American Medical Association. *Principles of medical ethics*. AMA 2001. http://www.ama-assn.org/ama/pub/category/2512.html/ (accessed 14 December 2007).
4. General Medical Council. *Tomorrow's doctors*. London: GMC, 1993. http://www.gmc-uk.org/education/documents/Tomorrows_Doctors_1993.pdf/.
5. General Medical Council. *Tomorrow's Doctors*. London: GMC, 2003. http://www.gmc-uk.org/education/undergraduate/undergraduate_policy/tomorrows_doctors.asp
6. Consensus stations by teachers of medical ethics and law in UK medical schools. Teaching medical ethics and law within medical education: a model for the UK core curriculum. *J Med Ethics* 1998; **24**(3): 188-92.
7. Eckles RE, Meslin EM, Gaffney M, Helft PR. Medical ethics education: where are we? Where should we be going? A review. *Acad Med* 2005; **80**(12): 1143–52.
8. Rhodes R. Two concepts of medical ethics and their implications for medical ethics education. *J Med Philos* 2002; **27**(4): 493–508.
9. Goldie J, Schwartz L, McConnachie A, Morrison J. The impact of a modern medical curriculum on students' proposed behaviour on meeting ethical dilemmas. *Med Educ* 2004; **38**(9): 942–9.

10. Roff S, Preece P. Helping medical students to find their moral compasses: ethics teaching for second and third year undergraduates. *J Med Ethics* 2004; **30**(5): 487–9.

11. Roberts LW, Warner TD, Hammond KA, Geppert CM, Heinrich T. Becoming a good doctor: perceived need for ethics training focused on practical and professional development topics. *Acad Psychiatry* 2005; **29**(3): 301–9.

12. Calman KC. *Medical education: past present and future*. Edinburgh: Elsevier, 2007; p. 7.

13. Cahn SM. *Saints and scamps: ethics in academia*. Maryland: Rowman and Littlefield, 1994.

14. Recupero PR, Cooney MC, Rayner C, Heru AM, Price M. Supervisor-trainee relationship boundaries in medical education. *Med Teach* 2006; **27**(6): 484–8.

15. Wagner P, Hendrich J, Hudson V. Defining medical professionalism: a qualitative study *Med Educ* 2007; **41**: 288–94.

16. Bonke B. Unprofessional or problematic behaviour of medical students outside the learning environment. *Med Teach* **28**(5): 440–2.

17. General Medical Council. *Medical students: professional behaviour and fitness to practise*. London: GMC, 2007.

18. Ibid paragraph 58.

19. Korzun A, Winterburn PJ, Sweetland H, Tapper Jones L, Houston H. Assesement of professional attitude and conduct in medical undergraduates *Med Teach* 2005; **27**(8): 704–8.

20. Kenny NP, Mann KV, MacLeod H. Role modelling in physician's professional formation: reconsidering an essential but untapped educational strategy. *Acad Med* 2003; **78**(12): 1203–10.

21. Grant J. Learning needs assessment assessing the need. *Br Med J* 2002; **324**: 156–9.

22. Le Morvan P Stock B. Medical learning curves and the Kantian ideal. *J Med Ethics* 2005; **31**: 513–18.

23. Brecher B. Why the Kantian ideal survives medical learning curves, and why it matters. *J Med Ethics* 2006; **32**: 511–12.

24. Ives J. Kant, curves and medical learning practice: a replyto Le Morvan and Stock. *J Med Ethics* 2007; **33**: 119–22.

25. General Medical Council. *Seeking patients' consent: the ethical issues*. London: GMC, 1998.

26. Hope T, Frith P, Craze J, Mussai F, Chadha A, Noble D. Developing guidelines for medical students about the examination of patients under 18 years old. *BMJ* 2005; **331**: 1384.

27. Coldicott Y, Pope C, Roberts C. The ethics of intimate examinations-teaching tomorrow's doctors. *BMJ* 2003; **326**: 97–101.

28. Schniederjan S, Donovan GK. Ethics versus education: pelvic exams on anesthetized women. *J Okla State Med Assoc* 2005; **98**(8): 386.

29. Office of Public Sector Information. Human Tissue Act 21004. http://www.england-legislation.hmso.gov.uk/acts/acts2004/ukpga_20040030_en_1/ (accessed 14 December 2007).

30. Office of Public Sector Information. Data Protection Act 1998. http://opsi.gov.uk/acts/acts1998/ukpga_19980029_en_1/ (accessed 14 December 2007).

31. Moraq RM DeSouza S, Steen PA, Salem A, Harris M, Ohnstan O, Fosen JT, Brenner BE. Performing procedures on the newly deceased for teaching purposes: what if we were to ask? *Arch Intern Med* 2005; **165**: 92–6.

32. Denny CJ, Kollek D. Practicing procedures on the recently dead. *J Emerg Med* 1999; **17**(6).

33. Office of Public Sector Information. Mental Capacity Act 2005 (section 30) http://www.england-legislation.hmso.gov.uk/acts/acts2005/ukpga_20050009_en_3#pt1-pb8–11g30/.

34. Christakis DA, Feudtner C. Ethics in a short white coat: the ethical dilemmas that medical students confront. *Acad Med* 1993; **68**: 249–54.

35. Caldicott CV, Faber-Langendoen K. Deception, discrimination, and fear of reprisal: lessons in ethics from third-year medical students. *Acad Med* 2005; **80**(9): 866–73.

36. Cordingley L, Hyde C, Peters S, Vernon B, Bundy C. Undergraduate medical students_ exposure to clinical ethics: a challenge to the development of professional behaviours? *Med Educ* 2007; **41**(12): 1202–9.

37. McLachlan JC, McHarg J. Ethical permission for the publication of routinely collected data. *Med Educ* 2005; **39**(9): 944–8.

38. Eva KW. The yin and yang of education research. *Med Educ* 2007; **41**(8): 724–5.

39. Principles of Good Medical Education and Training Board. http://www.pmetb.org.uk (accessed 14 December 2007).

40. St David's College, Lampeter v Ministry of Education [1951] All ER 559.

41. Further and Higher Education Act. s77[4].

42. Oxford Centre for Higher Education Policy Studies. http://oxcheps.new.ox.ac.uk/ (accessed 14 December 2007).

Index